T0257733

Cancer Treatment: Conventional and Modern Approaches

Cancer Treatment: Conventional and Modern Approaches

Edited by **Karen Miles and Richard Gray**

hayle medical

New York

Published by Hayle Medical,
30 West, 37th Street, Suite 612,
New York, NY 10018, USA
www.haylemedical.com

Cancer Treatment: Conventional and Modern Approaches
Edited by Karen Miles and Richard Gray

© 2015 Hayle Medical

International Standard Book Number: 978-1-63241-073-3 (Hardback)

This book contains information obtained from authentic and highly regarded sources. Copyright for all individual chapters remain with the respective authors as indicated. A wide variety of references are listed. Permission and sources are indicated; for detailed attributions, please refer to the permissions page. Reasonable efforts have been made to publish reliable data and information, but the authors, editors and publisher cannot assume any responsibility for the validity of all materials or the consequences of their use.

The publisher's policy is to use permanent paper from mills that operate a sustainable forestry policy. Furthermore, the publisher ensures that the text paper and cover boards used have met acceptable environmental accreditation standards.

Trademark Notice: Registered trademark of products or corporate names are used only for explanation and identification without intent to infringe.

Printed in the United States of America.

Contents

Permissions

List of Contributors

Preface

Currently, there is an increase in the use of modern techniques and mechanisms for cancer treatment. However, an ultimate treatment has not yet been found, and it needs more time and research to develop more effective methods for cancer treatment. This book will serve not just physicians but also patients with an overview on new research and developments in this area. This book is a comprehensive and valuable account discussing various therapeutic methods in cancer treatment comprising of new modalities of cancer therapy like xenovaccinotherapy for cancer; antiangiogenic treatment concepts in gynecologic oncology; NKG2D-based cancer immunotherapy; photodynamic therapy in combination with antiangiogenic approaches; and electrotherapy on cancer experiment and mathematical modeling.

All of the data presented henceforth, was collaborated in the wake of recent advancements in the field. The aim of this book is to present the diversified developments from across the globe in a comprehensible manner. The opinions expressed in each chapter belong solely to the contributing authors. Their interpretations of the topics are the integral part of this book, which I have carefully compiled for a better understanding of the readers.

At the end, I would like to thank all those who dedicated their time and efforts for the successful completion of this book. I also wish to convey my gratitude towards my friends and family who supported me at every step.

Editor

New Modalities of Cancer Therapy

Harnessing the Immune System to Fight Cancer: The Promise of Genetic Cancer Vaccines

Luigi Aurisicchio[1,2] and Gennaro Ciliberto[1,3]

[1]Takis, via di Castel Romano, 100, 00128 Rome
[2]Biogem scarl, via Camporeale, 83131 Ariano Irpino (AV),
[3]Dipartimento di Medicina Sperimentale e Clinica, Università degli studi di Catanzaro
"Magna Graecia" Campus Germaneto, 88100 Catanzaro
Italy

1. Introduction

In spite of significant progress in recent years towards the development of new targeted therapies Cancer is still a largely unmet medical need and the leading cause of death in industrialized countries (Globocan Project, 2008). Cancer is continuously increasing and is associated with a variety of factors, including genetic predisposition, infectious agents, exposure to mutagens, as well as lifestyle factors (Minamoto et al, 1999). Cancer is linked to the occurrence of genetic and epigenetic changes (Heng et al, 2010) and indeed tumour cells harbor hundreds of these modifications as also witnessed by the recent results of genome wide analyses of cancer genomes (Sastre, 2011). This feature of cancer cells implies that they can be recognized as foreign entities and eliminated by our immune system, and is at the basis of the theory of immunosurveillance (Dunn et al, 2004).

Several studies have shown that it is possible to establish clear correlates between the nature, density and location of immune cells within distinct tumour regions and the risk of disease relapse (reviewed in Mleknic et al, 2011). Compelling data have recently led to propose that an immune classification of patients, based on the density and the immune location within the tumour may have a prognostic value even superior to the standard TNM classification (Bindea et al, 2011; Fridman et al, 2011). In recent years a better knowledge of the immune system has led to an evolution of the initial concept of immunosurveillance into a more articulated theory of immunoediting (Schreiber et al, 2011). Cancer immunoediting acts as an intrinsic tumour suppressor mechanism that engages after cellular transformation has occurred and intrinsic tumour suppressor mechanisms have failed. One can envisage the existence of three sequential steps during clinical tumour evolution: elimination, equilibrium, and escape. In the first step, innate and adaptive immunity are capable of destroying transformed cells before they give rise to tumour masses. If this process is maximally efficient, then the host remains tumour free. If, however, cancer cell variants are not destroyed, they can enter into an equilibrium phase, in which their outgrowth is held in check by immunological mechanisms, which are principally due to the activation of IL-12/IFNγ-dependent adaptive immunity, mainly driven by antigen-specific CD8[+] and CD4[+]

T cells. Equilibrium may still represent the end stage of the process and may restrain outgrowth of occult cancers for the lifetime of the host. However, as a consequence of constant immune selection pressure placed by the host on genetically/epigenetically unstable tumour cells, cancerous cells that are no longer recognized by adaptive immunity may emerge, become insensitive to immune effectors mechanisms and in addition they can induce the creation of an immunosuppressive environment. When tumour cells enter the escape phase in which their growth is no longer blocked by immunity, equilibrium is lost and disease becomes apparent. Re-establishing this equilibrium is the realistic goal of cancer immunotherapy.

In spite of being the object of intensive efforts over the past decades, Cancer Immunotherapy has seen many more clinical failures than successes. However, very recently major breakthroughs have been achieved, and these have led us to believe that this approach may become an established platform for the therapy of cancer within the next decade. One can envisage three distinct avenues for Cancer immunotherapy: a) Adoptive Cell Therapy (ACT); b) systemic immune-modulators; c) therapeutic cancer vaccines. ACT is based upon the possibility to isolate, *in vitro* expand and re-inject in immunodepleted hosts, tumour-specific T cells. This approach has seen its best demonstration in the treatment of patients with advanced metastatic melanoma. Superb clinical results have been obtained with objective response rates of up to 49-72% and disease control in some cases lasting several years (Rosenberg and Dudley, 2009). Although evolution of this approach such as genetic modification of T cells to redirect their effector cell specificity may open up to broader applications (Morgan et al, 2010), this strategy has several limitations that currently limit its wide applicability: it is patient specific, very expensive, requires hospitalization and can only be executed in highly specialized clinical centers. In contrast, systemic immunomodulators such as monoclonal antibodies against CTLA-4 or PD-1/PD-L1, do not suffer the manufacturing and delivery problems shown by ACT. On March 2011, FDA approved Ipilimumab (Yervoy® - BMS) (Culver et al, 2011), a human monoclonal antibody against CTLA-4 for the treatment of metastatic melanoma, based on the results of a randomized, controlled Phase III, where Ipilimumab showed statistically increased overall survival compared with controls (Hodi et al, 2010). Although the clinical development of anti PD-1 antibodies is at an earlier stage as compared to anti CTLA-4, results are highly promising both for efficacy and tolerability (Kline and Gajewski, 2010). Finally cancer vaccines recently gained increased visibility due to the demonstration that Sipuleucel-T, a immune cell vaccine for the treatment of hormone refractory prostate cancer, is capable of increasing overall survival of cancer patients (Kantoff et al, 2010). These results led to FDA approval as Provenge® (Dendreon) in year 2010 (Cheever and Higano, 2011). This recent approval has acted as a strong injection of enthusiasm in an area that has long suffered major setbacks.

In this review we will focus mainly on recent developments for therapeutic cancer vaccines and will not discuss in detail ACT and systemic immunomodulators (Klebanoff et al, 2011). Major emphasis will be given to aspects that are critical to increase vaccine immunogenicity and probability of success in the clinic. We believe these are mainly: a) efficient vaccine delivery systems, b) development of response biomarkers, c) modified clinical endpoints and d) combinatorial treatments with chemotherapy or other agents. In analyzing vaccine delivery systems a greater attention will be given to genetic vaccines which we believe represent the most promising methods to elicit immune responses against a wide variety of tumour antigens especially when administered in combined immunization protocols (heterologous prime/boost). We invite the reader to other recent excellent reviews for aspects of tumour immunology and cancer immunotherapy that we may have missed in our work (Steer et al, 2010; Klebanoff et al, 2011; Palucka et al, 2011; Vergati et al, 2010; Aldrich et al, 2010) .

2. Tumour immunology

Our immune system has the intrinsic capability of recognizing tumour cells as foreign entities and to mount responses capable of impacting upon disease evolution. In this section of the chapter we review the main evidences for this spontaneous response, what are the targets of this response, which are the principal components of the immune system involved and what is curtailing this response leading to tumour escape and lack of control of the immune system over cancer.

2.1 Immunosurveillance and Immunoediting
The key studies that unequivocally demonstrated the role of the immune system in the control of cancer development date back to about a decade ago when mouse models of immunodeficiency on pure genetic backgrounds became available. These studies showed that interferon-γ (IFN-γ) is a key factor responsible for the immunological rejection of transplanted tumour cells (Dighe et al, 1994). Furthermore, mice lacking IFN-γ response (either as a consequence of IFN-γ receptor or STAT1 inactivating mutations) or adaptive immunity as a whole (RAG2 -/- deficient mice) are more susceptible to carcinogen induced or spontaneous tumours (Kaplan et al, 1998; Shankaran et al, 2001, Street et al, 2002). These evidences collectively demonstrated that the immune system can function as an extrinsic tumour suppressor. However, as mentioned in the introduction section, a new emerging concept in cancer immunology is that the immune system is not simply a component that protects the host against tumour development, but rather an agent that shapes tumour quality. In other words, tumours that develop in an immunocompetent organism are the resultant of a selection process imposed by the host and by the type of immune response that the host immune system is capable to mount. This concept was originated by pivotal studies that demonstrated that tumours developing in immunocompetent mice have a different molecular profile, are less immunogenic than tumours developing in immunodeficient hosts and progress more rapidly when implanted into naïve wt recipient mice (Dunn et al 2002).

Although both natural and acquired immunity are required to fully exert this control mechanism, the principal contribution comes from adaptive immunity and in particular from the development of tumour-antigen-specific T cells, mainly CD8+, but also CD4+. Indeed the fundamental principle of cancer immunology is that tumour cells express antigens (TAAs – tumour associated antigens) that differentiate them from normal cells. The existence of tumour antigens has been abundantly demonstrated both in mouse and human studies (Novellino et al, 2005). In the case of human cancers, identification of tumour antigens was made possible *via* the development of methods that used as probes antibodies and CD8+ T cells derived from patients and capable of reacting with the autologous tumours (Sahin et al, 1997; Coulie et al, 1997). In the next section we will describe in more detail the types and nature of TAAs under study.

What is happening in the tumour cells that makes them "invisible" or "poorly visible" to the immune system? Certainly the most common mechanism is believed to be loss of tumour antigen expression, which can occur in at least three possible ways: a) downmodulation of tumour antigen gene expression consequent mainly to epigenetic changes; b) downregulation of MHC class I protein expression and antigen presentation to the cell surface; c) alterations in tumour cells of the machinery responsible for antigen processing and peptide loading onto MHC molecules. In addition to this, it has to be taken into account that tumour cells develop mechanisms of resistance to apoptosis and to the cytotoxic effects of immunity through, for instance, upregulation of anti-apoptotic BCL-2 proteins or activation of transcription factors such as STAT-3. All these processes are strongly favoured by the genetic/epigenetic instability intrinsic of tumour cells, which in the presence of a continuous selection favors the emergence of "immune stealth" clones.

If we analyze in detail the three phases of immunosurveillance/immunoediting, namely Elimination, Equilibrium and Escape, the phase where we have more direct proof of the activity of the immune system is the Equilibrium phase. This phase can represent a type of tumour dormancy where growth of tumour cells is kept at bay for a long period of time, even for the entire life of an organism. Strong evidence for this phenomenon first came when immunocompetent mice treated with low dose carcinogens such as methylcolantrene, were shown to harbor occult cancers for an extended period of time (Koebel et al, 2007). Intriguingly, when these mice were subjected to treatments that selectively affected adaptive immunity, but not innate immunity, tumours rapidly developed, thus demonstrating that equilibrium is established only when a Tumour Antigen Specific CD8+ and CD4+ response has occurred. This may explain the clinical findings of aggressive tumour arising in organs from a donor apparently cured from cancer, when transplanted into a patient (MacKie et al, 2003).

Although studies of tumour development in mice served as the main driver for the formulation of the cancer immunosurveillance/immunoediting hypothesis, strong demonstration has also been obtained in humans by three different types of evidence. As mentioned before, the first is the demonstration that cancer patients develop detectable levels of antibodies and T cell responses to tumour antigens (Dougan and Dranoff, 2009). The second one is that patients affected by immunodeficiencies are at higher risk of developing cancers (Dunn et al, 2002). The third and strongest one is that intratumoural infiltration by cells of the immune system correlates with disease evolution. In this respect several studies have shown that the quantity, quality, and spatial distribution of tumour infiltrating lymphocytes correlate with patients survival. In fact, tumour infiltration by IFN-γ producing CD8+ and CD4+ T cells has been associated with an improved prognosis for patients with several different cancer types, including melanoma (Clemente et al, 1996; van Houdt, 1998), colorectal cancer (Chiba et al, 2004) and ovarian cancer (Nelson, 2008). More recent studies in colorectal cancer have extended these findings and have shown, through a global analysis of the tumour microenvironment from both a morphological standpoint and from a system biology approach, that the nature, functional orientation, density and location of cells of the adaptive immune system within distinct tumour regions influence the risk of relapse (Mlecnik et al, 2011). The same authors have come to the conclusion that the density and the immune cell location within the tumour may have a prognostic value superior to the standard TNM classification, and that tumour spread is statistically dependent upon the extent of the host-immune reaction (Bindea et al, 2011).

2.2 Tumour associated antigens (TAAs)

In the past years, several TAAs have been identified having unique expression patterns or being overexpressed by cancer cells. These antigens, under appropriate conditions, can be

recognized by components of the immune system (Campi et al, 2003; Frenoy et al, 1987; Kawashima et al, 1998). Therefore, many current vaccination strategies are designed to induce antibody as well as cell-mediated immune responses against the antigen of interest. A high number of TAAs has been discovered and evaluated in pre-clinical and clinical studies with different results. A list of well-known TAAs subdivided in four main categories is provided in Table 1. Among the most studied and validated TAAs, vaccinations against CEA (Marshall et al, 2003), HER-2/*neu* (Shumway et al, 2009), TERT (Vonderheide, 2008), EpCAM (Chaudry et al., 2007), survivin (Andersen and Thor, 2002), prostate-specific antigens (Doehn et al., 2008) provided good immunologic results. In light of the increasing interest and potential for cancer immunotherapy, the National Cancer Institute recently conducted an interesting pilot project to prioritize cancer antigens and to develop a priority-ranked list of cancer vaccine target antigens based on predefined and pre-weighted objective criteria (Cheever et al., 2009). **Shared TAAs**
Among the shared TAAs, the following three main groups can be identified: (1) cancer-testis (CT) antigens, (2) differentiation antigens, and (3) widely occurring overexpressed antigens. Among shared tumour-specific antigens, *cancer-testis (CT)* antigens are expressed in histologically different human tumours and, among normal tissues, in spermatocytes/spermatogonia of the testis and occasionally in placenta. CT antigens result from the reactivation of genes which are normally silent in adult tissues but are transcriptionally activated in different tumour histotypes (De Smet et al., 1999). Many CT antigens have been identified and used in clinical trials, although little is known about their specific functions, especially with regard to malignant transformation. This group of TAAs includes MAGE-A1 (Chaux et al., 1999) and NY-ESO-1 (Jager et al., 1998). *Differentiation antigens* are shared between tumours and the normal tissue of origin and found mostly in melanomas and normal melanocytes (Gp100, Melan-A/Mart-1, and Tyrosinase), although they are also found in epithelial tissues and tumours such as prostate tumours (prostate-specific antigen [PSA]). To variable extent, normal tissues can be target of the elicited immunity against shared TAAs. An example is the vitiligo developing as a consequence of the immune response in melanoma patients undergoing immunotherapy. Vaccine-induced T cells recognizing gp100 and tyrosinase are present at the *vitiligo* lesions and normal melanocytes are eliminated by the immune system (Jacobs et al., 2009). Importantly, this effect has been associated to a clinical response. Additionally, expression of several oncofetal antigens appears to be increased in many adult cancer tissues, including carcinoembryonic antigen (CEA), which is highly expressed in colon cancer (Tsang et al., 1995).
TAAs from this group, despite representing self-antigens, have been and still are commonly used in current cancer vaccination trials, often together with CT antigens. Widely occurring, overexpressed TAAs have been detected in different types of tumours as well as in many normal tissues, and their overexpression in tumour cells can reach the threshold for T cell recognition, breaking the immunological tolerance and triggering an anticancer response. Among the most interesting TAAs of this group are the antiapoptotic proteins (survivin) (Schmidt et al., 2003), hTERT (Vonderheide et al., 2008), and tumour suppressor proteins (e.g., p53) (Umano et al, 2001).
Unique tumour antigens. Unique TAAs are products of random somatic point mutations induced by physical or chemical carcinogens and therefore expressed uniquely by individual tumours and not by any normal tissue, representing the only true tumour-specific antigens (Ags) (reviewed in Parmiani et al., 2007). Such Ags characterize each single

neoplasm and were shown to be diverse between tumours induced in the same animal or even in different tissue fragments from the same tumour nodule. A relevant feature of unique Ags is their potential resistance to immunoselection if the mutated protein is crucial to the oncogenic process and thus indispensable for maintaining the neoplastic state. As a consequence, unique Ags should elicit an immune response clinically more effective than that of shared Ags. However, identification of unique tumour antigens for solid human tumours requires sequencing of the whole genome of each individual tumour in order to identify mutated genes and select peptides whose motifs are predicted to be presented by the patient's HLA alleles. Moreover, each tumour bears highly heterogeneous sets of defects in different genes which need to be further verified for their substantial contribution to the tumour development and progression and, consequently, for their relevance as vaccine targets (Fox et al., 2009). An interesting class of potential TAAs is associated with fusions between different proteins. Best example is the Bcr–Abl fusion protein, the driving force in chronic myelogenous leukemia (CML) (Daley et al., 1990). By establishing a causal link between a specific chromosomal lesion and a specific malignancy, BCR–ABL also pioneered cancer therapy: the TK inhibitor, imatinib (Gleevec), was introduced as the first widely used targeted therapeutic (Druker et al., 2001). Similar discoveries led to the characterization of causative fusions in other hematological malignancies. A variety of prostate cancer gene fusions have been identified so far (reviewed in Shah and Chinnaiyan, 2009), characterized by 5'-genomic regulatory elements, most notably the androgen-controlled prostate specific gene, transmembrane protease serine 2 (TMPRSS2), fused to members of the erythroblastosis virus E26 transforming sequence family of transcription factors, most notably ERG, leading to the overexpression of oncogenic transcription factors. This class of potential TAAs is matter of extensive studies and holds promise for personalized vaccine applications.

Viral Antigens. Some viruses, such as human papillomavirus (HPV) and hepatitis B virus (HBV) can induce cancer. As a matter of fact, HBV vaccination in newborns has eradicated hepatocellular carcinoma (HCC) in populations at high risk (McMahon et al, 2011; Blumberg et al., 2010). The high-risk HPV types (e.g., HPV16) are causally related to the development of anogenital lesions, including vulvar intraepithelial neoplasia (VIN), and their subsequent progression to invasive squamous cell carcinoma. The expression of viral antigens (hence non-self proteins) such as HPV E6 and E7 proteins by cancer cells can represent the mechanism through which the tumour becomes visible to the immune system. Recently, promising results have been obtained by vaccination of patients with HPV16 E6/E7 synthetic long-peptide vaccine (Van der Burg and Melief, 2011), providing an important proof of concept for the development of therapeutic cancer vaccines against cervical and anal cancers.

Stromal Antigens. During transformation, reciprocal interactions occur between neoplastic and adjacent normal cells, i.e. fibroblasts, endothelial, and immunocompetent cells. In general, stroma cells contribute 20–50% to the tumour mass, but the stromal compartment may account for up to 90% in several carcinomas. In contrast to cancer cells, tumour stroma cells are genetically more stable so that at least some immune evasion mechanisms of tumours do not apply to these cells. Nevertheless, stroma cells differ from their normal counterparts by upregulation or induction of various antigens (reviewed in Hofmeister et al., 2006). Some of the tumour stroma-associated antigens (TSAAs) are highly selective for the tumour microenvironment. TSAAs are also expressed by a broad spectrum of solid tumours, thus therapies designed to target tumour stroma are not restricted to a selected tumour type. Cancer-associated fibroblasts (CAFs) are reactive fibroblasts with a phenotype differing from that of quiescent fibroblasts in normal adult tissue. CAFs contribute to the development of cancer by secreting growth promoting factors such as TGF-β, matrix degrading enzymes, and angiogenic factors, e.g. MMPs or vascular endothelial growth factor (VEGF). Endothelial cells have a major part in tumour progression since they are necessary for angiogenesis. Tumour endothelial cells (TECs) express surface receptors and secrete factors that sustain their own growth by an autocrine pathway. Another target cell population for immune intervention present in the tumour microenvironment are tumour-associated macrophages (TAMs, see also paragraph 2.3). Among the proteins explored as promising stromal immunotherapy targets it is worth mentioning Fibroblast Activation Protein a (FAPα, seprase), a surface glycoprotein selectively expressed in reactive stromal fibroblasts of solid tumours, Carbonic Anhydrase IX (CAIX) an important pH regulator, Matrix Metalloproteases (MMP) such as MMP11 (Peruzzi et al., 2009), extracellular angiogenic factors, such as Vascular Endothelial Growth factor (VEGF) and its receptor VEGFR2 and basic Fibroblast Growth Factor (bFGF). Tumour endothelial markers (TEMs), among them TEM1 and TEM8, are overexpressed during tumour angiogenesis and prostate-specific membrane antigen (PSMA) is another endothelial cell surface molecule of particular interest for vascular targeting. In conclusion, ideal target stromal proteins are those selectively induced or upregulated in the tumour *micromilieu*, and confer a growth or survival advantage to the tumour.

Shared Antigens	Features	Type of Tumour	Examples
Cancer Testis (CT) Ags	Expressed only by tumours and testis	Melanoma, lymphoma, bladder, breast, colon, lung	BAGE, GAGE, MAGE, NY-ESO-1
Differentiation Ags	Expressed also by normal cells	Melanoma,prostate, colon, breast	Gp100, MART-1, tyrosinase, CEA, PSA
Overexpressed Ags	Expressed by tumor cells prevalently	Liver, colon, breast, ovary, bladder, prostate, esophagus, lymphoma	p53, Her2/*neu,* survivin, hTERT
Unique Antigens	Features	Type of Tumour	Examples
Unique	Expressed by a single tumor	Melanoma, NSCLC, RCC	CDα-actin-m, K-4/m, β-actin-m, Myosin-m
Viral Antigens	Features	Type of Tumour	Examples
Viral	Encoded by genome of oncogenic viruses	HCC, anogenital lesions	HBV, HPV E6 and E7
Stromal Antigens	Features	Type of Tumour	Examples
Fibroblast TSAA	Expressed by CAFs	Ubiquitous	FAPα, CAIX, MMP11
Endothelial TSAA	Expressed by TECs	Ubiquitous	VEGF, VEGFR2, TEMs, PSMA

Table 1. Classification and examples of TAAs and TSAAs.

2.3 Immune suppression mechanisms

A strong and persistent immune response against cancer is necessary but not sufficient to controlling tumour growth in the escape phase. For example, while robust T cell responses generated by vaccinations against HPV are capable of successfully controlling pre-malignant intraepithelial neoplasias (Welters et al, 2010), in clinical trials of tumour vaccines against large, invasive malignancies the effective generation of tumour antigen-specific T cells is not predictive of clinical efficacy (Radoja et al, 2001). Although this discrepancy may be due in part to differences in the affinity/avidity of effector T cells developing against self *vs* exogenous antigens, the principal cause is believed to be the establishment of an immunosuppressive state within the tumour microenvironment (reviewed by Gajewski et al, 2006). This immunosuppression is not due to a single mechanism but to the concerted action of several processes. In first instance the presence of regulatory T cells (Tregs) and Myeloid-derived suppressor cells (MDSCs), which play a direct inhibitory role on host-protective antitumour responses.

Tregs are CD4[+] T cells which constitutively express CD25 and the transcription factor FoxP3 (Nishikawa and Sakaguchi, 2010). It is unclear what proportion of intratumoural Tregs react with specific tumour antigens (Wang et al, 2005), or instead are recruited through the recognition of shared self-antigens co-expressed by tumour cells (Darrasse-Jeze et al, 2009). At any rate, their inhibitory function is exerted *via* the production of immunosuppressive cytokines such as IL-10 and TGFβ, the expression of negative co-stimulatory receptors such as CTLA-4 and PD-1, and the expression of IDO. IDO (indoleamine 2,3-dioxygenase) is an enzyme responsible for a rate-limiting step in tryptophan catabolism and is strongly induced in the tumour environment by IFN-γ. The immunosuppressive effect of IDO expression is due both to reduction of local levels of tryptophan and to the generation of cytotoxic catabolites kynurenins, which affect T cell activity and dendritic cell survival (Soliman et al, 2010). Several studies have shown that in several cancer types the presence of regulatory CD4[+]CD25[+] T cells in tumours inversely correlates with disease outcome (Woo et al, 2001; Curiel et al, 2004)

MDSCs or Tumour Associated Macrophages (TAMs) are a heterogenous group of myeloid progenitor cells and immature myeloid cells that inhibit lymphocyte function by inducing Tregs, producing TGFβ, depleting essential aminoacids as tryptophan, arginine and cysteine, and inducing down-regulation of L selectin on T cells (Ostrand-Rosenberg, 2010; Lindenberg et al, 2011). T cells must have an L-selectin phenotype to home to lymphnodes and inflammatory sites where they encounter antigens and are activated. TAMs therefore, perturb T cell trafficking and inhibit T cell activation. Furthermore, immunosuppression appears to be enhanced by active angiogenesis and angiogenic cytokines like VEGF (Johnson et al, 2007), also through a possible direct effect on dendritic cells.

Recent studies have shown that a symbiotic relationship exists between tumour cells and TAMs, in which tumour cells attract TAMs and sustain their survival, with TAMs responding to microenvironmental factors in tumours such as hypoxia by producing important mitogens, growth factors and enzymes that stimulate tumour growth angiogenesis (Bingle et al, 2002). Actually it seems that in response to different stimuli, TAMs differentiate into subsets capable of stimulating different pro-tumourigenic functions. For example in areas of invasion TAMs promote cancer cell motility, in perivascular areas they promote metastasis, and in avascular and perinecrotic areas hypoxic TAMs stimulate angiogenesis (Lewis and Pollard, 2006). Finally in a very recent study it has been shown that macrophage infiltration in tumours is able to affect chemotherapy (De Nardo et al, 2011). Indeed these authors have shown that TAM depletion in highly infiltrated tumours increased the antitumour efficacy of paclitaxel, and this was at least in part due to their suppression of the antitumour functions of cytotoxic T cells. This study therefore confirms the high complexity of the immune cell interactions in tumours (DeNardo et al, 2010) and shows that cross-talk between TAMs and cytotoxic T cells impairs effective tumour eradication by immune mechanisms.

Unraveling the mechanisms at the basis of immunosuppression in the tumour microenvironment has led to the definition of novel targets for therapeutic intervention. Agents directed against these new targets, such as for example IDO or PD-1, may act in concert with cancer vaccines to enhance their efficacy, in particular in conditions of advanced tumour development. We believe that the clinical efficacy of anti CTLA-4 antibody Ipilimumab is in part linked to the inhibition of immunosuppressive processes. Indeed recent studies have demonstrated that maximal anti-tumour effects of CTLA-4 blockade are due to the concomitant blockade not only of effector T cells, but also of Tregs (Peggs et al, 2009). Also, it cannot be excluded that at least in part the clinical efficacy of the anti-VEGF antibody Bevacizumab is due to inhibition of the immunosuppressive function of VEGF (Chouaib et al, 2010).

3. Types of cancer vaccines

Different technologies have been employed to develop cancer immunotherapies. These include passive immunotherapy, based on the adoptive transfer of *ex-vivo* activated immune cells, immunomodulators (including cytokines) or tumour specific antibodies; and active immunotherapy, aimed at activating the patient's own immune system via the administration of a therapeutic vaccine. To date, active cancer immunotherapy trials have included therapeutic vaccination with recombinant viral vectors encoding TAAs, recombinant proteins with appropriate adjuvants, antigen-loaded Dendritic Cells (DCs), DNA encoding tumour-associated antigens, heat shock proteins and synthetic peptides (see next paragraphs). However, apart from melanoma, in which impressive clinical responses have been observed in a small proportion of patients, the recent success of Sipuleucel-T (see paragraph 3.1.2.1) and the promise of PROSTVAC-VF (see paragraph 3.2.1), most results have been disappointing. Therefore, the continuous development of novel vaccine strategies and technologies is needed to improve recognition, immune response, effector functions, and trafficking of T cells induced by vaccination. These goals may be achieved by the concurrent administration of novel immunotherapeutics with an immunopotentiating profile (see section 4.3).

3.1 Cell-based vaccines

A first category of cancer vaccines under evaluation is based on delivery of cells. As pointed out before, we will not discuss in this chapter ACT but only Whole Tumour Cell Vaccines and Dendritic Cells vaccines.

3.1.1 Whole cell vaccines

Autologous tumour cells are an obvious source of TAAs for vaccination purposes, since, by definition, all relevant candidate TAAs should be contained within them. In early clinical trials, individualized tailor-made vaccines prepared from whole tumour cells were associated with limited activity, presumably due to the already biased nature of the host immune response to specific TAAs (Vermorken et al. 1999; Jocham et al., 2004). However, due to the mechanism of immunologic tolerance, this approach has resulted in poor immunogenicity and different categories of adjuvants have been evaluated in the past years (de Gruijl et al., 2008).

Perhaps the most explored approach in the clinic is GVAX (Cell Genesys). Autologous tumour cells, transduced with GM-CSF were shown to induce tumour-specific immunity and durable anti-tumour responses in a number of trials. The efficacy of GVAX depends on the cross-presentation of vaccine-derived TAAs to specific cytotoxic T lymphocytes (CTLs) *in vivo* (Hege et al., 2006). This process of cross-priming is facilitated by the activation of Dendritic Cells (DC), by GM-CSF. This finding led to the realization that allogeneic cells would also present a viable source of TAAs, which would be taken up by DCs and then presented in the context of appropriate MHC alleles to autologous CTLs. Advantages of the use of allogeneic cells are obvious: (1) through the use of antigenically well-defined cell lines one has access to a sustained and virtually limitless source of material, (2) the use of cell lines allows for a highly standardized and large-scale production of vaccine, (3) the use of a single batch of allo-vaccines for all vaccinees, independent of HLA haplotype, eliminates variability in the quality and composition of the vaccines and facilitates reliable comparative analysis of clinical outcome. Eliminating the need for the continuous production of tailor-made individual vaccines simplifies the logistics, reduces the laboriousness of vaccine production and distribution, and increases its cost-effectiveness.

3.1.2 Dendritic cell vaccines

Dendritic Cells (DCs) collect antigens from various tissues and carry them to secondary lymphoid organs to ultimately activate antigen-specific T cells. Myeloid DCs and plasmacytoid DCs are the 2 main subsets of DCs (Palucka et al, 2011. Through toll-like receptors (TLRs) 7 and 9, plasmacytoid DCs recognize viral nucleic acids and secrete type I interferon (IFN). Three myeloid DC subsets localize to the skin. Langerhans cells (LCs) are found in the epidermis, while CD1α+DCs and CD14+DCs are found in the dermis. CD14+DCs produce interleukin (IL)-1β, IL-6, IL-8, IL-10, IL-12, GM-CSF, membrane cofactor protein-1, and tumour growth factor-β. LCs produce IL-15, which is a growth and maintenance factor for CD8+ T cells and natural killer cells. LCs are more efficient in cross presentation and prime higher avidity T cells with reported greater capacity for cell kill. Although DC biology is complicated, it is clear that these cells are the critical regulators of adaptive T-cell and B-cell responses. These findings have provided the rationale for *ex vivo* antigen loading of DCs for the preparation of vaccines. DCs have been loaded with tumour antigens in the form of peptides, proteins, tumour lysates, and mRNAs. Alternatively, they have been fused with tumour cells or infected with viral vectors encoding tumour-associated antigens (reviewed in Le et al., 2010).

Clinical development of DC-based cancer vaccines has several aspects that make this technology not ideal for application on a large scale. The first aspect is the difficulty to set up standardized procedures for the reliable production of functioning DCs. Currently, it is difficult to demonstrate that each preparation has the same levels of processed and presented antigen, and can induce an equivalent degree of immune response after administration. Quality control in the processing of cellular products is critical to the integrity of the product. Large amounts of autologous peripheral blood mononuclear cells must be cultured in the presence of several cytokines making their off-the-shelf marketability challenging. There are critical issues not only in ensuring the proper maturation status of the DCs but also in the precise selection of appropriate subsets of DCs required to elicit the desired response. Other aspects include the significant costs of manufacturing the product and the huge amount of labor required to produce a viable product within a short time frame.

3.1.2.1 The Sipuleucel-T (Provenge) experience

Despite the above described technical hurdles, a immune cell-based vaccine, Sipuleucel-T, recently received Food and Drug Administration approval based on a successful phase III trial showing improvement in overall survival (OS) in men with asymptomatic or minimally symptomatic metastatic advanced castrate resistant prostate cancer (CRPC). The key to manufacturing feasibility of Sipuleucel-T is the absence of DC purification in the preparation. The preparation of a Sipuleucel-T product involves a leukapheresis to obtain the peripheral blood of the patient. The leukapheresed specimen is then transferred to the company manufacturing facility. The cell pellet containing DCs (CD54+), T lymphocytes (CD3+), B lymphocytes (CD19+), monocytes (CD14+), and natural killer cells (CD56+) is exposed to PA2024, an engineered antigen-cytokine fusion protein consisting of Prostate Acidic Protein (PAP) and GM-CSF. GM-CSF facilitates uptake of the fusion protein by DCs and promotes DC stimulation. PAP is the tumour antigen used in this vaccine. The final product is transported to the patient at 4°C and infused intravenously within 8 hours of formulation. Because the product is a mixture of cell types, the precise mechanism of action has not been established. It is not clear it is not clear if induction of anti-prostate cancer responses involves *in vivo* activation of T cells by the loaded DCs in the preparation. It is also possible that T cells in the preparation are activated by *ex vivo* manipulations and that this therapy actually represents an alternative form of adoptive T-cell therapy. The paucity of available immunologic data to date precludes mechanicistic dissection of this drug.

Phase I and II trials of Sipuleucel-T demonstrated T-cell and antibody responses to the antigen (Burch et al., 2004). Immune responses correlated with improved time to progression (TTP). Two sequential phase III placebo-controlled studies were subsequently conducted in patients with metastatic CRPC, with a primary end point of TTP. Integrated data again suggested a survival benefit but failed to show significance for the predetermined clinical end point. In this combined data set, a total of 225 patients were randomized to Sipuleucel-T (n = 147) or placebo (n = 78). There was a 33% reduction in the risk of death (HR 1.50; 95% CI 1.10– 2.05; P = 0.011). There was only a 4.8% PSA response in the combined analysis. Median survival was 23.2 versus 18.9 months and the percentage alive at 36 months was 33% versus 15% in favor of the treatment groups. Cumulative CD54 up-regulation, a measure of product potency, correlated with Overall Survival (OS). As a result of these studies, Dendreon pursued a new study, known as the IMmunotherapy for Prostate Adeno Carcinoma Treatment (IMPACT) trial. OS was the primary end point. Five hundred twelve patients were enrolled in this study. Despite absence of clinical response to Sipuleucel-T or effect on TTP, the study met its primary end point of survival benefit. Subjects in the treatment group experienced a statistically significant increase in median survival vs controls (25.8 vs. 21.7 months respectively) and greater OS at 36 months (31.7% vs. 23%). The final analysis after 349 events demonstrated a median OS benefit of 4.1 months (HR 0.759; 95%CI 0.606–0.951; P = 0.017) (www.dendreon.com).

3.1.3 Heat shock proteins-based vaccines

Another interesting approach in cancer vaccine development is the use of heat shock protein (HSP)-peptide complexes, as natural host vector for vaccination (reviewed in di Pietro et al., 2009). Heat shock proteins are intracellular molecules of a family characterized by members of similar molecular mass (such as hsp70 and hsp90) that act as chaperones for a repertoire of peptides, including normal self-peptides and antigenic peptides. During both protein synthesis and breakdown, heat shock protein complexes are released from cells still associated non-covalently with peptides. Release by necrotic cells function as endogenous danger signals as well as a method to cross-present antigens to DCs. In fact, DCs have a specific receptor for heat shock proteins (CD91) and its engagement leads to their maturation. HSPs complexed with antigenic peptides have been shown to efficiently deliver peptides into the MHC class I processing pathway thus generating cellular immune responses. This phenomenon has been demonstrated in mouse and human tumours. In the latter, hsp70-peptide complexes extracted from melanoma cells have been found to contain well-known peptides on the basis of their ability to stimulate antigen-specific CD8$^+$ T cells from melanoma patients' peripheral blood mononuclear cells (PBMCs). This observation has led to the purification of HSP-complexes from the tumours of patients and their administration as vaccines. The immunogenicity of tumour-derived HSP-peptide complexes, like the immunogenicity of experimentally induced tumours of mice and rats, has been shown to be individually tumour specific and not tumour type specific. These observations have led to the conclusion that the relevant tumour-antigenic, immunoprotective peptides are derived from unique rather than from shared tumour antigens.

Heat shock proteins explored for clinical immunotherapy may contain a defined antigen (E7 antigen derived from the human papilloma virus, MAGE tumour antigen, etc) or nondefined tumour antigens, which require the individualized production of heat shock proteins from fresh tumour samples. This could be a limitation, since several grams of tumour tissue must be available for the patient to be eligible for the trial. Following a number of trials (http://www.agenusbio.com/prophage/past-trials.html) in a range of tumour types (pancreatic cancer, Kidney cancer, Non-Hodgkin's lymphoma, CRC, gastric cancer) the tumour specific HSP-complexes vaccine named HSP peptide complex-96 (HSPPC-96 or Oncophage® or Prophage; Agenus, Lexington, MA, USA) has been approved in Russia as Oncophage® for the adjuvant treatment of kidney cancer patients at intermediate risk for disease recurrence. Currently Agenus is planning a registration Phase III trial for recurrent and newly diagnosed glioblastoma (http://www.agenusbio.com/prophage/ongoing-trials.html) in order to obtain drug approval by EMA.

3.1.4 Peptide vaccines

Peptide-based cancer vaccines represent the most popular approach to direct the immune system against malignant cells, since they are usually made of single epitopes, the minimal immunogenic region of an antigen. Peptides can be synthesized in a standardized manner and their cost of production is relatively low. Thus peptide vaccines have been the technology of choice by several group. Despite the strong rationale, the promising preclinical results and the frequent induction of antigen-specific immune responses in patients, peptide-based cancer vaccines have yielded relatively poor results in the clinical setting and so far none of advanced clinical trials with peptide vaccines has resulted in statistically significant increase in survival. A particular mention deserve the results of the phase III clinical trial in 676 metastatic melanoma patients, which compared the efficacy of a gp100 peptide vaccine, with that of the fully human anti CTLA-4 antibody ipilimumab, or with the combined agents (Hodi et al, 2010). Ipilimumab when compared to gp100 alone improved median overall survival from 6.4 to 10.1 months (hazard ratio for death, 0.68; P < 0.001). More importantly no difference in survival was detected between the Ipilimumab alone vs Ipilimumab plus vaccine groups (median overall survival 10.1 vs 10.0 months, hazard ration with ipilumumab plus gp100, 1.04; P = 0.76). Based on these results ipilimumab was recently approved by FDA for the treatment of unresectable stage III and IV melanoma, with the name of Yervoy® (BMS). A possible interpretation for the lack of efficacy of a peptide vaccine in a patient population otherwise responsive to immunotherapy is the necessity to generate a polyclonal immune response directed simultaneously against several MHC class I epitopes. This could not be achieved in the Ipilimimab trial cited above because of the use of a single peptide. In order to overcome this limitation alternative approaches are being undertaken which make use of a combination of immunogenic peptides.

Advances in the engineering of peptides and in our understanding of the molecular mechanisms underlying an effective immune response against tumours have renewed the enthusiasm for peptide-based vaccination regimens in the setting of cancer and a variety of clinical trials are being conducted based on the use of peptides (Aurisicchio and Ciliberto, 2010). In this respect promising results in phase II studies have been obtained by Immatics (www.immatics.com) . This technology consists in the vaccination of patients with multiple tumour-associated peptides (TUMAPs) that can be isolated from tumour specimens and identified by mass spectrometry (Dengjel et al, 2006). The most advanced product, IMA901, a combination of several TUMAPs for the treatment of renal cell carcinoma, completed a Europe-wide multi-center Phase II clinical trial and has recently commenced a Phase III trial. Another advanced peptide vaccine is L-BLP25 (Stimuvax) currently under development by MerckSerono. L-BLP25 is a peptide vaccine that targets the exposed core peptide of MUC1, a mucinous glycoprotein which is overexpressed and aberrantly glycosylated in many human malignancies. MUC1 is associated with cellular transformation and can confer resistance to genotoxic agents. In preclinical studies, L-BLP25 induced a cellular immune response characterized by T-cell proliferation in response to MUC1 and production of IFN-γ (reviewed in Gridelli et al., 2009). Phase I and II trials have established the dose and schedule of the vaccine as well as its excellent safety profile. A randomized phase II trial of maintenance L-BLP25 versus best supportive care in patients with stage IIIB/IV non-small cell lung cancer showed a strong survival trend in favor of L-BLP25 (median survival, 30.6 versus 13.3 months) in a subgroup of patients with locoregional stage IIIB disease (Butts et al., 2011). These promising results are being tested in three phase III trials (START, INSPIRE and STRIDE). The START and the INSPIRE studies are Phase III, multi-center, randomized, double-blind, placebo-controlled clinical trial designed to evaluate the efficacy, safety and tolerability of Stimuvax in subjects suffering from unresectable, stage IIIA or IIIB non-small cell lung cancer (NSCLC) who have had a response or stable disease after at least two cycles of platinum-based chemo-radiotherapy. The primary endpoint of the START study is overall survival (OS). STRIDE is a randomized, double-blind, controlled, multi-center Phase III study designed to determine if Stimuvax can extend progression free survival in patients treated with hormonal therapy who have inoperable, locally advanced, recurrent or metastatic breast cancer. Overall survival, quality of life, tumour response and safety will also be assessed in this study.

3.1.5 Protein vaccines

Isolated recombinant proteins have been successfully employed for antiviral vaccines. However, soluble proteins are poorly immunogenic and require appropriate adjuvants and delivery systems to induce the desirable level and type of immune responses. For optimal performance, antigen delivery vehicles should closely mimic the composition and immunological processing of actual pathogens; they should actively or passively target APCs such as DCs; protect the antigenic protein from spontaneous degradation; direct the nature of the resulting immune response (i.e., cellular versus humoral responses) and, lastly, induce APC maturation by interacting with elements of the innate immune system such as Toll-like receptors (TLRs). Several strategies have been reported including directly conjugating TLR ligands to protein antigens or co-encapsulating immunostimulatory agents and proteins in liposomes or hydrophobic polymeric particles (Beaudette et al., 2009).

The most advanced approach is the one being pursued for the development of MAGE-A3 antigen specific immunotherapy (ASCI). MAGE-A3 ASCI is a therapeutic cancer vaccine directed against tumour antigen MAGE-A3, which is overexpressed in subset of patients affected by various cancers, and is being developed by GSK (Tyagi and Mirakhur, 2009). The vaccine is delivered as highly purified recombinant protein in conjunction wih GSK's own proprietary adjuvant System. The most advanced development for the MAGE-A3 vaccine is a Phase III trial called MAGRIT (MAGE-A3 as Adjuvant Non-Small Cell Lung Cancer Immunotherapy), which began in October 2007 aimed at recruiting 2270 patients randomized to ASCI or placebo. The objective of the MAGRIT trial is to investigate the efficacy of MAGE-A3 ASCI in preventing cancer relapse, when administered after tumour resection, in patients with MAGE-A3 positive stages IB, II and IIIA NSCLC and is going to be the largest-ever trial in the adjuvant treatment for NSCLC. Results of the MAGRIT trial are expected in late 2011 and may lead to registration of this product in the coming years.

3.2 Genetic vaccines

Genetic vaccines represent promising methods to elicit immune responses against a wide variety of antigens, including TAAs. A variety of vectors have been utilized in the past, each of them presenting advantages and drawbacks with respect to "classic" protein-based vaccines. The main advantage of genetic vaccines is that they allow a) endogenous expression of the antigen of interest by muscle and/or antigen-presenting cells, which maximize antigen processing through the endogenous pathway and epitope display on MHC class I molecules, and b) easy molecular engineering of the targeted tumour antigen which help to boost significantly self-antigen immunogenicity.

3.2.1 Viral vaccines

Viral infection results in the presentation of virus-specific peptides in association with both MHC class I and MHC class II on the surface of infected cells. Based on this observation, several strategies have been designed to use viruses as immunization vehicles to elicit antigen-specific immune responses. In this approach, the cDNA encoding one or more antigens, is inserted into a viral vector. The resulting recombinant viruses are used as vaccine, obtaining the *in vivo* expression of the selected antigen(s) and its presentation to the immune system. A variety of gene therapy viral vectors have been adapted to cancer immunotherapy. For vaccination purposes, the ideal viral vector should be safe with respect to disease-causing potential, transmissibility and long-term persistence in the host. It should enable efficient presentation of expressed antigens to the immune system while preferably exhibiting low intrinsic immunogenicity so that it can be administered repeatedly to boost relevant specific immune responses, often necessary to break immune tolerance to self antigens.

Tumour antigen DNA sequences have been inserted into attenuated pox viruses that are unable to replicate in mammalian hosts (such as modified vaccinia Ankara, fowlpox, or canarypox). Vaccinia poxvirus (VV) was demonstrated to be safe and very effective in the induction of potent cellular and humoral immune response in several tumour model systems (Gómez et al. 2011). For Carcinoembryonic Antigen (CEA), VV as well as ALVAC, a variant of the canary poxvirus, have been successfully used in colorectal cancer patients. As an avian virus, ALVAC has an advantage over vaccinia in that it is unable to replicate in human cells and thus has a very favorable safety profile. Combination of vaccinia followed by multiple injection of ALVAC revealed to be efficient in terms of elicited anti-CEA immune response and overall patient survival (Marshall et al., 2005). Another successful story of a vaccine based on this technology is PROSTVAC-VF (Bavarian Nordic, Kvistgård, Denmark). PROSTVAC-VF is a vaccine against Prostate Specific Antigen (PSA) that includes a number of costimulatory molecules. Three well-characterized costimulatory molecules were found to be synergistic when added to the poxvirus system. This triad, which includes B7.1 (CD80), ICAM-1 (CD54), and LFA-3 (CD58), is designated as TRICOM and has been added to both the vaccinia priming vector and the fowlpox boosting vector. With PSA as the encoded antigen, this configuration constitutes PROSTVAC-VF, vaccinia-PSA-TRICOM, and fowlpox-PSA-TRICOM. Interestingly, a randomized, controlled, and double-blinded phase II study was designed and powered for the short-term end point of PFS, and it failed to find an association between treatment arm and progression. However, a strong association between treatment arm and OS was observed (Kantoff et al., 2010). The estimated hazard ratio is 0.56 (95% CI, 0.37 to 0.85), and the observed difference in median survival of 8.5 months suggests a significant therapeutic benefit. PROSTVAC-VF immunotherapy is, therefore, a promising approach, and a larger pivotal phase III trial is being planned. Another Poxvector based vaccine is Trovax, a vector directed against a tumour enriched surface marker named 5T4 (Kim et al, 2010). Clinical trials with Trovax showed good safety profile, immunologic responses to the target antigen and efficacy in relation to a defined biomarker strategy (see section 4.2). TG4010 is an MVA vector developed by Transgene (Strasbourg, France) that incorporates the MUC1 antigen, which is overexpressed in the majority of cancers. A second gene, interleukin-2 is also incorporated as an immune stimulus. The vaccine has been tested in breast, kidney, prostate and lung cancers with encouraging results in phase II. For RCC, thirty-seven patients with progressive, MUC1-positive tumours received TG4010 10^8 pfu/inj weekly for 6 weeks, then every 3 weeks until progression, when TG4010 was continued in combination with interferon-α2a and interleukin-2. Assessments included clinical response (primary endpoint), safety, time to treatment failure (TTF), OS, and immune response. No objective clinical responses occurred, but median OS was 19.3 months for all patients and 22.4 months for combination therapy recipients. MUC1-specific CD8$^+$ T cell responses were associated with longer survival (Oudard et al., 2011).

Another emerging viral system for vaccination is Adenovirus (Ad). Ads are very efficient vehicles for gene delivery and have been extensively characterized for gene therapy purposes (reviewed in Dharmapuri et al., 2009). Ad gene therapy products have recently been demonstrated to be safe, well-tolerated and capable of successful gene transfer to target cells. The high immunogenicity of E1-deleted first generation Ad recombinants has largely excluded their use for somatic gene therapy but re-directed their development as vaccine carriers. Ad vaccines have been shown to induce the highest degree of B- and CD8$^+$ T-cell responses in experimental animals, including rodents, canines, and primates against a variety of immunogens derived from a variety of infectious agents (e.g., viruses, parasites, or bacterial pathogens) and tumour cells, including tumour-associated antigens (TAAs). Most clinical trials with Ad vectors have been conducted in oncology. Among the others, intratumour (IT) injections of Ad containing the wild-type p53 tumour suppressor gene showed clinical efficacy when combined with chemotherapy and led to the clinical development of Advexin® and Gendicine®. Advexin and Gendicine® are recombinant Ad5 vectors with an E1 region that is replaced by a human wild type p53 expression cassette containing a Cytomegalovirus (CMV) or Rous sarcoma virus (RSV) promoter, respectively. In October 2003, the State Food and Drug Administration (SFDA) of China approved Gendicine as the first commercialized gene therapy product in the world. Another example is Onyx-015, the first engineered replication-selective virus to be used in humans. It is an Ad2/Ad5 hybrid with deletions in E1B and E3B region and replicates exclusively in cells with inactive p53, activated p14ARF and late viral mRNA transport. Onyx-015 has been tested in more than 15 clinical trials by direct IT injection (up to 5×10^9 vp) and resulted in transient antitumoural effects (objective response rate 14%).

For development of cancer vaccines, several groups are currently assessing the immunologic and clinical activity of Ad vectors expressing TAAs, such as prostate serum antigen (PSA), HER-2/*neu*, carcinoembryonic antigen (CEA) and telomerase (hTERT) (see www.clinicaltrials.gov). It will be of great interest to verify how local and systemic suppression exerted by the tumour itself as well as pre-existing immunity to Ad will impact the outcome of these studies.

In conclusion, viral vectors appear promising tools for cancer vaccines. From a practical standpoint, viral vectors also meet criteria that enable their large scale industrialization. These include; efficient growth on a cell substrate acceptable to regulatory authorities; total genetic stability with respect to attenuation and presence of the foreign gene(s), scalability to large doses; easy purification of the vector virus away from cellular debris, and stability in the final formulation.

3.2.2 DNA plasmid vaccines

The inoculation of plasmid DNA coding for a protein antigen by means of a simple intramuscular or intradermal injection currently represents an easily performed vaccine approach that is safe for host and relatively inexpensive. DNA delivery vehicles contain a gene expression cassette bearing the coding region of an antigen gene regulated by a promoter usually with constitutive activity (like the cytomegalovirus early enhancer-promoter). Simple injection of naked DNA sequences results in gene expression and the generation of immune responses. A possible mechanism of how DNA immunization works is the following: the protein antigen is produced by the target cells (usually skeletal myocytes or dermal fibroblasts, depending upon the injection route) that usually lack the co-stimulatory molecules needed as part of the CTL activation process. Subsequently, the antigen is taken up by host APCs, processed, and cross-presented to the immune system in the draining lymph nodes, although direct transfection of rare APCs residing at the injection site has also been demonstrated (Liu, 2011).

In mouse models, DNA vaccines have been successfully used to generate strong cellular immune responses against a wide variety of tumour antigens and to exert a preventive or therapeutic effect on tumour growth (Liu, 2011). However, clinical trials for DNA vaccines have shown that, albeit immune responses can be generated in humans, there is a need for increased potency if this vaccine technology is to be effective. The reasons for the failure of DNA vaccines to induce potent immune responses when scaled up from mice to man have not been fully elucidated. However, it is reasonable to assume that low levels of antigen production, inefficient cellular delivery of DNA plasmids and insufficient stimulation of the innate immune system have roles in low potency of DNA vaccines (Ulmer et al., 2006). In the design of more potent DNA vaccines, clearly regimens, plasmid dose, timing, adjuvants, alternative delivery systems and/or routes of vaccination are being considered. Methods for enhancing DNA plasmid delivery include tattooing, Gene gun, Ultrasound, Laser and DNA electroporation (reviewed in Bolhassani et al., 2011). In particular, here we will focus our attention on DNA electroporation.

3.2.3 DNA electroporation

In vivo electroporation of plasmid DNA (DNA-EP) has emerged as a safe method resulting in greater DNA uptake leading to enhanced protein expression in the treated muscle, and in a concomitant increase in immune responses to the target antigen in a variety of species (Aurisicchio et al., 2007; Peruzzi et al., 2010a). For its properties, DNA-EP is a desirable vaccine technology for cancer vaccines since it is repeatable several times, as required for the maintenance of anti-tumour immunity (Peruzzi et al., 2010b). This approach uses brief electrical pulses that create transient "pores" in the cell membrane, thus allowing large molecules such as DNA or RNA to enter the cell cytoplasm. Immediately following cessation of the electrical field, these pores close and the molecules are trapped in the cytoplasm (Andre et al., 2010). Typically, milli- and microsecond pulses have been used for EP. In addition to the increased permeability of target cells, EP may also enhance immune responses through increased protein expression, secretion of inflammatory chemokines and cytokines, and recruitment of APCs at the EP site (Liu, 2011). As a result, both antigen-specific humoral and cellular immune responses are increased by EP mediated delivery of plasmid DNA in comparison with levels achieved by intramuscular injection of DNA alone. Indeed, the addition of *in vivo* EP has been associated with a consistent enhancement of cell-mediated and humoral immune responses in small and large animals, supporting its use in humans.

Several devices have been developed for DNA-EP. Cytopulse has developed two clinical vaccine delivery systems: DermaVax™ and Easy Vax™. Easy Vax™ primarily targets the epidermis layer of skin and has been used in mass-scale prophylactic virus vaccination. In contrast, Derma Vax™ primarily targets the dermis layer of skin. Clinical trials in progress and planned using DermaVax™ include Prostate cancer (Phase I/II) and Colorectal cancer (Phase I/II). In this study, DNA vaccine was delivered by intradermal electroporation to treat colorectal cancer (El-porCEA; ID: NCT01064375). The purpose of this study was to evaluate the safety and immunogenicity of a CEA DNA immunization approach in patients with colorectal cancer. Altogether, the electroporation with DNA vaccines has been investigated in several clinical trials for cancer therapy. They include: (1) Intratumoural IL-12 DNA plasmid (pDNA) [ID: NCT00323206, phase I clinical trials in patients with malignant melanoma]; (2) Intratumoural VCL-IM01 (encoding IL-2) [ID: NCT00223899; phase I clinical trials in patients with metastatic melanoma]; (3) Xenogeneic tyrosinase DNA vaccine [ID: NCT00471133, phase I clinical trials in patients with melanoma]; (4) VGX-3100 [ID: NCT00685412, phase I clinical trials for HPV infections], and 5) IM injection prostate-specific membrane antigen (PSMA)/pDOM fusion gene [ID: UK-112, phase I/II clinical trials for prostate cancer] (Bodles-Bakhop et al., 2009). Inovio (Oslo, Norway) has developed electroporators suitable for muscle DNA-EP, such as MedPulser®. Plasmid V930 is DNA vaccine candidate being developed by Merck. This vaccine is designed to target cancers expressing the antigens HER-2/*neu* and/or CEA, which include breast, colorectal, ovarian, and non-small cell lung cancer (ID: NCT00250419). V934 is a DNA plasmid that encodes human Telomerase (hTERT). The biologic is a Merck proprietary, therapeutic DNA vaccine candidate designed to target cancers expressing the antigen hTERT (ID: NCT00753415), including non-small cell lung carcinoma; breast cancer; melanoma; upper GI tract (e.g. esophagus, stomach, gallbladder) in collaboration with Geron Corp. (Menlo Park, CA, USA). Both vaccines are undergoing Phase I studies using MedPulser® DNA Delivery System in combination with Ad vectors.

Attempts to further enhance immune responses elicited by DNA vaccines are focusing on the use of codon optimization in order to enhance expression in eukaryotic cells. In fact, the potency of current gene delivery methods that include plasmid DNA and viral vectors can also be improved through increasing the expression efficiency of the encoded antigens. Elevated percentages of AU in human mRNA have been shown to result in instability, increased turnover, and low expression levels of the encoded proteins. These findings have prompted modification of the target gene coding sequence through reduction of the AT content with the assumption that these modifications could result in improved mRNA stability and increased expression. These changes have been justified by the observation that for highly expressed genes, G or C is generally preferred over A or T. In fact, optimization of the codon usage of the target gene has been shown in a variety of experimental systems to lead to enhanced expression and increased immunogenicity (Aurisicchio et al., 2007; Peruzzi et al., 2010a, b).

Another strategy to enhance the efficacy of DNA vaccine is the development of gene fusions in which antigens are linked to various immunoenhancing elements (reviewed in Stevenson et al., 2004). The enhancement of immune responses is particularly relevant for cancer vaccines because of the limited immunogenicity of tumour antigens and the need to overcome tolerance. Enhancement of immune response to target antigens has been demonstrated in animal models by vectors encoding antigens fused to heat shock protein 70 (HSP70), the Fc portion of IgG1, lysosome-associated membrane protein (LAMP), the universal helper T (Th) epitope from tetanus toxin (DOM) (Facciabene et al., 2006) and Heat labile enterotoxin B from *E. Coli* (Facciabene et al., 2007). A DOM-PSMA fusion DNA vaccine delivered *via* DNA-EP resulted in highest antibody response to DOM in prostate cancer patients (Low et al., 2009), while LTB fusions are currently being evaluated in the clinical trials for CEA and hTERT cited above.

In conclusion, DNA vaccines have several promising features. They are simpler and cheaper to produce. DNA immunization is not associated with anamnestic immune responses against the vector. On the other hand, it appears that efficacy must be improved, especially for cancer vaccines targeting 'self' antigens.

3.3 Heterologous prime/boost
There are emerging evidences that vaccination schedules comprising more than one delivery method against the same antigen(s) (i.e., genetic vectors, genetic vector/protein, genetic vector/peptides, etc.) may be beneficial to overcome the 'therapeutic immunity' threshold and adequately harness the immune system to fight cancer. In particular, genetic vectors, if appropriately combined with each other and with other agents (immunomodulators and/or chemotherapy) hold promise for clinical development (reviewed in Lu et al., 2009).

The sequential administration of DNA and a viral vector in different combinations may result in synergistic immune activation. Preclinical murine and primate models have shown that this heterologous prime-boost regimen induces 10- to 100-fold higher frequencies of T cells than do naked DNA or recombinant viral vectors alone (Ribas et al., 2003). In addition to the enhanced immune response, the therapeutic proof of concept of DNA/viral vector combination has recently been achieved in dogs affected by B cell lymphoma (Peruzzi et al., 2010b). In this study, the best performing vaccination schedule consisted of Ad followed by DNA-EP boosters, concurrently with chemotherapy (see also section 4.1). Another strategy is the sequential administration of two different viral vectors carrying the same tumour antigen gene, which bypasses the limitation of the development of neutralizing antibodies to the viral backbone by boosting with a different vector without shared viral epitopes (see paragraph 3.2.1).

4. Cancer vaccines clinical development

Due to the complexity of tumour immunology, the success of cancer vaccines points to important considerations for clinical development: (1) evaluation of vaccines in predictive preclinical animal models. (2) Biomarker strategies for patient selection. This turns to be a crucial aspect as revealed by the experience of different cancer vaccine products under evaluation (see next paragraph); (3) value of vaccinating at early stages of cancer progression. Advances in early cancer detection methods and the development of efficacious cancer vaccines will allow vaccination of patients with various types of cancer at early stages of disease, when they still have an intact immune system. This may become the most promising strategy for preventing tumour progression. (4) use of heterologous prime-boost technologies (see previous paragraph). (5) combination with other therapies. Some classes of chemotherapy drugs could act as immunomodulators by affecting antigen cross-presentation, inducing a cytokine storm, reducing the number of regulatory T cells and activating homeostatic lymphoid proliferation. (6) autoimmunity as a possible side effect of cancer immunotherapy. In those instances when intense immunotherapy is necessary the incidence of autoimmunity in early or especially in advanced cancer should be evaluated in the short or long term following immunotherapy.

4.1 Pre-clinical models
Cancer immune therapy and its translation to the clinic are strictly dependent on efficient vaccine technology, delivery systems and evaluation in appropriate pre-clinical models. For

cancer vaccines the most widely used models for immunologic and anti-tumoural studies are transgenic rodents expressing the human TAA which show central and/or peripheral tolerance to the antigen of interest (see Fig. 1). The mouse is an excellent and reproducible system: mice from a given strain are inbred, with same MHC-I, allow experimentation on a large number of subjects. The mouse immune system is well-known and all reagents are available. Nevertheless, the translational relevance of cancer vaccines additionally needs a suitable, outbred therapeutic large animal model. In fact, scaling up experimental protocols from rodents to humans is often not a straightforward procedure, and this particularly applies to cancer vaccines, where vaccination technology must be especially effective to overcome a variety of immune suppressive mechanisms.

Nonhuman primates such as macaques are valid models to determine the safety and immunogenicity of candidate vaccines that are being developed for implementation in humans. In fact, the immune response is similar to that expected in humans. In the last two decades numerous immunogenicity studies have been performed in nonhuman primates utilizing pre-clinical candidate vaccines, most of them utilizing recombinant proteins of bacterial or viral origin as immunogen or genetic vectors coding for viral antigens (Shiver et al., 2002; Montgomery et al., 1993; Jeong et al., 2004). This is a reasonable approach when dealing with bacterial or viral diseases, where the organism recognizes the antigen as an exogenous protein and consequently the elicited immune-response is generally strong and effective against the target pathogen. Similarly, other studies involving the use of TAAs have been conducted with human proteins or vectors encoding for human TAAs: in these reports, the elicited immune response is not expected to be fully predictive of the possible outcome in human patients, since the antigen is recognized as a non-self protein. Therefore, the evaluation of the immune response against the 'self' antigen requires cloning of the nonhuman primate ortholog gene and evaluation of a technology able to break immune tolerance (Aurisicchio et al., 2007; Fattori et al., 2009). Still, evaluation of antitumour efficacy cannot be performed in nonhuman primates.

Another emerging model in oncology is the dog. The dog is extensively used in drug discovery and development because of its similarities to human anatomy and physiology. Compared with other animal models, dogs naturally develop cancers that share many characteristics with human malignancies (Paoloni et al., 2008). Cancers in pet dogs are characterized by tumour growth over long periods of time in the setting of an intact immune system, interindividual and intra-tumoural heterogeneity, the development of recurrent or resistant disease, and metastasis to relevant distant sites. Thanks to their large population size, cancer rate in pets is sufficient to power clinical trials, including assessment of new drugs. Examples include non-Hodgkin lymphoma, osteosarcoma, melanoma, prostate carcinoma, lung carcinoma, head and neck carcinoma, mammary carcinoma and soft tissue sarcoma, which share similar histological appearance, tumour genetics, biological behavior and response to conventional therapies with human cancers. With the recent release of the canine genome sequence, the dog is now also amenable to comparative genomic and expression analysis, including tumour samples (Uva et al., 2009) . However, to date the application of cancer vaccines in dogs has been poorly explored. A xenogeneic DNA-based vaccine strategy for melanoma is the only example in the setting of minimal residual disease in dogs (Bergman et al., 2006) that led to the successful approval and the commercial launch of a veterinary biological (Merial US). Furthermore, recently we have been able to successfully evaluate a heterologous prime-boost Ad-vector /DNA-EP based vaccine against telomerase in canine subjects affected by B cell lymphoma (Peruzzi et al., 2010b). Unfortunately, the canine immune system is not deeply characterized and there are not many tools available to further evaluate the impact of a vaccination strategies. However, we expect that pet dog nonclinical studies will increasingly gain interest to help a better definition of the safety and activity of new anticancer agents and the identification of relevant biomarkers associated with response or exposure to these drugs.

Animal Models for Cancer Vaccines

Basic requirements:
- Appropriate expression of the antigen
  - Tissue distribution
  - Expression level
- Immunologically tolerant to the antigen
- Spontaneous tumorigenesis

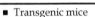

▪ Transgenic mice	▪ Rhesus monkey	▪ Dogs
– Immune system well characterized – Ease of manipulation – Can develop spontaneous tumors – Small size	– Larger size – Immune system similar to Humans – Efficacy studies difficult to perform	– Similar tumor gene expression profile to humans – Large number of cancer patients – Immune system less characterized

Fig. 1. Animal models for Cancer Vaccines. Advantages and drawbacks of each model are indicated.

4.2 Biomarker strategies

Drug failures in Oncology often originate from a lack of understanding of the biology of the drug, its mechanism of action (MOA), the complexity of patient physiology, and inadequate characterization of patient tumours. Poor understanding of the criteria required for patient selection for the drug may lead to misapprehensions of the drug's potential for safety and efficacy. It is these misapprehensions that can persist through to late development until the clinical program crashes in a late and costly failure. Clearly, there is an urgent need for detailed information on new anticancer drugs to help make critical development decisions at the earliest possible point, speeding up the development process and enabling valuable time and resources to be placed where they can do the most good.

Molecular biomarkers are widely recognized as being integral to this solution. They provide a set of tools which can provide invaluable information to support two major development concerns:

1.   Does the drug perform according to the expected mechanism of action?
2.   Which patients will experience benefit in disease management utilizing the drug?

Thus, appropriately selected biomarkers can be used to confirm the MOA, while patient selection biomarkers can be used to guide the selection of the most appropriate patients for therapies. Correct use of biomarkers for patient selection can enrich the treatment population by identifying those most likely to benefit from the treatment. This reduces the risk to the non-responder population and, by allowing earlier assessment of therapeutic efficacy, substantially shrinks the costs of development.

Over the past two decades molecular biomarkers have become established components of clinical research in a way few could have foreseen. Today > 50% of new molecular entities are estimated to have a biomarker element also in development (Carden et al, 2010).

Nowadays the most successful examples of biomarkers for patient selection are HER2 positivity for treating breast cancer patients with Herceptin® and lack of KRAS mutations for treatment of colorectal cancer patients with Erbitux® or Vectibix®. They have completely different histories. The development of Herceptin was guided from its earliest stages by the use of the selection biomarker – HER2 – as an integral part of the original development plan for the product (Pietras et al, 1998). However, in the case of Erbitux® (cetuximab) and Vectibix® (panitumumab) in colorectal cancer, the original hypothesis that the level of epidermal growth factor receptor (EGFR) expression was critical for success of the antibody turned out to be wrong. Only recently the crucial role of KRAS wild type (or non-KRAS mutant carrying) tumour cells has been found to be a necessary element for Erbitux functioning and thus has been introduced into the drug's label (http://www.fda.gov/AboutFDA/CentersOffices/CDER/ucm172905.htm).

All the considerations above need to be applied also to the development of cancer vaccines and cancer immunotherapeutics in general. It is inconceivable nowadays to imagine that a new immunotherapy will be efficacious when administered to all patients affected by a given cancer pathology. Therefore a rigorous biomarker strategy is absolutely essential to avoid failures in cancer vaccines development (Gajewski et al, 2010; Disis, 2011). As a corollary, we believe that one of the main reasons for the several failures of previous cancer vaccines in phase III is the lack of biomarkers for patients selection, and this in spite of radiological evidences of direct anti-tumour efficacy observed in subsets of patients during precedent Phase II trials. Therefore, several attempts are currently being made to rescue vaccines "failed" in Phase III trials through a rigorous retrospective analysis of data collected in Phase III in order to identify biomarkers that can allow to predict patients who will most benefit from treatment, and then to restart Phase II and Phase III development.

This is the case for example of Trovax (see paragraph 3.2.1). Trovax was developed through a series of Phase I an II trials, until it was brought into a Phase III trial called TRIST (TroVax Renal Immunotherapy Trial) in patients with advanced or metastatic renal cell carcinoma. The study enrolled 733 patients divided in two arms: 1) Trovax + IL2 or IFNα or sunitinib; 2) Placebo + IL2 or IFNα or sunitinib (Amato et al, 2010). The primary predefined endpoint, namely survival (80% power, HR= 0.725; α= 0.05), was not met. However , subsequent analysis showed survival advantage in certain subsets of patients, and this opened up to studies aiming at identifying factors which could maximize benefit. In particular immunological monitoring suggested that 5T4 antibody responses were associated with increased survival (Harrop et al, 2011). However, it was necessary to show that 5T4 antibody responses was not simply linked to the general health status of the patients. This was possible through the identification of an "immune response surrogate", capable of predicting antibody responses with a reasonable level of accuracy. This was indeed identified in baseline platelet levels. In fact elevated platelet levels inversely correlate with anti 5T4 antibody responses and therapeutic efficacy. This new biomarker is currently being analyzed in additional ongoing trials and will likely be used to inform future strategies for renewed Phase II/III development of TroVax.

As mentioned in the introduction section, ipilimumab, the fully human monoclonal antibody directed against CTLA-4 has had a luckier developmental fate and was recently approved by FDA for the treatment of metastatic melanoma. A 3.7-month survival benefit was observed in the registration PhaseIII trial in the ipilimumab arm vs control gp-100 peptide vaccine arm was achieved (hazard ratio 0.68; P = 0.003), which met the predefined primary endpoint (Hodi et al, 2010). However if we look only at tumour responses only a minority of patients treated with ipilimumab or with the other anti CTLA-4 antibody under development, tremelimumab, achieve radiographic responses (Sarnaik and Weber, 2009). In the search of biomarkers capable of predicting early efficacy of these two antibodies immunological monitoring has been an integral part of their clinical development. Approaches to immunological monitoring have included: 1) monitoring the frequency of specific populations of cells in peripheral blood or tumour; 2) monitoring changes in expression levels of specific markers on immune cells; 3) quantifying antigen specific immune responses including antibody and CD8+ or CD4+ T cell responses; 4) monitoring changes in peripheral cytokine levels of cytokines produced by specific immune cell populations. This has led to the identification of several endpoints that may correlate with a variety of clinical parameters (reviewed in Callahan et al, 2010). The most robust correlation to date is with the rate of absolute lymphocyte counts (ALC), which was shown to correlate with clinical benefit (Berman et al, 2009). Also, inducible costimulator (ICOS) a member of the immunoglobulin gene family, seems to be involved. In some studies a correlation between increased frequency of circulating CD4+ICOShigh T cells and Overall Survival has been shown (Chen et al, 2009; Vonderheide et al, 2010; Charton et al, 2010). Promising biomarkers also appear to be increases in CD54RO and HLA-DR on circulating CD4+ and CD8+ T cells (Comin-Anduix et al, 2008), poly-epitope antigen specific immune responses (Yuan et al, 2008) and degree of intratumoural Treg infiltration (Ribas et al, 2009). Finally perhaps the most recent but probably most promising biomarker appears to be the change in circulating levels of Th17 as shown in a recent study on 75 patients (Sarnaik et al, 2011), where higher changes in Th-17 inducible frequency was a surrogate marker of freedom from relapse (p=0.047). These biomarkers have been so far identified in small retrospective trials, but their validation awaits larger prospective studies. Also, another present limitation of these biomarkers is that they belong more to the category of efficacy biomarkers than to that of stratification biomarkers and therefore, do not look as promising tools to stratify patients that are expected to better respond to therapy.

A clever biomarker strategy has been applied for MAGE-A3 ASCI by GSK (see paragraph 3.1.5). The MAGRIT study applies stringent patient stratification criteria based upon the level of expression of MAGE-A3 in patients' tumours (approximately 40% of NSCLC patients), which are believed to have greater chances of responding to therapy, mirroring the same strategy adopted during Herceptin® development. Furthermore, during the early phases of MAGE-A3 ASCI clinical development a multiple gene signature predictive of response to therapy was derived with an unbiased approach from microarray analysis of RNA extracted from peripheral lymphocytes of treated patients, in the attempt to establish a correlation between gene expression and disease relapse. The MAGRIT trial will have as an additional objective the validation of this predictive signature in a prospective manner.

4.3 Combination therapies

The greatest potential for cancer vaccines will derive from the possibility to combine these treatments with existing and forthcoming therapeutics in order to create synergies while mitigating side effects (Andersen et al, 2010). Understanding the molecular basis for synergies poses significant scientific challenges, together with the definition of the best protocols for combinations. The establishment and optimization of dosing and scheduling of multiple treatments will require intensive pre-clinical studies as well as the conduct of well designed clinical study protocols with the consequence of significantly increasing development costs. Furthermore, for the combination of experimental drugs the ability to conduct combination studies will require that Companies that are commercially pursuing different drugs and vaccine candidates must come to specific agreements.

4.3.1 Combining vaccines with chemotherapy

It is now clear that chemotherapy, instead of having a general immunodepressant effect, when given in particular combination schedules, can have a potent immunostimulatory effect and may enhance cancer vaccine efficacy. Several pre-clinical studies have been at the basis of what is now called chemoimmunotherapy, a strategy which is structured upon the possibility to enhance cancer vaccine efficacy through well studied combinations with available chemotherapeutic agents. Promising clinical results have been obtained, which are waiting for confirmation in larger randomized trials (Zitvogel et al, 2008).

A leading example is that of cyclophosphamide (CTX), an alkylating agent that has been used for a long time at high dosages as a potent cytotoxic and lymphoablative drug. In recent years careful studies have shown that low doses CTX (also called metronomic CTX) have instead immunostimulatory and antiangiogenic effects, opening up new applications for cancer immunotherapy. By promoting IFNα secretion, CTX influences dendritic cells homeostatis, leading to preferential expansion of CD8α+ DCs, i.e. the main subset involved in cross-presentation of cell-derived antigens (Schiavoni et al, 2011; Moschella et al, 2011). Furthermore CTX induces tumour cell death with consequent DCs uptake of tumour apoptotic material, and CD8+ T-cell cross priming. Finally CTX induces a T-helper 17 (Th17) status, capable of shifting the Treg/Teffector equilibrium in favor of tumour regression (Sistigu et al, 2011). Another drug that is being combined with cancer vaccines with promising results is dacarbazine, due to its known effect in stimulating cytokine production, modulating Treg numbers and favouring homeostatic proliferation of effector T cells (Nisticò et al, 2009).

Chemotherapy-induced cell death can also be qualitatively immunogenic through upregulation of surface calreticulin. This process, called immunogenic apoptosis has been observed with chemotherapeutic agents such as oxaliplatin and anthracyclines and is activated by pre-apoptotic ER stress. Calreticulin, a protein usually residing in the endoplasmic reticulum is translocated onto the plasma membrane surface and triggers cell engulfment by dendritic cells and tumour associated antigens presentation (Zitvogel et al, 2010). Finally, other chemotherapeutic agents such as gemcitabine have been shown to favor depletion of TAMs and may enhance vaccine efficacy through removal of their negative regulation on effector T cells (Suzuki et al, 2007).

4.3.2 Combining vaccines with immunomodulators

From the mechanistic standpoint these are the combinations that should work best. Depending upon their mechanism of action immunomodulators are expected either to increase vaccine immunogenicity by potentiating antigen-specific CD8+ and/or CD4+ T cell responses, or to increase vaccine effectiveness by impairing one or more of those immunosuppressive mechanisms that operate at the level of tumour microenvironment. It was unfortunate that these expectations were not met in the Phase III trial that led to registration of Ipilimumab. In that 3 arms trial, Ipilimumab alone was as effective at increasing OS as the combination of Ipilimumab plus a peptide gp100 vaccine (Hodi et al, 2010). In other words, adding a therapeutic melanoma vaccine on top of Ipilimumab did not provide additional advantage. Several are the possible explanations of this failure, but we believe, as discussed above (see section 3.1.4) that peptide vaccines, especially those monospecific, i.e. directed against a single epitope, are not potent enough to show efficacy, in particular in large trials like this one, where no patients stratification criteria are being applied.

Nevertheless, we believe that vaccines plus immunomodulators combinations hold a great potential; however, they need to be studied in detail starting from rigorous preclinical studies. Furthermore, success of the same immunomodulators in one combination cannot be automatically extrapolated to another combination, because this may be affected by the combined vaccine/immunomodulators mechanism of action, and by the disease under study. For example we have observed that the same immunomodulators, namely an IMO TLR9 agonist exerts different effects when co-delivered with two genetic vaccines targeting different tumour antigens in two distinct pre-C models. In the BALB/*NeuT* model repeated vaccinations against HER2 with DNA electroporation plus systemic IMO administration proved to be the most effective treatment in the eradication of advanced mammary tumours (Aurisicchio et al, 2009). In contrast this was not the case when the same systemic IMO was co-delivered together with a genetic telomerase vaccine in an immunocompetent mouse model of melanoma (Conforti et al, 2010). We believe this discrepancy is due to the fact that in the first case the anti-HER2 vaccine acts primarily through the induction of antitumoural antibody responses that are strongly enhanced by systemic IMO in mice (Aurisicchio et al, 2009). In contrast, the telomerase vaccine mechanism of action is exerted via the induction of antigen-specific cytotoxic CD8+ responses (Mennuni et al, 2008) which are not increased by systemic IMO delivery.

Among the most promising approaches to combinations is the one with agents capable to target Tregs (Golovina and Vonderheide, 2010). For example, in a transgenic CEA preclinical model we have observed that administration of an anti CEA vaccine plus an antibody against CD25 strongly enhanced CEA specific CD4+ and CD8+ antigen-specific immunity and exerted a strong tumour protection (Elia et al , 2007). Indeed a single infusion of daclizumab (Zenapax), a monoclonal antibody against CD25, in patients with metastatic breast cancer is associated with a strong and prolonged decrease of circulating CD25+ FoxP3+ Tregs. When a peptide vaccine was administered after Zenapax infusion, at the nadir of circulating Tregs, a strong generation of antigen-specific immunity was observed.

In a very recent study, the administration of an agonistic CD40 antibody was shown, when combined with gemcitabine in a small cohort of patients with pancreatic ductal adenocarcinoma to induce tumour regressions (Beatty et al, 2011). Although in theory antibodies against CD40 are believed to act through reversion of immune suppression and induction of antitumour T cell responses, this was shown not to be the case in this trial and in a relevant mouse model. Surprisingly the antibody seemed to act via a new and unsuspected mechanism of action, which consisted in the stimulation of macrophages which infiltrated the tumours, became tumouricidal and facilitated depletion of tumour stroma.

In conclusion, we believe that combinations of immunomodulators like Zenapax, TLR agonists, anti-CTLA4 antibodies, anti-PD1 antibodies, IDO inhibitors, etc. together with cancer vaccines, may have great potential to increase vaccine effectiveness and to prolong survival, but careful mechanistic studies have to be conducted to identify the best combination and the most appropriate delivery schedule for the two agents.

4.3.3 Combining vaccines with other targeted therapies

The availability of an expanding repertoire of targeted therapies against cancer opens up tremendous possibility for combinations with therapeutic cancer vaccines. This is still a largely unexplored area. However we believe that, in parallel with the clinical progress and the increasing number of FDA and EMA approved vaccines, this area will be the object of extensive investigations. Based on the mechanism of action for example anti-angiogenic agents are expected to act synergically with cancer vaccines. The same concept can be applied to combinations with anti-apoptotic agents targeting Bcl-2 members. Finally we have to be aware that some cancer targeted therapies may exert a negative effect on immune responses. This is for example the case of sorafenib, which has been shown in a preclinical model to significantly affect the immunostimulatory capacity of DCs (Hipp et al, 2008), or of HDAC inhibitors which are able to increase the suppressive functions of Tregs (Akimova et al, 2010)

4.3.4 Adverse effects of cancer Immunotherapy

Cancer Immunotherapy has been initially advocated as being very specific for cancer cells and to have fewer side effects than conventional therapies. This concept is confirmed by reports from cancer vaccines clinical trials of cases of patients experiencing complete responses in the absence of any serious adverse event (Suso et al, 2011). An even more significant example is the very benign toxicity profile of Sipuleucel-T (Plosker, 2011). It has to be pointed out however, when examining large trials, that vaccine-related adverse events, albeit rare and usually mild, are being observed. For example in a recent meta-analysis of 500 cases of advanced cancer patients treated with therapeutic peptide vaccines, 6 severe adverse events (SAEs) were related to the vaccine itself (Yoshida et al, 2011). They consisted mainly in local skin reactions or cellulitis around the injection sites. In some cases, more systemic effects such as edemas of the head and neck regions, colitis, rectal bleeding and bladder-vaginal fistulae were reported.

The occurrence of autimmuninty is particularly evident in the case of therapies with systemic immunomodulators more than with cancer vaccines. Indeed, Immune-related adverse events (IRAEs) are being commonly observed in patients after CTLA-4 blockade and most likely reflect the drug mechanism of action and corresponding effects on the immune system (Weber, 2007). Immunotoxicities resulting from Ipilimumab treatment can range from relatively minor conditions, such as skin depigmentation, to severe toxicities against crucial organ systems, such as liver, heart and lung. In the Ipilimumab registration trial Grade 3 or 4 IRAEs occurred in 10 to 15% of patients treated and seven deaths were associated with IRAEs (Hodi et al, 2010). Treatment-related toxicity correlates with better responses in some cases, and it is likely that serious adverse events from immune-mediated reactions will increase in frequency and severity as immunotherapeutic approaches become more effective (Amost et al, 2011). Hence, scientists and physicians should be on guard for SAEs associated with augmented immune responses and strategies will have to be developed to avoid or circumvent these side effects.

The use of viral vectors in past gene-therapy trials has been shown to cause the occurrence of leukemogenesis (Dunbar, 2007). This phenomenon has been linked to the use of retroviral vectors and is due to their integration into the host genome and the activation of adjacent proto-oncogenes. It is, therefore, important to carefully analyze whether genetic vaccines that make use of either naked DNA or viral vectors may raise similar issues. It has to be pointed out, however, that genetic vaccines bear two significant differences when compared to gene therapy with retroviral vectors. In first instance DNA, also following electroporation (Wang et al, 2004), as well as Adenoviral (Jager and Ehrhardt, 2007) or Pox vectors used for cancer vaccines have a very low or null chromosomal integration respectively in the host genome. The second aspect is that vaccines are inoculated at peripheral sites in the body such as dermal tissue or skeletal muscles which are mainly composed of terminally differentiated and mitotic quiescent cells. At any rate, Regulatory Agencies require the inclusion of genome integration and genotox studies for any new genetic vaccine as part of the documentation to be included in IND filings.

5. Clinical endpoints

Cancer Vaccines and Cancer Immunotherapy in general act via a gradual build up of immune responses in the body that eventually are expected to affect cancer growth and propagation. The realization that the kinetics of this process are relatively slow as compared to the more immediate effects of chemotherapy have led to the conclusion that the conventional clinical trial endpoints cannot be applied as such also to Cancer Immunotherapy trials, and that there was a need for the establishment of new and specific criteria. Several initiatives in this direction were started over the past years and were coordinated by the Cancer Immunotherapy Consortium of the Cancer Research Institute (CIC-CRI) in collaboration with the International Society for Biological Therapy of Cancer in USA and with the Association for Cancer Immunotherapy (C-IMT) in Europe. They led to the issuance in year 2009 of a guidance document by FDA (see next paragraph)whose principles are summarized below (for a detailed description, please refer to Hoos et al, 2010).

Essentially three novel endpoint considerations, which require extensive validation by prospective assessment in clinical studies, were formulated: 1) Harmonize assays directed to assess cellular immune response to tumour antigens in order to minimize assay variability among clinical sites. The goal is to obtain a reproducible biomarker that eventually will allow to establish more precise correlations between immune response and clinical efficacy; 2) Adopt new criteria for antitumour response which are adapted from the standard Response Evaluation Criteria in Solid Tumours (RECIST) criteria; 3) Use different statistical methods for trial design and assessment of survival outcomes.

The Cancer Vaccine Clinical Trial Working group first proposed that immunoassays should be performed at least at three different time points, one baseline and two follow up. At least two assays should be used in parallel to provide relevant data to inform go/nogo decision for further development. Furthermore, the cutoff values for an immune response should be established prospectively both to define a positive vs negative response and to define the proportion of patients needed to conclude for a positive outcome. With respect to assay harmonization it was soon realized that several assays are being used (ELISPOT, IFN-γ intracellular staining, HLA-peptide multimer-staining, etc) with principles and procedures different in different laboratories. This hampers data reproducibility and comparisons among studies. Immunomonitoring proficiency panels were launched to address these issues for individual assays. These panels have worked by accrual of patients' samples and preparation of peripheral blood mononuclear cells, which were then shipped and tested across multiple laboratories, using their respective protocols. Results were then centrally analyzed. The ELISPOT panel has been the longest running panel, and its results have led to initial ELISPOT harmonization guidelines (Janetzki et al, 2007), which are directed to address key variables across different laboratories that influence assay outcome, but do not impose assay standardizations (Hoos et al, 2010).

Investigators rely on RECIST criteria to assess clinical activity of anticancer agents (Eisenhauer et al, 2009). These criteria nicely capture the effects of chemotherapeutic agents and measure tumour shrinkage. These criteria are used to distinguish Progressive Disease (PD) vs Stable Disease (SD), Partial Response (PR) or Complete Response (CR) and inform about trial continuation or discontinuation of experimental new therapies. However, it has become evident with time that RECIST criteria do not offer a complete description of the response to immunotherapeutic agents and need to be adjusted. This is due to the fact that the dynamics of antitumour effects of immunotherapeutic agents are in general much slower then chemotherapies and that in some cases patients with a stable disease, or a progressive disease at early time points, experience tumour regression at a later time. The Cancer Vaccine Clinical Trial Working Group addressed this issue, concluded that the appearance of measurable clinical activity for immunotherapies may take longer than for cytotoxic therapies (also after conventional progressive disease has been declared) and that application of standard RECIST criteria, may lead to inappropriate trial discontinuation (Hoos et al, 2007). By analyzing data from several different immunotherapy trials on a large number of patients a set of four distinct patterns were detected: immediate response, durable stable disease, response after tumour increase, and response in the presence of new lesions. While the first two patterns are included in conventional RECIST criteria, the other two are not. Therefore, in order to capture all patterns observed, the so called immune related Response Criteria (irRC) were formulated (Wolchok et al, 2009); irPD (immune-related Progressive Disease), irSD (immune-related Stable Disease), irPR (immune-related Partial Response), irCR (immune-related Complete Response) using the same thresholds to distinguish between categories as in the standard RECIST criteria. However, there are two substantial differences: a) Progressive Disease is declared not simply upon the appearance of new tumour lesions but upon the measure of total tumour burden according to a precise formula (Hoos et al, 2010); b) that measure should be confirmed at least at two consecutive time points. Using irRC the appearance of new tumour lesions alone does not constitute therefore irPD if they do not add to the total tumour burden measured at the initiation of the treatment by at least 25%, and if they are not confirmed at the subsequent time point. These new criteria are meaningful because they have received extensive validation in clinical trials with ipilimumab and have shown to correlate with favorable patients survival. However, their prospective evaluation in new trials is required to confirm their clinical utility.

Finally, at variance with chemotherapy, where early clinical effects are possible, immunotherapies often show delayed clinical effects. This is evident when analyzing

Kaplan-Meier survival curves of Provenge trials (Kantoff et al, 2010), where delayed separation of survival curves between active treatment vs control is observed. If this delayed separation is a general phenomenon for immunotherapeutic agents, then the statistical power to differentiate the curves is reduced. Therefore new statistical paradigms need to be established which take this into account in order to avoid miscalculations in the number of patients to be accrued in Phase III registration trials, and in the number of events required to calculate Hazard Ratio and Confidence Interval. It is highly recommended in this case that the quantification to compute the required events comes from previous randomized well designed Phase II trials.

In conclusion to this section we anticipate that the application of these new clinical endpoints is going to positively enhance the probability of success of cancer vaccines, allow faster and more informed GO/NOGO decisions in early clinical development and to prioritize agents that have the best profile to show statistically meaningful survival benefit.

6. Regulatory perspectives

Sipuleucel-T (Provenge®,Dendreon) is the only therapeutic cancer vaccine approved by FDA. However several promising vaccines such as M-Vax, (AVAX Technologies, Inc.) OncoVax (Vaccinogen), TroVax (Oxford Biomedica), ASCI MAGE-A3 (GSK), Oncophage® (Agenus) are in late stage development and are preparing for regulatory review in the United States, Europe, Canada, or other international regions (www.MarketResearch.com). Many of the products with potential approval status over the coming years are already in Phase III development, have orphan drug status, SPA status, or Fast Track status. As a signal of a new open attitude towards cancer vaccines, the FDA has recently issued new draft clinical trial guidelines for makers of therapeutic cancer vaccines intended to treat patients with existing disease (http://www.fda.gov/BiologicsBlood Vaccines /GuidanceComplianceRegulatoryInformation/Guidances/Vaccines/ucm182443.htm). Most notably, the draft guidance, in line with the new criteria described in section 5. advises that time-to-tumor-progression may not be an appropriate endpoint for cancer vaccines and that immune response launched against the tumour may take longer than the time it takes for it to progress. As the mechanism of action for most cancer vaccines is thought to be mediated through amplifying a native T-cell response, especially cytotoxic T cells, regulators explained that development of a cancer vaccine can present different considerations for clinical trial design than development of a traditional cytotoxic drug or biological product for the treatment of cancer. Consequently, developers of cancer vaccines are now encouraged to move forward with new products, although they need to weigh the advantages and disadvantages of testing their agents in patients with metastatic diseases vs. patients with no evidence of residual disease or minimal burden of disease.

7. Future directions

We believe that therapeutic cancer vaccines have a bright future and that within the next ten years they will become an established therapeutic modality for cancer, in a manner similar to what have now become monoclonal antibodies. This success will strictly depend upon the respect of the four major principles listed below (see also Fig 2);

The "Key" to successful cancer vaccine development

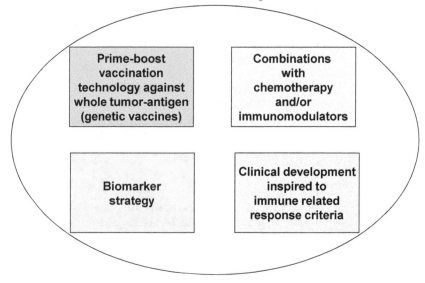

Fig. 2. Components and requirements for successful cancer vaccines development.

1. Use of a well established vaccination technology capable of inducing strong multi-epitope antigen-specific T and B cell responses, while using reproducible and easily scalable technologies. In this respect we believe that the most promising platforms for vaccination are those based on the use of genetic vectors, primarily when used in heterologous prime-boost combinations;
2. Appropriate combinations of vaccines with chemotherapy and/or with immunomodulators;
3. Development of an articulated biomarker strategy, which allows in parallel with clinical development to reproducibly quantify antigen-specific T cell responses as a pharmacodynamic measure of vaccine immunogenicity, and to pre-select the best responders to treatment;
4. A development paradigm that takes into account the evolving scenario and that is constantly inspired to the improved endpoints for cancer immunotherapy trials

8. Acknowledgements

G.C. work was supported in part by a grant AIRC IG 10334. L.A. work was supported in part by a grant AIRC IG 10507.

9. References

Akimova T, Ge G, Golovina T et al (2010) Histone/protein deacetylase inhibitors increase suppressive functions of human FOXP3 + Tregs , *Clin Immunol* Sep; 136 (3): 348-63

Aldrich JF, Lowe DB, Shearer MH et al (2010) Vaccines and Immunotherapeutics for the Treatment of Malignant Disease, *Clin. Dev. Immunol.* 697158 Epub 2010 Sep26

Amato RJ, Hawkins RE, Kaufman HL et al (2010) Vaccination of metastatic renal cancer patients with MVA-5T4: a randomized, double-blind, placebo-controlled phase III study, *Clin Cancer Res* Nov 15; 16(22): 5539-47

Amos SM, Duong CP, Westwood JA, Ritchie DS, Junghans RP, Darcy PK, Kershaw MH (2011) Autoimmunity associated with immunotherapy of cancer. Blood. 2011 Apr 29.

Andersen MH, Thor SP (2002). Survivin--a universal tumour antigen. *Histol Histopathol;*17(2):669-75.

Andersen MH, Junker N, Ellebaek E et al (2010) Therapeutic cancer vaccines in combination with conventional therapy , *Journal of Biomedicine an Biotechnology* 237623. Epub 2010 Jun 29

Andre FM, Mir LM (2010). Nucleic acids electrotransfer in vivo: mechanisms and practical aspects. *Curr Gene Ther.* Aug;10(4):267-80.

Ascierto PA, Simeone E, Sznol M et al (2010) Clinical experiences with anti-CD137 and anti-PD1 therapeutic antibodies, *Semin Oncol* Oct; 37(5): 508-16

Aurisicchio L, Mennuni C, Giannetti P, Calvaruso F, Nuzzo M, Cipriani B, Palombo F, Monaci P, Ciliberto G, La Monica N. (2007). Immunogenicity and safety of a DNA prime/adenovirus boost vaccine against rhesus CEA in nonhuman primates. *Int J Cancer.* Jun 1;120(11):2290-300.

Aurisicchio L, Peruzzi D, Conforti A et al (2009) Treatment of mammary carcinomas in HER-2 transgenic mice through combination of genetic vaccine and an agonist of Toll-like receptor 9, *Clin Cancer Res* Mar 1; 15(5): 1575-84

Aurisicchio L, Ciliberto G. (2010). Patented cancer vaccines: the promising leads. *Expert Opin Ther Pat.* May;20(5):647-60

Beatty GL, Chiorean EG, Fishman MP et al (2011) CD40 agonists alter tumour stroma and show efficacy against pancreatic carcinoma in mice and humans, *Science* Mar 25; 331(6024): 1612-6

Bei R, Scardino A (2010) TAA polyepitope DNA-based vaccines: a potential tool for cancer therapy, *J Biomed Biotechnol;*102758. Epub 2010 Jun 17

Beaudette TT, Bachelder EM, Cohen JA, Obermeyer AC, Broaders KE, Fréchet JM, Kang ES, Mende I, Tseng WW, Davidson MG, Engleman EG. (2009). *In vivo* studies on the effect of co-encapsulation of CpG DNA and antigen in acid-degradable microparticle vaccines. *Mol Pharm.;*6(4):1160–1169.

Bergman PJ, Camps-Palau MA, McKnight JA, Leibman NF, Craft DM, Leung C, et al. (2006). Development of a xenogeneic DNA vaccine program for canine malignant melanoma at the Animal Medical Center. *Vaccine;*24(21):4582-5

Bindea G , Mlecnik B, Fridman WH et al (2011) The prognostic impact of anti-cancer immune response: a novel classification of cancer patients, *Semin Immunopathol* 33(4):335-40.

Bingle L, Brown NJ, Lewis CE (2002) The role of tumour-associatted macrophages in tumour progression : implications for new anticancer therapies, *J Pathol* Mar; 196(3): 254-65

Blumberg BS. (2010). Primary and secondary prevention of liver cancer caused by HBV. *Front Biosci (Schol Ed).* Jan 1;2:756-63.

Bodles-Bakhop AM, Heller R, Draghia-Akli R (2009) Electroporation for the Delivery of DNA-based Vaccines and Immunotherapeutics: Current Clinical Developments, *Mol Ther* Apr; vol 17 n.4 : 585-592

Bolhassani A, Safaiyan S, Rafati S (2011) Improvement of different vaccine delivery systems for cancer therapy, *Mol Cancer* Jan 7; 10:3

Bozic I, Antal T, Ohtsuki H et al (2010) Accumulation of driver and passenger mutations during tumour progression, *Proc Natl Acad Sci U S A* Oct 26; 107(43); 18545-50

Burch PA, Croghan GA, Gastineau DA, et al. (2004) Immunotherapy (APC8015, provenge) targetingprostatic acid phosphatase can induce durable remission of metastatic androgen-independent prostate cancer: A phase 2 trial. *Prostate.*; 60:197–204

Butts C, Maksymiuk A, Goss G, Soulières D, Marshall E, Cormier Y, Ellis PM, Price A, Sawhney R, Beier F, Falk M, Murray N. (2011). Updated survival analysis in patients with stage IIIB or IV non-small-cell lung cancer receiving BLP25 liposome vaccine (L-BLP25): phase IIB randomized, multicenter, open-label trial. *J Cancer Res Clin Oncol.* Jul 9.

Callahan MK, Wolchok JD, Allison JP (2010) Anti-CTLA-4 Antibody Therapy: Immune Monitoring During Clinical Development of a Novel Immunotherapy, *Semin Oncol.* October; 37(5): 473-484

Campi G CM, Consogno G, et al. (2003) CD4+ T cells from healthy subjects and colon cancer patients recognize a carcinoembryonic antigen-specific immunodominant epitope. *Cancer Res*; 63:8481-6.

Carden CP, Sarker D, Postel-Vinay S et al (2010) Can molecular biomarker-based patient selection in Phase I trials accelerate anticancer drug development?, *Drug Discov Today* Feb; 15(3-4): 88-97

Cecco S, Muraro E, Giacomin E et al (2011) Cancer vaccines in phase II/III clinical trials: state of the art and future perspectives, *Curr Cancer Drug Targets* Jan: 11(1): 85-102

Chaudry MA, Sales K, Ruf P, et al. (2007). EpCAM an immunotherapeutic target for gastrointestinal malignancy: current experience and future challenges. *Br J Cancer*;96(7):1013-9.

Chaux, P., R. Luiten, N. Demotte, V. Vantomme, V. Stroobant, C. Traversari, V. Russo, E. Schultz, G. R. Cornelis, T. Boon, and B. P. van der. (1999). Identification of five MAGE-A1 epitopes recognized by cytolytic T lymphocytes obtained by in vitro stimulation with dendritic cells transduced with MAGE-A1. *J. Immunol.* 163:2928-2936.

Cheever MA, Allison JP, Ferris AS, Finn OJ, Hastings BM, Hecht TT, Mellman I, Prindiville SA, Viner JL, Weiner LM, Matrisian LM. (2009). The prioritization of cancer antigens: a national cancer institute pilot project for the acceleration of translational research. *Clin Cancer Res.* Sep 1;15(17):5323-37

Cheever MA, Higano C (2011) PROVENGE (Sipuleucel-T) in Prostate Cancer: The First FDA Approved Ther Cancer Vaccine, *Clin Cancer Res* Jun; 17(11):3520-6

Chen H, Liakou CI, Kamat A et al (2009) Anti-CTLA-4 therapy results in higher CD4+ICOShi T cell frequency and IFN-gamma levels in both nonmalignant and malignant prostate tissue, *Proc Natl Acad Sci U S A* Feb 24; 106(8):2729-34

Chiba T, Ohtani H, Mizoi T et al (2004), Intraepithelial CD8+ T-cell-count becomes a prognostic factor after a longer follow-up period in human colorectal carcinoma: possible association with suppression of micrometastasis, *Br J Cancer.* Nov 1;91(9):1711-7

Chouaib S, Kieda C, Benlalam H (2010), Endothelial cells as key determinants of the tumour microenvironment: interaction with tumour cells, extracellular matrix and immune killer cells, *Crit Rev Immunol.*;30(6):529-45

Clemente CG, Mihm MC Jr, Bufalino R et al (1996), Prognostic value of tumour infiltrating lymphocytes in the vertical growth phase of primary cutaneous melanoma, *Cancer.* Apr 1;77(7):1303-10

Comin-Anduix B, Lee Y, Jalil J et al (2008) Detailed analysis of immunologic effects of the cytotoxic T lymphocyte-associated antigen 4-blocking monoclonal antibody tremelimumab in peripheral blood of patients with melanoma, *J Transl Med* May 1; 6:22

Conforti A, Cipriani B, Peruzzi D et al (2010) A TLR9 agonist enhances therapeutic effects of telomerase genetic vaccine, *Vaccine* Apr 30; 28(20):3522-30

Coulie PG, Van den Eynde BJ, van der Bruggen P et al (1997), Antigens recognized by T-lymphocytes on human tumours, *Biochem Soc Trans.* May;25(2):544-8

Couzin-Frankel J (2010) Immune Therapy Steps Up the Attack, *Science* Oct; vol 330 n. 6003: 440-443

Culver ME, Gatesman ML, Mancl EE et al (2011) Ipilimumab : a novel treatment for metastatic melanoma, *Ann Pharmacother* Apr; 45 (4) : 510-9

Curiel TJ, Coukos G, Zou L et al (2004) Specific recruitment of regulatory T cells in ovarian carcinoma fosters immune privilege and predicts reduced survival, *Nat Med* Sep; 10(9) :942-9

Daley GQ, Van Etten RA, Baltimore D. (1990). Induction of chronic myelogenous leukemia in mice by the P210bcr/abl gene of the Philadelphia chromosome. *Science*;247(4944):824-30.

Darrasse-Jèze G, Bergot AS, Durgeau A et al (2009), Tumour emergence is sensed by self-specific CD44hi memory Tregs that create a dominant tolerogenic environment for tumours in mice, *J Clin Invest.* Sep; 119(9):2648-62.

de Gruijl TD, van den Eertwegh AJ, Pinedo HM, et al. (2008). Whole-cell cancer vaccination: from autologous to allogeneic tumour- and dendritic cell-based vaccines. *Cancer Immunol Immunother* ;57(10):1569-77

DeNardo DG, Andreu P, Coussens LM (2010) Interactions between lymphocytes and myeloid cells regulate pro-versus anti-tumour immunity, *Cancer Metastasis Rev* Jun; 29(2):309-16

Dengjel J, Nastke MD, Gouttefangeas C, Gitsioudis G, Schoor O, Altenberend F, Müller M, Krämer B, Missiou A, Sauter M, Hennenlotter J, Wernet D, Stenzl A, Rammensee HG, Klingel K, Stevanović S (2006). Unexpected abundance of HLA class II presented peptides in primary renal cell carcinomas. *Clin Cancer Res.* Jul 15;12(14 Pt 1):4163-70.

De Palma M, Lewis CE (2011) Cancer: Macrophages limit chemotherapy, *Nature* Apr 21; 472(7343): 303-4

De Smet, C., C. Lurquin, B. Lethe, V. Martelange, and T. Boon. (1999). DNA methylation is the primary silencing mechanism for a set of germ line- and tumour-specific genes with a CpG-rich promoter. *Mol. Cell. Biol.* 19:7327-7335

di Pietro A, Tosti G, Ferrucci PF, Testori A (2009). Heat shock protein peptide complex 96-based vaccines in melanoma: How far we are, how far we can get. Hum Vaccin. 2009 Nov 23;5(11).

Dharmapuri S, Peruzzi D, Aurisicchio L. Engineered adenovirus serotypes for overcoming anti-vector immunity. *Expert Opin Biol Ther.* 2009 Oct;9(10):1279-87.

Disis ML (2011) Immunologic biomarkers as correlates of clinical response to cancer immunotherapy, *Cancer Immunol Immunother* Mar; 60(3): 433-42

Doehn C, Bohmer T, Kausch I, et al. (2008). Prostate cancer vaccines: current status and future potential. *BioDrugs*;22(2):71-84

Dougan M, Dranoff G.(2009) Immune therapy for cancer, *Ann Rev Immunol.* ;27:83-117

Druker BJ, Talpaz M, Resta DJ, et al. (2001). Efficacy and safety of a specific inhibitor of the BCR-ABL tyrosine kinase in chronic myeloid leukemia. *N Engl J Med*;344(14):1031-7.

Dunbar CE. (2007). The yin and yang of stem cell gene therapy: insights into hematopoiesis, leukemogenesis, and gene therapy safety. *Hematology Am Soc Hematol Educ Program*.: 460-5

Dunn GP, Bruce AT, Ikeda H, Old LJ, Schreiber RD (2002) Cancer immunoediting: from immunosurveillance to tumour escape, *Nat Immunol*. Nov;3(11):991-8

Elia L, Aurisicchio L., Facciabene A et al (2007) CD4+CD25+regulatory T-cell-inactivation in combination with adenovirus vaccines enhances T-cell responses and protects mice from tumour challenge, *Cancer Gene Ther* Feb; 14(2): 201-10

Facciabene A, Aurisicchio L, Elia L, Palombo F, Mennuni C, Ciliberto G, La Monica N. (2006) DNA and adenoviral vectors encoding carcinoembryonic antigen fused to immunoenhancing sequences augment antigen-specific immune response and confer tumour protection. *Hum Gene Ther*. 2006 Jan;17(1):81-92.

Facciabene A, Aurisicchio L, Elia L, Palombo F, Mennuni C, Ciliberto G, La Monica N. (2007). Vectors encoding carcinoembryonic antigen fused to the B subunit of heat-labile enterotoxin elicit antigen-specific immune responses and antitumour effects. *Vaccine*. Dec 21;26(1):47-58

Fattori E, Aurisicchio L, Zampaglione I, Arcuri M, Cappelletti M, Cipriani B, Mennuni C, Calvaruso F, Nuzzo M, Ciliberto G, Monaci P, La Monica N (2009). ErbB2 genetic cancer vaccine in nonhuman primates: relevance of single nucleotide polymorphisms. *Hum Gene Ther*. Mar;20(3):253-65.

Fox, E. J., J. J. Salk, and L. A. Loeb. (2009). Cancer genome sequencing—an interim analysis. *Cancer Res*. 69:4948-4950

Fridman WH, Mlecnik B, Bindea G et al (2011) Immunosurveillance in human non-viral cancers, *Curr Opin Immunol* Apr; 23(2): 272-8

Frenoy N SJ, Cahour A, Burtin P (1987). Natural antibodies against the carcinoembryonic antigen (CEA) and a related antigen, NCA, in human sera. *Anticancer Res*;7:1229-33.

Gajewski TF, Louahed J, Brichard VG (2010) Gene signature in melanoma associated with clinical activity: a potential clue to unlock cancer immunotherapy, *Cancer J* Jul-Aug; 16(4): 399-403

Gajewski TF, Meng Y, Blank C et al (2006), Immune resistance orchestrated by the tumour microenvironment, *Immunol Rev*. Oct; 213:131-45

Globocan Project by International Agency for Research on Cancer (2008), Cancer Incidence and Mortality Worldwide in 2008, Available from http: http://globocan.iarc.fr

Golovina TN, Vonderheide RH (2010) Regulatory T cells: overcoming suppression of T-cell immunity, *Cancer J* Jul-Aug; 16(4): 342-7

Gómez CE, Nájera JL, Krupa M, Perdiguero B, Esteban. M. (2011). MVA and NYVAC as vaccines against emergent infectious diseases and cancer. *Curr Gene Ther*. Jun 1;11(3):189-217.

Gonzalez G, Crombet T, Lage A (2011) Chronic vaccination with a therapeutic EGF-based cancer vaccine: a review of patients receiving long lasting treatment, *Curr Cancer Drug Targets* Jan; 11 (1): 103-10

Gridelli C, Rossi A, Maione P, Ferrara ML, Castaldo V, Sacco PC. (2009). Vaccines for the treatment of non-small cell lung cancer: a renewed anticancer strategy. *Oncologist*. Sep;14(9):909-20

Harrop R, Shingler WH, McDonald M et al (2011) MVA-5T4-induced immune responses are an early marker of efficacy in renal patients , *Cancer Immunol Immunother* Jun; 60(6):829-37

Hege KM, Jooss K, Pardoll D. (2006). GM-CSF gene-modifed cancer cell immunotherapies: of mice and men. *Int Rev Immunol* 25(5-6):321-52.

Heng HH, Liu G, Stevens JB et al (2010) Genetic and epigenetic heterogeneity in cancer: the ultimate challenge for drug therapy, *Curr Drug Targets* Oct; 11(10): 1304-16

Hipp MM, Hilf N, Walter S et al (2008) Sorafenib, but not sunitinib, affects function of dendritic cells and induction of primary immune responses, *Blood* Jun 15; 111(12): 5610-20

Hodi FS, O'Day SJ, McDermott DF et al (2010) Improved Survival with Ipilimumab in Patients with Metastatic Melanoma, *N Engl J Med* Aug; 363(8): 711-23

Hofmeister V, Vetter C, Schrama D, Bröcker EB, Becker JC. (2006). Tumour stroma-associated antigens for anti-cancer immunotherapy. *Cancer Immunol Immunother*. May;55(5):481-94.

Hood A, Eggermont AMM, Janetzki S et al (2010) Improved Endpoints for Cancer Immunotherapy Trials , *JNCI* vol 102 Issue 18, Sept,2010 : 1388-97

Hoos A, Parmiani G., Hege K et al (2007) A clinical development paradigm for cancer vaccines and related biologics, *J. Immunother* Jan; 30(1) : 1-15

Huang RR, Jalil J, Economou JS et al (2011) CTLA4 blockade induces frequent tumour infiltration by activated lymphocytes regardless of clinical responses in humans, *Clin Cancer Res* Jun; 17 (2):4101-9

Jacobs JF, Aarntzen EH, Sibelt LA, et al. (2009). Vaccine-specific local T cell reactivity in immunotherapy-associated vitiligo in melanoma patients. *Cancer Immunol Immunother*;58(1):145-51

Jager, E., Y. T. Chen, J. W. Drijfhout, J. Karbach, M. Ringhoffer, D. Jager, M. Arand, H. Wada, Y. Noguchi, E. Stockert, L. J. Old, and A. Knuth. (1998). Simultaneous humoral and cellular immune response against cancer-testis antigen NY-ESO-1: definition of human histocompatibility leukocyte antigen (HLA)-A2-binding peptide epitopes. *J. Exp. Med*. 187:265-270

Jager L, Ehrhardt A (2007). Emerging adenoviral vectors for stable correction of genetic disorders. *Curr Gene Ther*. Aug;7(4):272-83

Jeong SH, Qiao M, Nascimbeni M, Hu Z, Rehermann B, Murthy K, Liang TJ. (2004). Immunization with hepatitis C virus-like particles induces humoral and cellular immune responses in nonhuman primates. *J Virol*;78(13):6995-7003

Jocham D, Richter A, Hoffmann L, et al. (2004). Adjuvant autologous renal tumour cell vaccine and risk of tumour progression in patients with renal-cell carcinoma after radical nephrectomy: phase III, randomised controlled trial. *Lancet*;363(9409):594-9

Johnson BF, Clay TM, Hobeika AC et al (2007) Vascular endothelial growth factor and immunosuppression in cancer: current knowledge and potential for new therapy, *Expert Opin Biol Ther*. Apr;7(4):449-60

Kantoff PW, Schuetz TJ, Blumenstein BA, Glode LM, Bilhartz DL, Wyand M, Manson K, Panicali DL, Laus R, Schlom J, Dahut WL, Arlen PM, Gulley JL, Godfrey WR. (2010). Overall survival analysis of a phase II randomized controlled trial of a Poxviral-based PSA-targeted immunotherapy in metastatic castration-resistant prostate cancer. *J Clin Oncol*. Mar 1;28(7):1099-105.

Kantoff PW, Higano CS, Shore ND et al (2010) Sipuleucel-T immunotherapy for castration-resistant prostate cancer, *N.Engl J Med* Jul 29; 363 (5): 411-22

Kaplan DH, Shankaran V, Dighe AS et al (1998), Demonstration of an interferon gamma-dependent tumour surveillance system in immunocompetent mice, *Proc Natl Acad Sci U S A*. Jun 23;95(13):7556-61

Kawashima I HS, Tsai V et al. (1998). The multiepitope approach for immunotherapy for cancer: identification of several CTL epitopes from tumour-associated antigens expressed on solid epithelial tumours. *Hum Immunol* ;59:1-14.

Kim DW, Krishnamurthy V, Bines SD et al (2010) TroVax, a recombinant modified vaccinia Ankara virus encoding 5T4: lessons learned and future development, *Hum Vaccine* Oct; 6 (10): 784-91

Klebanoff CA, Acquavella N, Yu Z et al (2011) Therapeutic cancer vaccines : are we there yet?, *Immunol Rev* Jan; 239 (1) 27-44

Kline J, Gajewski TF (2010) Clinical development of mAbs to block the PD1 pathway as an immunotherapy for cancer, *Curr Opin Investig Drugs* Dec; 11(12): 1354-9

Koebel CM, Vermi W, Swann JB et al (2007), Adaptive immunity maintains occult cancer in an equilibrium state, *Nature.* Dec 6;450(7171):903-7

Le DT, Pardoll DM, Jaffee EM. (2010) Cellular vaccine approaches. *Cancer J.* Jul-Aug;16(4):304-10

Lewis CE, Pollard JW (2006) Distinct role of macrophages in different tumour microenvironments, *Cancer Res* Jan 15; 66(2): 605-12

Lindenberg JJ, Fehres CM, van Cruijsen H et al (2011), Cross-talk between tumour and myeloid cells: how to tip the balance in favor of antitumour immunity, *Immunotherapy.* Jan;3(1):77-96

Liu MA. (2011) .DNA vaccines: an historical perspective and view to the future. *Immunol Rev.*Jan;239(1):62-84.

Low L, Mander A, McCann K, Dearnaley D, Tjelle T, Mathiesen I, Stevenson F, Ottensmeier CH. (2009). DNA vaccination with electroporation induces increased antibody responses in patients with prostate cancer. *Hum Gene Ther.* Nov;20(11):1269-78.

Lu S. (2009). Heterologous prime-boost vaccination. *Curr Opin Immunol.* Jun;21(3):346-51

MacKie RM, Reid R, Junor B, (2003) Fatal melanoma transferred in a donated kidney 16 years after melanoma surgery, *N Engl J Med.* 2003 Feb 6;348(6):567-8

McMahon BJ, Bulkow LR, Singleton RJ, Williams J, Snowball M, Homan C, Parkinson AJ (2011) Elimination of hepatocellular carcinoma and acute hepatitis B in children 25 years after a hepatitis B newborn and catch-up immunization program. *Hepatology.* 2011 May 26. doi: 10.1002/hep.24442.

Marshall JL (2003). Carcinoembryonic antigen-based vaccines. *Semin Oncol*;30(3 Suppl 8):30-6.

Marshall JL, Gulley JL, Arlen PM, Beetham PK, Tsang KY, Slack R, Hodge JW, Doren S, Grosenbach DW, Hwang J, Fox E, Odogwu L, Park S, Panicali D, Schlom J. (2005) Phase I study of sequential vaccinations with fowlpox-CEA(6D)-TRICOM alone and sequentially with vaccinia-CEA(6D)-TRICOM, with and without granulocyte-macrophage colony-stimulating factor, in patients with carcinoembryonic antigen-expressing carcinomas. *J Clin Oncol.* Feb 1;23(4):720-31.

Mennuni C, Ugel S, Mori F et al (2008) Preventive vaccination with telomerase controls tumour growth in genetically engineered and carcinogen-induced mouse models of cancer. *Cancer Res* Dec 1; 68(23): 9865-74

Minamoto T, Mai M, Ronai Z. (1999) Environmental factors as regulators and effectors of multistep carcinogenesis. *Carcinogenesis* Apr;20(4):519-27.

Mlecnik B, Bindea G, Pagès F et al (2011) Tumour immunosurveillance in human cancers , *Cancer Metastasis Rev* 30:5-12

Mlecnick B, Sanchez-Cabo F., Charoentong P et al (2010) Data integration and exploration for the identification of molecular mechanisms in tumour-immune cells interaction, *BMC Genomics* Feb 10; 11 Suppl 1:S7

Montgomery DL, Shiver JW, Leander KR, Perry HC, Friedman A, Martinez D, Ulmer JB, Donnelly JJ and Liu MA (1993). Heterologous and homologous protection against influenza A by DNA vaccination: optimization of DNA vectors. *DNA Cell Biol.*;129:777-83.

Morgan RA, Dudley ME, Rosenberg SA (2010) Adoptive cell therapy: genetic modification to redirect effector cell specificity, *Cancer J.* Jul-Aug; 16(4): 336-41

Moschella F, Valentini M, Aricò E et al (2011) Unraveling cancer chemoimmunotherapy mechanisms by gene and protein expression profiling of responses to cyclophosphamide, *Cancer Res* May 15; 71(10): 3528-39

Moschella F, Proietti E, Capone I et al (2010) Combination strategies for enhancing the efficacy of immunotherapy in cancer patients, *Ann N Y Acad Sci* Apr; 1194: 169-78

Nelson BH (2008) , Impact of T-cell immunity on ovarian cancer outcomes, *Immunol Rev.* Apr;222:101-16

Nishikawa H, Sakaguchi S.(2010), Regulatory T cells in tumour immunity, *Int J Cancer.* Aug 15;127(4):759-67

Nisticò P, Capone I, Palermo B et al (2009) Chemotherapy enhances vaccine-induced antitumour immunity in melanoma patients, *Int J Cancer* Jan 1; 124(1): 130-9

Novellino L, Castelli C, Parmiani G (2005) A listing of human tumour antigens recognized by T cells: March 2004 update, *Cancer Immunol Immunother.* Mar;54(3):187-207

Ostrand-Rosenberg S (2010) Myeloid-derived suppressor cells: more mechanisms for inhibiting antitumour immunity, *Cancer Immunol Immunother.* Oct;59(10):1593-600

Oudard S, Rixe O, Beuselinck B, Linassier C, Banu E, Machiels JP, Baudard M, Ringeisen F, Velu T, Lefrere-Belda MA, Limacher JM, Fridman WH, Azizi M, Acres B, Tartour E. (2011). A phase II study of the cancer vaccine TG4010 alone and in combination with cytokines in patients with metastatic renal clear-cell carcinoma: clinical and immunological findings. *Cancer Immunol Immunother.* Feb;60(2):261-71

Palucka K, Ueno H, Banchereu J (2011) Recent developments in cancer vaccines, *J. Immunol* Feb 1; 186(3): 1325-31

Paoloni M, Khanna C. (2008). Translation of new cancer treatments from pet dogs to humans. *Nat Rev Cancer*;8(2):147-56.

Parmiani G, De Filippo A, Novellino L, Castelli C (2007). Unique human tumour antigens: immunobiology and use in clinical trials. *J Immunol.* Feb 15;178(4):1975-9.

Pedicord VA, Montalvo W, Leiner IM et al (2011) Single dose of anti-CTLA-4 enhances CD8+ T-cell memory formation, function , and maintenance, *PNAS* Jan 4; vol 108 n.1: 266-271

Peggs KS, Quezada SA, Chambers CA et al (2009), Blockade of CTLA-4 on both effector and regulatory T cell compartments contributes to the antitumour activity of anti-CTLA-4 antibodies, *J Exp Med.* Aug 3;206(8):1717-25

Peled N, Oton AB, Hirsch FR et al (2009) MAGE A3 antigen-specific cancer immunotherapeutic, *Immunotherapy* Jan; 1(1):19-25

Peruzzi D, Mesiti G, Ciliberto G, La Monica N, Aurisicchio L (2010). Telomerase and HER-2/neu as targets of genetic cancer vaccines in dogs.*Vaccine.* Feb 3;28(5):1201-8.

Peruzzi D, Mori F, Conforti A, Lazzaro D, De Rinaldis E, Ciliberto G, La Monica N, Aurisicchio L. MMP11: a novel target antigen for cancer immunotherapy. *Clin Cancer Res.* Jun 15;15(12):4104-13.

Peruzzi D, Gavazza A, Mesiti G, Lubas G, Scarselli E, Conforti A, Bendtsen C, Ciliberto G, La Monica N, Aurisicchio L (2010). A vaccine targeting telomerase enhances survival of dogs affected by B-cell lymphoma. *Mol Ther.* Aug;18(8):1559-67.

Pietras RJ, Pegram MD, Finn RS et al (1998) Remission of human breast cancer xenografts on therapy with humanized monoclonal antibody to HER-2 receptor and DNA-reactive drugs, *Oncogene* Oct 29 ; 17(17): 2235-49

Plosker GL (2011), Sipuleucel-T: in metastatic castration-resistant prostate cancer, *Drugs* Jan 1; 71(1): 101-8

Potebnya GP, Symchych TV, Lisovenko GS (2010) Xenogenic cancer vaccines, *Exp Oncol* Jul; 32(2): 61-5

Quezada SA, Peggs KS, Simpson TR et al (2011) Shifting the equilibrium in cancer immunoediting: from tumour tolerance to eradication, *Immunol Rev* May; 241(1); 104-18

Radoja S, Saio M, Schaer D et al (2001), CD8(+) tumour-infiltrating T cells are deficient in perforin-mediated cytolytic activity due to defective microtubule-organizing center mobilization and lytic granule exocytosis, *J Immunol.* Nov 1;167(9):5042-51

Rech AJ, Vonderheide RH (2009) Clinical use of anti-CD25 antibody daclizumab to enhance immune responses to tumour antigen vaccination by targeting regulatory T cells , *Ann N Y Acad Sci* Sep; 1174: 99-106

Ribas A, Butterfield L, Glaspy JA, Economou JS (2003). Current Developments in Cancer Vaccines and Cellular Immunotherapy *Journal of Clinical Oncology,* Vol 21, 12: 2415-2432

Ribas A, Comin-Anduix B, Economou JS et al (2009) Intratumoural immune cell infiltrates, FoxP3, and indoleamine 2,3-dioxygenas patients with melanoma undergoing CTLA4 blockade, *Clin Cancer Res* Jan 1; 15(1): 390-9

Rodriguez-Paredes M, Esteller M (2011) Cancer epigenetics reaches mainstream oncology, *Nat Med* Mar; 17(3): 330-9

Rosenberg SA, Dudley ME (2009) Adoptive cell therapy for the treatment of patients with metastatic melanoma , *Curr Opin Immunol* Apr; 21(2):233-40

Rosenblatt J, Glotzbecker B, Mills H et al (2011) PD-1 Blockade by CT-011, Anti-PD-1 Antibody, Enhances Ex Vivo T-cell Responses to Autologous Dendritic Cell/Myeloma Fusion Vaccine, *J.Immunother* Jun: 34(5); 409-18

Sahin U, Türeci O, Pfreundschuh M. (1997) , Serological identification of human tumour antigens, *Curr Opin Immunol.* Oct;9(5):709-16

Sarnaik AA, Yu B, Morelli D et al (2011) Extended dose ipilimumab with a peptide vaccine: immune correlates associated with clinical benefit in patients with resected high-risk stage IIIc/IV melanoma, *Clin Cancer Res* Feb 15;17(4): 896-906

Sarnaik AA, Weber JS (2009) Recent advances using anti-CTLA-4 for the treatment of melanoma, *Cancer J* May-Hun; 15(3) :169-73

Sastre L (2011) New DNA sequencing technologies open a promising era for cancer research and treatment , *Clin Transl Oncol* May; 13(5):301-6

Shah RB, Chinnaiyan AM. (2009). The discovery of common recurrent transmembrane protease serine 2 (TMPRSS2)-erythroblastosis virus E26 transforming sequence (ETS) gene fusions in prostate cancer: significance and clinical implications. *Adv Anat Pathol*;16(3):145-53.

Schiavoni G, Sistigu A, Valentini M et al (2011) Cyclophosphamide synergizes with type I interferons through systemic dendritic cell reactivation and induction of immunogenic tumour apoptosis, *Cancer Res* Feb 1; 71(3): 768-78

Shiver JW, Fu TM, Chen L, Casimiro D, Davies ME, Evans RK, Zhang ZQ, Simon AJ, Trigona WL, Dubey SA, Huang L,. Harris VA, et al. (2002). Replication-incompetent adenoviral vaccine vector elicits effective anti-immunodeficiency-virus immunity. *Nature*;415:331-35.

Schmidt, S. M., K. Schag, M. R. Muller, M. M. Weck, S. Appel, L. Kanz, F. Grunebach, and P. Brossart. (2003). Survivin is a shared tumour-associated antigen expressed in a broad variety of malignancies and recognized by specific cytotoxic T cells. *Blood* 102:571-576

Schreiber RD, Old LJ, Smyth MJ (2011) Cancer Immunoediting: Integrating Immunity's Roles in Cancer Suppression and Promotion, *Science* March 25, vol 331 : 1565-70

Shumway NM, Ibrahim N, Ponniah S, et al. (2009) Therapeutic breast cancer vaccines: a new strategy for early-stage disease. *BioDrugs*;23(5):277-87.

Sistigu A, Viaud S, Chaput N et al (2011) Immunomodulatory effects of cyclophosphamide and implementations for vaccine design, *Semin Immunopathol* May 25,

Soliman H, Mediavilla-Varela M, Antonia S (2010) Indoleamine 2,3-dioxygenase: is it an immune suppressor? *Cancer J.* Jul-Aug;16(4):354-9

Steer HJ, Lake RA, Nowak AK et al (2010) Harnessing the immune response to treat cancer , *Oncogene*, 29, 6301-6313

Stevenson FK, Rice J, Ottensmeier CH, Thirdborough SM, Zhu D. (2004). DNA fusion gene vaccines against cancer: from the laboratory to the clinic. *Immunol Rev.* Jun;199:156-80.

Street SE, Trapani JA, MacGregor D et al (2002), Suppression of lymphoma and epithelial malignancies effected by interferon gamma, *J Exp Med.* Jul 1;196(1):129-34

Suso EM, Dueland S, Rasmussen AM, Vetrhus T, Aamdal S, Kvalheim G, Gaudernack G. (2011). hTERT mRNA dendritic cell vaccination: complete response in a pancreatic cancer patient associated with response against several hTERT epitopes. *Cancer Immunol Immunother.* Jun;60(6):809-18.

Suzuki E, Sun J, Kapoor V et al (2007) Gemcitabine has significant immunomodulatory activity in murine tumour models independent of its cytotoxic effects, *Cancer Biol Ther* Jun; 6 (6) : 880-5

Tsang, K. Y., S. Zaremba, C. A. Nieroda, M. Z. Zhu, J. M. Hamilton, and J. Schlom. (1995). Generation of human cytotoxic T cells specific for human carcinoembryonic antigen epitopes from patients immunized with recombinant vaccinia-CEA vaccine. *J. Natl. Cancer Inst.* 87:982-990

Tyagi P, Mirakhur B (2009) MAGRIT: The largest-Ever Phase III Lung Cancer Trial Aims to Establish a Novel Tumour-Specific Approach to Therapy, *Clinical Lung Cancer* Vol 10,n.5, 371-374;

Ulmer JB, Wahren B, Liu MA: Gene-based vaccines: recent technical and clinical advances.(2006) *Trends in Molecular Medicine*, 12:216-222.

Umano, Y., T. Tsunoda, H. Tanaka, K. Matsuda, H. Yamaue, and H. Tanimura. (2001). Generation of cytotoxic T cell responses to an HLA-A24 restricted epitope peptide derived from wild-type p53. *Br. J. Cancer* 84:1052-1057

Uva P, Aurisicchio L, Watters J, Loboda A, Kulkarni A, Castle J, et al. (2009). Comparative expression pathway analysis of human and canine mammary tumours. *BMC Genomics* ;10(1):135

Van der Burg SH, Melief CJ (2011). Therapeutic vaccination against human papilloma virus induced malignancies. *Curr Opin Immunol.* Apr;23(2):252-7. Epub 2011 Jan 13.

Van Houdt IS, Sluijter BJ, Moesbergen LM et al (2008), Favorable outcome in clinically stage II melanoma patients is associated with the presence of activated tumour infiltrating T-lymphocytes and preserved MHC class I antigen expression, *Int J Cancer.* Aug 1;123(3):609-15

Vergati M, Intrivici C, Huen NY et al (2010) Strategies for Cancer Vaccine Development, J Biomed Biotechnol 596432.Epub 2010 Jul 11

Vermorken JB, Claessen AM, van Tinteren H, et al. (1999). Active specific immunotherapy for stage II and stage III human colon cancer: a randomised trial. *Lancet*;353(9150):345-50.

Vonderheide RH (2008). Prospects and challenges of building a cancer vaccine targeting telomerase. *Biochimie*;90(1):173-80

Vonderheide RH, LoRusso PM, Khalil M et al (2010) Tremelimumab in combination with exemestane in patients with advanced breast cancer and treatment-associated modulation of inducible costimulator expression on patient T cells, *Clin Cancer Res*, Jul 1; 16(13): 3485-94

Wang Z, Troilo PJ, Wang X, Griffiths TG, Pacchione SJ, Barnum AB, Harper LB, Pauley CJ, Niu Z, Denisova L, Follmer TT, Rizzuto G, Ciliberto G, Fattori E, Monica NL, Manam S, Ledwith BJ. (2004). Detection of integration of plasmid DNA into host genomic DNA following intramuscular injection and electroporation. *Gene Ther.* Apr;11(8):711-21.

Wang HY, Peng G, Guo Z et al (2005), Recognition of a new ARTC1 peptide ligand uniquely expressed in tumour cells by antigen-specific CD4+ regulatory T cells, *J Immunol.* Mar 1;174(5): 2661-70

Weber J. (2007). Review: anti-CTLA-4 antibody ipilimumab: case studies of clinical response and immune-related adverse events. *Oncologist.* Jul;12(7):864-72.

Welters MJ, Kenter GG, de Vos van Steenwijk PJ et al (2010), Success or failure of vaccination for HPV16-positive vulvar lesions correlates with kinetics and phenotype of induced T-cell responses, *Proc Natl Acad Sci U S A*, Jun 29;107(26):11895-9

Wolchok JD, Hoos A, O'Day S et al (2009), Guidelines for the evaluation of immune therapy activity in solid tumours: immunerelated response criteria, *Clin Cancer Res*, Dec 1; 15(23):7412-20

Wolchok JD, Weber JS, Hamid O et al (2010) Ipilimumab efficacy and safety in patients with advanced melanoma: a retrospective analysis of HLA subtype from four trials, *Cancer Immun.* Oct 10; 10:9

Woo EY, Chu CS, Goletz TJ et al (2001), Regulatory CD4+CD25+T Cells in Tumours from Patients with Early-Stage Non-Small Cell Lung Cancer and Late-Stage Ovarian Cancer, *Cancer Research*, June 15; 61 : 4766-4772

Yoshida K, Noguchi M, Mine T, Komatsu N, Yutani S, Ueno T, Yanagimoto H, Kawano K, Itoh K, Yamada A. (2011) Characteristics of severe adverse events after peptide vaccination for advanced cancer patients: Analysis of 500 cases. *Oncol Rep.* Jan;25(1):57-62.

Yuan J, Gnjatic S, Li H et al (2008) CTLA-4 blockade enhances polyfunctional NY-ESO-1 specific T cell responses in metastatic melanoma patients with clinical benefit, *Proc Natl Acad Sci USA* Dec 23; 105(51): 20410-5

Zitvogel L, Apetoh L, Ghiringhelli F et al (2008) Immunological aspects of cancer chemotherapy, *Nat Rev Immunol* Jan; 8(1): 59-73

Zitvogel L, Kepp O, Senovilla L et al (2010) Immunogenetic tumour cell death for optimal anticancer therapy: the calreticulin exposure pathway, *Clin Cancer Res* Jun 15; 16(12): 3100-4

Xenovaccinotherapy for Cancer

V.I. Seledtsov[1], A.A. Shishkov[2] and G.V. Seledtsova[2]
[1]Immanuel Kant Baltic Federal University, Kaliningrad,
[2]Institute of Clinical Immunology SB RAMS, Novosibirsk,
Russia

1. Introduction

Up to date, a systemic treatment of cancer is based mainly on the use of chemotherapy. However, in the majority of cases, chemotherapy is not a radical treatment. In initially identified tumors there already exist cells that are resistant to toxic drug action, due to their biochemical properties. Furthermore, the proportion of such cells is progressively increased throughout the treatment period because they receive selective growth advantages over the cytotoxic drug-susceptible cells. It should also be noted that cytotoxic action of antineoplastic drugs is not selective: the drugs affect not only tumor, but also normal cells. Hence, there may be serious side effects of chemotherapy, which, by themselves, may be life-dangerous and frequently requiring further medical interventions. An appearance of the drugs with selective cytotoxic activity seems improbable in the near future because the vital biochemical processes in tumor and normal cells are similar in their basis.

Nevertheless, tumor cells are distinguished from normal ones by quantitative and qualitative expression on their surfaces of potentially immunogenic structures (antigens). It is generally accepted that the immune responses induced by these structures can cause destruction of tumor cells, and that reactivity of the immune system can define an outcome of disease. All of the tumor-associated antigens (TAA) can be divided into two groups: the first one involves the differentiation antigens that can be expressed in not only tumor, but also normal cells, whereas the second one comprises of the products of mutated or viral genes, which can be expressed exclusively in malignant cells. The vast majority of TAA belongs to the first group. These TAA can be expressed in a variety of tumors, due to commonality in the intracellular mechanisms involved in malignizeition of various types of cells. There is considerable interest in developing therapeutic vaccines for cancer, as they hold the promise of delaying or preventing cancer recurrence, particularly in early-stage disease patients. However, there exists a general problem with cancer vaccine application, because most of the TAA are represented by self, nonmutated proteins which are poorly immunogenic for the immune system [reviewed in 1]. Hence, overcoming the immune tolerance toward TAA is indeed a key task of cancer immunotherapy. The use of vaccines based on xenogenic TAA seems to be a promising approach to resolving this problem. Since TAA are typically evolutionarily conservative molecules, there is a strong homology between human and animal TAA. On the other hand, small interspecific structural differences of TAA can be advantageously used in constructing cancer vaccines because xenoantigens may potentially represent an "altered self", with sufficient differences from self-antigens to render them immunogenic, but with sufficient similarities to allow reactive T cells to maintain recognition of self [1].

2. Xenovaccinotherapy in animal models

The majority of studies concerning xenogenic vaccines have been carried out on animals with melanoma, the tumor that expresses a whole number of potentially immunogenic antigens. There is compelling evidence that xenogenic melanoma- associated antigens are much more effective in inducing antitumor immune responses in mice than are their murine analogs. For example, multiple immunizations of mice with human glycoproteins gp75 and gp-100 were reported [2-6] to be effective in preventing the growth of the syngeneic melanoma cells expressing the appropriate mouse analogs [6]. Interestingly, the murine gp75 being initially non-immunogenic became immunogenic in mice when it was administered in the form expressed on a membrane of insect cells [7]. This suggests that the membrane-bound xenoantigens that are not related to tumorogenesis are capable of contributing to self TAA-driven immune responses. The related melanosomal antigens appear to differ in immune response patterns which they induce. For example, the DNA vaccination of mice with human tirosinase-related protein-1 (TRP-1/gp75) induced antibody- mediated responses and autoimmune depigmentation, whereas the DNA vaccination with human TRP-2 resulted in the generation of tumor-specific CD8+ cytotoxic T lymphocytes (CTL) and failed to elicit depigmentaion [8].

As surgery is essential for any melanoma treatment, experiments have been performed to evaluate antitumor effects of xenovaccination in the postoperative period. It was shown that the postoperative DNA vaccination of mice with human TRP-2 could prevent the development of melanoma metastasis in the lungs [4]. These data suggest that xenovaccinotherapy can be the most effective when applied in addition to surgical treatment.

The polyantigenic vaccination has apparent advantages over the monoantigenic one in achieving clinically relevant antitumor responses, thank to its ability to simultaneously induce immune reactions directed against different TAA. We demonstrated that the survival in the melanoma-bearing mice vaccinated with destroyed human melanoma cells was noticeably superior than that in the control mice immunized with murine tumor cells. Surprisingly, the antitumor effect in this experimental model was associated with the rise of serum interleukin (IL)-4, but not interferon (IFN)-γ [9].

As already mentioned, the differentiation antigens are expressed not only in tumor but also in normal cells. This raises the possibility of obtaining such antigens from normal tissues in which they are highly expressed. Placenta is well known to express a whole range of differentiation antigens, including those shared by different tumors including melanoma [10]. Therefore, placental tissue, could be a suitable source of the xenoantigens applicable for breaking the immunological tolerance to a number of TAA. In fact, the mice that received the soluble proteins derived from the porcine placenta as a vaccine, demonstrated the immune protection from melanoma where both CD4+ and CD8+ T lymphocytes were involved [10].

The xenovaccination aimed at breaking the tolerance to a melanosomal antigen gp 100 has been applied in the treatment of 34 melanoma dogs [11]. Canine melanoma cells 17CM98 transfected with a DNA fragment encoding human gp 100 were used as a vaccine. With such vaccinotherapy, a complete or partial response was achieved in 17% animals, and disease stabilization with a duration of not shorter than 6 weeks was recorded in 35% vaccinated dogs. The clinical responses correlated with delayed-type hypersensitivity (DTH) skin reactivity to vaccinal antigens but was independent both of the functional activity of vaccine-specific CTL and of the serum level of antivaccinal antibodies [11]. In this study the animals that responded to vaccination, survived significantly longer compared to those which did not [11]. An objective antitumor effect in certain dogs with the stage IV melanoma could be also achieved by their vaccinating DNA encoding human tyrosinase [12,13]. This effect was immediately related to occurrence of canine tyrosinase-binding antibodies in the sera [14]. No autoimmune complications and serious side effects of the xenovaccinotherapy were noted in the dogs [12,13]. Noteworthy is also that this therapy could be effectively used in combination with surgical treatment [15].

The ability of xenovaccination to break the immunological tolerance to TAA has been demonstrated in a murine model of breast cancer [16]. Protooncogene HER-2/neu is a self-antigen expressed by tumors and nonmalignant epithelial tissues. DNA vaccination of mice with human HER-2/neu was found to overcome the immunological tolerance to that protein and to induce the antibody-mediated, immune responses directed against both cancer and normal breast cells [16]. Yet, vaccinations of mice with a fragment of human HER-2/neu (435-443) induced generation of the CTL able to effectively recognize the syngeneic, HER-2/neu-positive tumor cells. Importantly, the CTL generation in these experiments depended on the age of vaccinated mice [17].

Survivin, a member of the inhibitors of apoptosis, is considered as an ideal vaccinal TAA, due to its broad expression pattern in many types of human malignancies. Dendritic vaccination of mice with human survivin was shown to induce the T-helper 1-mediated, immune responses, which were markedly enhanced by depleting CD25 +, Foxp3+, CD4 + regulatory T cells. Noteworthy is that the generation of survinin-specific CTLs lacked in this model [18]. The antitumor effect of administrating human survinin in mice was also reported in the models of lymphoma [19], glioma [20, 21], and pancreatic cancer [19].

A high expression of epidermal growth factor receptor (EGFr) is attributable to different tumors including lung carcinoma and breast cancer [22]. It is likely that EGFr may be involved in autocrine and paracrine stimulation of tumor cell growth. Vaccination of mice with DNA encoding a extracellular part of EGFr was found to break the tolerance to murine EGFr and to induce immune responses directed against EGFr –positive tumor cells. The antitumor effect observed in this model was mediated both by IgG antibodies and by CTL and associated with elevation of the serum concentration of IFN-γ , as well as of IL-4 [22].

Prostate-specific membrane antigen (PSMA) is a prototypical differentiation antigen expressed on normal and neoplastic prostate epithelial cells, and on the neovasculature of many solid tumors]. Immunizations of mice with human recombinant PSMA or DNA encoding PSMA were shown to induce the production of antibodies able to bind to murine PSMA; an effective vaccination was also demonstrated with administrating the xenoantigens prepared from the tumor prostate [23, 24].

A high expression of mesothelin is attributed to pancreas cancer. Therapeutic vaccination of mice with human mesothelin was found to result in inhibition of pancreatic cancer disseminating. Such a antitumor effect was associated with the rise in serum antimesothelin antibodies, as well as with an increase in the functionality of mesothelin-specific CTL [25].

Glioma membrane proteins (HGP) are typically expressed in the cells of malignant glioma. Therapeutic vaccination of rats with human HGP was demonstrated to result in the glioma growth inhibition that was mediated by the HGP-specific Th1 cells and characterized by a pronounced infiltration of tumor tissues with CD4+ and CD8+ T cells. In contrast to the human HGP, its murine analog lacked any antitumor activity [26].

Alfa-fetoprotein (AFP) is highly expressed in liver cancer. Vaccination with the recombinant rat, but not mouse AFP was found to provide a significant prolongation of survival in hepatocarcinoma -bearing mice. The antitumor effect of such vaccination depended on functional activity of both CD4+ and CD8+ T-lymphocytes [27].

Unlike other cancers, the neuroendocrine tumors, such as a gastrinoma, insulinoma, and medullar thyroid carcinoma, do not demonstrate any clear association with expression of defined classes of membrane-bound TAA. Therefore, for generating antitumor immune responses in such cases, the approach has been offered based on breaking the immune tolerance to tumor-derived, soluble products. In a model of thyroid carcinoma it was demonstrated that therapeutic vaccination of mice with the human (but not murine) calcitonin resulted in a significant inhibition of tumor growth. The antitumor affect of this vaccination was associated with infiltrating the tumor by calcitonin-specific CTLs, as well as with a sharp decline in the serum level of calcitonin [28].

Tumor development requires neoangiogenesis. Therefore, the therapeutic approaches aimed at preventing growth of tumor-feeding vessels are in the focus of experimental and clinical studies. Theoretically, breaking the immunological tolerance to molecules involved in angiogenesis could restrain tumor growth. A fibroblast growth factor receptor-1 (FGFr-1) is one of such molecules. Vaccination of mice with recombinant chicken FGFr-1 was reported to be able to overcome the tolerance to endogenic FGFr-1, eliciting production of FGFr-1-specific, IgG autoantibodies [29].

Matrix metalloproteinase-2 (MMP-2) is well known to play an important role in angiogenesis and to promote tumor cell expansion in the body. Immunizations of mice with the LLC or CT26 tumor cells expressing chicken MMP-2 was found found to induce antiangiogenic immune responses, resulting in the appearance of MMP-2- binding autoantibodies [30, 31].

Endoglin is a marker of angiogenesis in solid malignancies, including liver cancer. Therapeutic vaccination of mice with an extracellular portion of porcine endoglin was shown to induce immune responses directed against colorectal and lung cancers. The generation of such responses depended on functional activity of CD4+ T-lymphocytes and resulted in the appearance of endoglin-binding autoantibodies [32, 33]. A significant enhancement of antitumor effect was achieved when protein vaccination was combined with DNA vaccination. Such a combined vaccination induced not only the synthesis of endoglin-binding autoantibodies, but also the generation of endoglin-specific CTL [34]. An antitumor effect of DNA vaccination with porcine endoglin was also demonstrated in a murine model of liver cancer. This effect was mediated by both cellular and humoral immune reactions [35].

Tie-2 is an endothelium-specific receptor tyrosine kinase known to play a key role in tumor angiogenesis. Therapeutic vaccination of mice with human Tie-2 was found to be capable of exerting a negative effect on the growth of melanoma and hepatic cancer. This effect was dependent on functional activity of CD4+ T-lymphocytes and mediated by antibodies binding murine Tie-2 [36].

A pronounced antiangiogenic effect can be induced by vaccination with xenogenic whole endothelial cells [37]. This effect may be associated with overall tumor growth inhibition [38].

An antiangiogenic effect can be also achieved by inactivating soluble angiogenic molecules. For example, the vaccination of 9 dogs with spontaneous sarcomas by human endothelial cell growth factor (VEGF) resulted in the production of autoantibodies capable of binding both human and canine VEGF. The antitumor effect was observed in 3 (30%) vaccine-treated dogs. No complications of the vaccinotherapy were noted [39] .

It appears that antiangiogenic immunotherapy can be effectively combined with breaking the tolerance to differentiation antigens in order to induce clinically relevant antitumor responses. For example, the administration of DNA encoding tumor endothelial marker 8 (TEM8) was able to enhance the tumor immunity in melanoma mice, induced either by rat neu or by human tyrosinase-related protein 1 (TYRP1/hgp75) [40]

3. Clinical application of xenovaccinotherapy

Prostate cancer, melanoma, colorectal cancer and renal cancer are usually resistant to the standard cytotoxic therapy, including highly toxic combinations. On the other hand, all of these cancers express TAA which are capable of inducing antitumor immune responses. Hence, immunotherapy has to become the mainstay in treating those cancers.

Prostatic acid phosphatase (PAP) is a differentiation antigen expressed by normal and malignant cells of prostate. Patients (n=21) with metastatic prostate cancer were multiply vaccinated with autological dendritic cells loaded with mouse PAP. Such vaccinations were found to be safe to use, with no serious side effects being observed. An increased T-cell reactivity to murine PAP was observed in all of the vaccine-treated patients. Only 8 of 21 evaluable patients exhibited enhanced immune responses to human PAP. These responses associated with the enhanced production of IFN-γ and tumor necrosis factor (TNF)-α, but not IL-4 [41]

Immunologic effects of DNA vaccination with mouse tyrosinase have been assessed in 18 patients with melanoma, and the generation of tyrosinase-specific CD8+ memory T cells was found in 7 of them No serious complications of such a treatment were noted [42]

It should be noted that immunizations with one or several tumor-associated, antigenic peptides frequently fail to control overall tumor development, creating favorable conditions for growth of the tumor cell clones lacking vaccinal determinants. Moreover, due to a high lability of cancer genome, there is an antigenic diversity even in tumor cells of the same origin [43]. Since whole tumor cells express a variety of TAA and are able to elicit a broad spectrum of immune responses, they could be more applicable to constructing cancer vaccines, compared to a single or just few antigenic peptides. However, immunizations with unmodified homologous (autological or allogeneic) tumor cells have demonstrated only limited therapeutic success in cancer patients. There are two major reasons for the low immunogenicity of homologous cell vaccines. Firstly, most of the homological TAA represents self-antigens, which are not inherently immunogenic. Secondly, antigen-presenting cells do not recognize the homologous tumor cells as potentially pathogenic targets that should be internalized and their antigens processed [43].

From the aforesaid, we favor a xenogenic cell-based vaccine . Because of their structural distinctions from homologous analogs, the xenoantigens are capable of effectively overcoming the immune tolerance to self-antigens, including TAA. Yet, all humans possess natural (preexisting) antibodies, which provide an acute rejection of any non-primate cells and function as a major barrier for the transplantation of animal organs to humans [44]. A significant part of these antibodies represents the Ig G specific to the a-gal epitope that is expressed abundantly on glycoproteins and glycolipids of non-primate mammals and New Word monkeys [45]. In our point of view, by the opsonization of xenogenic tumor cells, the natural antibodies could promote internalization of tumor material in antigen-presenting cells via a Fc-receptor-mediated mechanism, and thereby enhance greatly the immunogenic presentation of TAA to tumor-specific T lymphocytes. This proposition is consistent with the published data indicating a critical role of the FcR-receptors in generating an effective tumor immunity [46], as well as with the findings showing that the rejection of alpha-Gal positive tumor cells can efficiently boost the immune response to TAA present in alpha-Gal negative tumor cells [47].

A xenogenic polyantigenic vaccine (XPV) under study is composed of disrupted murine B16 melanoma and LLC carcinoma cells. The XPV is stored in the form of frozen-dried preparation and is suspended in physiological salt solution immediately before its administration. Since the XPV includes a wide spectrum of melanoma- and carcinoma-associated antigens, our opinion is that it may be applicable for treating different cancers.

The study with xenovaccination was performed in exact accordance with the protocol approved by the Scientific Council and Ethics Committee at the Institute of Clinical Immunology (Novosibirsk, Russia). Informed consent was obtained from every subject who underwent xenovaccinotherapy. Eligibility criteria included histologically proven, measurable disease, no prior immunosuppressive therapy for a minimum of 4 weeks, a good performance status (Karnofsky scale, 70% or more) and adequate marrow, renal and hepatic functions.

An inducing vaccinal course consisted of 10 subcutaneous immunizations (5 at weekly and 5 at fortnight intervals) and took about 3 months. Each vaccinal dose contained 75×10^6 (B16 + LLC) dead cells. Twenty-four hours following each of the first 5 vaccinations, a part of the patients was given subcutaneously a low dose of a non-oxidated recombinant IL-2. Since, when combined with XPV, IL-2 had no any significant effect on XPV-induced long-lasting immunoreactivity, its administration in the above- indicated way was recognized unpractical. Following an inducing course of the treatment each of the patients received supporting vaccinations monthly or less frequently. Throughout follow-up time the trial patients received no any systemic therapy other than immunotherapy.

A total of 152 patients with advanced forms of melanoma, colorectal or renal cancers have completed an inducing vaccinotherapy consisting of 10 immunizations and had adequate follow-up to monitor toxicity, immune responses and survival. No III-IV grade systemic toxicity associated with the vaccine administration was noted. During 24-to-48 h post vaccination only nearly 10% patients exhibited an influenza-like syndrome in the form of a small body temperature rise and musculoskeletal discomfort, which were usually self-limiting. Irritations at the injection sites were developed in the most patients in response to vaccination. Local manifestations usually disappeared within 72 h following vaccine injection. There were no treatment- related hospitalizations or mortalities.

Cell and biochemical blood parameters, as well as renal and hepatic functions, remained within the initial ranges throughout the inducing vaccinotherapy. Also there were no significant changes in subpopulation composition of PMBCs tested by immunofluorescence for expression of CD3, CD4, CD8, CD 20, and CD16 surface markers.

The development of systemic autoimmune disorders could not be excluded initially in XPV-treated patients because of the broad range of different antigens present in XPV. However, XPV-treated patients exhibited no evidence of any systemic autoimmune disorders. Their serum concentrations of a rheumatoid factor, but also of antibodies specific to DNA, cardiolipin, thyroglobulin, microsomal fraction of thyrocytes remained in the initial ranges throughout the inducing vaccinotherapy.

An inducing vaccinotherapy was found to increase detectably the serum concentrations both of IFN-γ and of IL-4. Yet it should be noted that an increase in the IFN-γ level was more common and greatly pronounced in the XPV-treated patients, compared with that in IL-4 level [48,49].

With inducing vaccinations, a remarkable increase in both T cell- and antibody-mediated immunoreactivity to vaccinal antigens was found in the majority of assessable patients. An important aim of our study was to determine whether or not murine TAA would be capable of contributing to the generation of immune responses specific to human TAA. Indeed, our data clearly indicated that inducing vaccinations were able to significantly enhance T cell-mediated reactivity to human melanoma-associated antigens, while not affecting that to the control alloantigens [50, 51]

In our study an overall survival in the XPV-treated patients (n=51) with metastatic melanoma was evaluated through 7 year follow-up period. The control group was composed retrospectively of the patients who received conventional therapy, and had the initial clinical characteristics similar to those of the trial group. The characteristics of the trial and control patients are presented in Table 1. If it was reasonable and possible, both trial and control patients underwent a cytoreductive palliative surgery. As shown in Figure 1, the median survival in the XPV-treated patients was significantly longer than that in the control patients (14 *vs.* 6 months, respectively; p< 0.05). Of note is that almost all of those trial patients, who have survived for 2 years after immunotherapy initiation, further survived as long as 7 years and longer. The overall 7-year survival rate in XPV-treated and control patients was 20% and 0%, respectively. More impressing results were obtained when a long-term overall survival has been analyzed in the stage III melanoma patients (n=48; 26 females and 22 males aged from 22 to 76 years). The control group was composed retrospectively of the clinically comparable patients (n=27; 12 females and 15 males aged from 35 to 77 years). Initially, each of assessable patients had a high risk of disease recurrence. As shown in Figure 2, an overall 6 year survival rate in the trial group was 54%, whereas that in the control group only 25%. It is important to note that a better survival in melanoma patients was associated with their increased DTH to the vaccinal B16 melanoma antigens [49,50].

Characteristic	Trial	Control
Number of patients	51	32
Males/females	25/26 (49%/51%)	10/22 (31%/69%)
Age, years (median, range)	51.8±2.4 (18-72)	48,2±2,3 (24-77)
Site of metastases:		
Lung	16 (31%)	6 (19%)
Liver	10 (20%)	7 (22%)
Lymph node, skin/soft tissue	34 (67%)	26 (81%)
Other organs	8 (15%)	8 (25%)

Table 1. Characteristics of stage IV melanoma patients assessable for survival.

We also evaluated a long-term overall survival in the 35 XPV-treated patients with stage IV colorectal cancer. The control group was composed retrospectively of the patients (n=35) who received conventional therapy. Since the trial patients were very heterogenous in their clinical characteristics, each control patient was randomly selected to be a clinically comparable counterpart of a trial patient, thus control and trial groups were evenly balanced by both prognostic and clinical parameters. The characteristics of colorectal cancer patients are presented in Table 2. As shown in Figure 3, the median survival in the XPV-treated patients was significantly longer when compared with that in the control patients (18 *vs* 8 months, respectively; p< 0.05). An overall 2-year survival rate in the trial and control group was 27% (10 patients) and 3% (1 patient), respectively. However, patients in the trial group almost completely lost their survival advantages as early as at 3.5 years after the immunotherapy initiation.

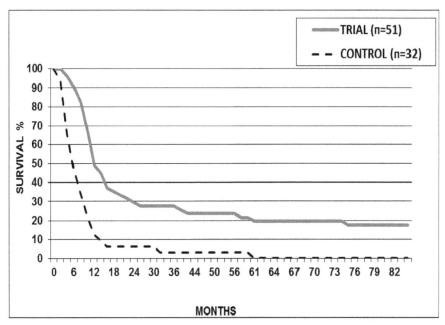

Fig. 1. Survival in the patients with stage IV melanoma. See text for further details.

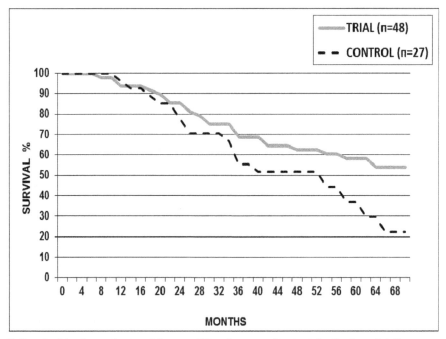

Fig. 2. Survival in the patients with stage III melanoma. See text for further details.

Characteristic	Trial	Control
Number of patients	35	35
Males/females	19/16 (54%/46%)	19/16 (54%/46%)
Age, years (median, range)	61.1 ± 1.4 (38- 79)	55.6 ± 1.7 (30 - 80)
Site of metastases:		
Lung	7 (20%)	6 (17%)
Liver	25 (71%)	19 (54%)
Lymph node,skin/soft tissue	17 (48%)	15 (43%)
Other organs	11 (31%)	8 (23%)

Table 2. Characteristics of stage IV colorectal cancer patients assessable for survival

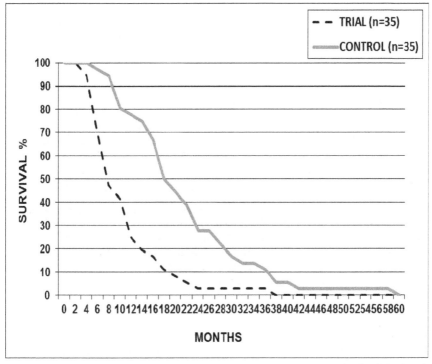

Fig. 3. Survival in the patients with stage IV colorectal cancer. See text for further details.

Figure 4 characterizes a long-term overall survival in the 16 XPV-treated patients (5 females and 11 males aged from 54 to 76 years) with stage IV renal cancer. The control group was composed retrospectively of clinically comparable patients (5 females and 11 males aged from 49 to 77 years) . The median survival in the trial patients was found significantly longer when compared with that in the control patients (20 vs 8 months, respectively; p<0.05). Noteworthy is that patients in the trial group maintained the certain survival benefits from the immunotherapy throughout 5 year follow-up period.

Overall, our results point out that the XPV-based therapy is safe for clinical use, and has no toxicity that is attributable to current standard treatments for cancer. It is also important that the XPV-treated patients exhibited no evidence of systemic autoimmune disorders, of which a risk of development could significantly limits clinical application of polyantigenic xenovaccination .

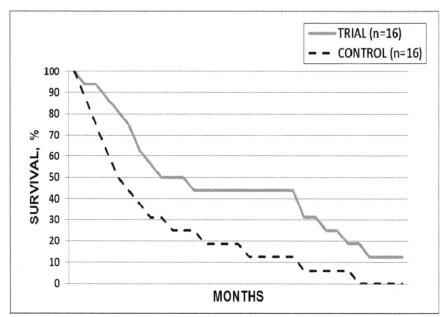

Fig. 4. Survival in the patients with stage IV renal cancer. See text for further details.

It appears that the xenogenic antigens, not only tumor-associated, but also those inherent to normal cells, can be involved in XPV-induced immune responses. As evidenced by both cell- and antibody-mediated reactions [50,51], the immune-mediated sensitization to murine TAA observed in the XPV-treated patients was detectably greater than that to murine spleen cells antigens. This may imply that the antigens associated with tumor cell phenotype might be more significant in generating XPV-driven immune processes than those being only expressed in fully differentiated cells.

Our data demonstrated that the xenovaccinations resulted in serum level elevations of not only of IFN-γ, but also of IL-4, suggesting intensification of both T helper 1- and T helper 2-mediated immune responses in XPV-treated patients [48, 49]. These findings are of great importance in the light of previously reported data that indicate a critical role for cooperating T cell- and antibody-mediated mechanisms in generating tumor cytotoxicity in vivo [46].

According to our experience [50, 51], the xenovaccinotherapy can result in generating complete or partial clinical responses in a certain portion of cancer patients. Nevertheless, stabilization of the disease appears to be the most common outcome of effective immunotherapy in advanced cancer patients. The XPV-based therapy is not an exception in this regard. Unlike the cytotoxic chemotherapy, tumor vaccine-based approaches may permit the host to reach a state of balance with the tumor, in which the net result of tumor growth and destruction is zero. That might lead to more significant survival benefits than a rapid destruction and rapid regrowth of the tumor following cytotoxic therapy.

Actually, our results suggest that the polyantigenic xenovaccinotherapy can significantly affect survival in cancer patients. It should be noted that the majority of patients entered into our investigations were with very advanced (stage IV) disease. It is reasonable to anticipate that, as with other immunotherapies, the XPV-based therapy might be maximally effective when being applied as early as possible following surgical resection of the prime tumor. Consistent with this assertion, the most survival benefits from immunotherapy were noted in the group of stage III melanoma patients when xenovaccinotherapy was initiated before appearing distant metastasis lesions.

4. Conclusion

From the data mentioned above it appears that there are two main ways of using cancer xenovaccinotherapy: the first approach is directed on activation of the immune system against membrane-bound and soluble TAA, and the second one is aimed at overcoming the immune tolerance to the proteins that promote tumor progression. The most antitumor effects are likely to be expected when vaccinal xenogenic TAA elicitit both cellular and humoral immune reactions. The present paper is the first demonstration of the positive effect of polyantigenic xenovaccinotherapy on a long–term survival patients with advanced cancers. Although the results are extremely encouraging, they must be interpreted with caution because they are based on a small number of patients with very advanced disease.

5. Acknowledgements

This study is supported by research grants № П804 and № 02.740.11.0090 from the Russian government. The authors thank Elena Atochina- Vasserman (the University of Pennsylvania School of Medicine, Philadelphia, USA) and Dmitry Logunov (the University of Manchester, Manchester, UK) for reading the paper.

6. References

[1] Potebnya GP, Symchych TV, Lisovenko G.S. Xenogenic cancer vaccines. *Experimental Oncology* 2010; 32: 61-65.

[2] Bowne WB, Srinivasan R, Wolchok JD, Hawkins WG, Blachere NE, Dyall R, Lewis JJ, Houghton AN. Coupling and uncoupling of tumor immunity and autoimmunity. *J Exp Med*. 1999; 190:1717-1722.

[3] Houghton AN, Gold JS, Blachere NE. Immunity against cancer: lesions learned from melanoma. *Curr Opin Immunol*. 2001; 13: 134-140.

[4] Hawkins WG, Gold JS, Blachere NE, Bowne WB, Hoos A, Lewis JJ, Houghton AN. Xenogeneic DNA immunization in melanoma models for minimal residual disease. *J Surg Res*.2002; 102:137-143.

[5] Hawkins WG, Gold JS, Dyall R, Wolchok JD, Hoos A, Bowne WB, Srinivasan R, Houghton AN, Lewis JJ.Immunization with DNA coding for gp100 results in CD4 T-cell independent antitumor immunity. *Surgery* 2000; 128: 273-280.

[6] Weber LW, Bowne WB, Wolchok JD, Srinivasan R, Qin J, Moroi Y, Clynes R, Song P, Lewis JJ, Houghton AN. Tumor immunity and autoimmunity induced by immunization with homologous DNA . *J Clin Invest*. 1998; 102: 1258-1264.

[7] Naftzger C, Takechi Y, Kohda H, Hara I, Vijayasaradhi S, Houghton AN. Immune response to a differentiation antigen induced by altered antigen: a study of tumor rejection and autoimmunity. *Proc Natl Acad Sci USA*.1996; 93:14809-14814.

[8] Wolchok JD, Srinivasan R, Perales MA, Houghton AN, Bowne WB, Blachere NE.Alternative roles for interferon-gamma in the immune response to DNA vaccines encoding related melanosomal antigens . Cancer Immun. 2001; 1: 9.

[9] Kaschenko E.A., Belogorodtsev S.N., Seledtsova G.V., Samarin D.M., Mayborodin I.V., Seledtsov V.I., Shishkov A.A., Savkin И.V., Kozlov V.A. Xenovaccinotherapy for melanoma in experiment. Siberian Oncological Journal (Russian). 2009; №1: 28-31.

[10] Zhong Z, Kusznieruk KP, Popov IA, Riordan NH, Izadi H, Yijian L, Sher S, Szczurko OM, Agadjanyan MG, Tullis RH, Harandi A, Reznik BN, Mamikonyan GV, Ichim TE. Induction of antitumor immunity through xenoplacental immunization . J Transl Med. 2006; 4:22.

[11] Alexander AN, Huelsmeyer MK, Mitzey A, Dubielzig RR, Kurzman ID, Macewen EG, Vail DM. Development of an allogeneic whole-cell tumor vaccine expressing xenogeneic gp100 and its implementation in a phase II clinical trial in canine patients with malignant melanoma. Cancer Immunol Immunother. 2006; 55: 433-442.

[12] Bergman PJ. Canine oral melanoma. Clin Tech Small Anim Pract.- 2007.- V.22.- P.55-60.

[13] Bergman PJ, McKnight J, Novosad A, Charney S, Farrelly J, Craft D, Wulderk M, Jeffers Y, Sadelain M, Hohenhaus AE, Segal N, Gregor P, Engelhorn M, Riviere I, Houghton AN, Wolchok JD // Long-term survival of dogs with advanced malignant melanoma after DNA vaccination with xenogeneic human tyrosinase: a phase I trial . Clin Cancer Res. -2003; 9: 1284-1290.

[14] Liao JC, Gregor P, Wolchok JD, Orlandi F, Craft D, Leung C, Houghton AN, Bergman PJ. Vaccination with human tyrosinase DNA induces antibody responses in dogs with advanced melanoma. Cancer Immun. 2006; 6: 8.

[15] Finocchiaro LM, Glikin GC. Cytokine-enhanced vaccine and suicide gene therapy as surgery adjuvant treatments for spontaneous canine melanoma. Gene Ther. 2008; 15: 267-276.

[16] Pupa SM, Iezzi M, Di Carlo E, Invernizzi A, Cavallo F, Meazza R, Comes A, Ferrini S, Musiani P, Ménard S. Inhibition of mammary carcinoma development in HER-2/neu transgenic mice through induction of autoimmunity by xenogeneic DNA vaccination. Cancer Res. 2005; 65:1071-1078.

[17] Pupa SM, Invernizzi AM, Forti S, Di Carlo E, Musiani P, Nanni P, Lollini PL, Meazza R, Ferrini S, Menard S. Prevention of spontaneous neu-expressing mammary tumor development in mice transgenic for rat proto-neu by DNA vaccination . Gene Ther. 2001; 8:75-79.

[18] Charalambous A, Oks M, Nchinda G, Yamazaki S, Steinman RM.Dendritic cell targeting of survivin protein in a xenogeneic form elicits strong CD4+ T cell immunity to mouse surviving. J Immunol. 2006; 177: 8410-8421.

[19] Zhu K, Qin H, Cha SC, Neelapu SS, Overwijk W, Lizee GA, Abbruzzese JL, Hwu P, Radvanyi L, Kwak LW, Chang DZ. Survivin DNA vaccine generated specific antitumor effects in pancreatic carcinoma and lymphoma mouse models. Vaccine 2007; 25: 7955-7961.

[20] Cho HI, Kim EK, Park SY, Lee SK, Hong YK, Kim TG. Enhanced induction of anti-tumor immunity in human and mouse by dendritic cells pulsed with recombinant TAT fused human survivin protein. Cancer Lett. 2007; 258:189-198.

[21] Ciesielski MJ, Apfel L, Barone TA, Castro CA, Weiss TC, Fenstermaker RA. Antitumor effects of a xenogeneic survivin bone marrow derived dendritic cell vaccine against murine GL261 gliomas. *Cancer Immunol Immunother*. 2006; 55:1491-1503.

[22] Lu Y, Wei YQ, Tian L, Zhao X, Yang L, Hu B, Kan B, Wen YJ, Liu F, Deng HX, Li J, Mao YQ, Lei S, Huang MJ, Peng F, Jiang Y, Zhou H, Zhou LQ, Luo F.Immunogene therapy of tumors with vaccine based on xenogeneic epidermal growth factor receptor. *J Immunol*. 2003; 170: 3162-3170.

[23] Suckow MA, Rosen ED, Wolter WR, Sailes V, Jeffrey R, Tenniswood M. Prevention of human PC-346C prostate cancer growth in mice by a xenogeneic tissue vaccine. *Cancer Immunol Immunother*. 2007; 56:1275-1283.

[24] Suckow MA, Wheeler J, Wolter WR, Sailes V, Yan M. Immunization with a tissue vaccine enhances the effect of irradiation on prostate tumors. *In Vivo*. 2008; 22:171-177.

[25] Li M, Bharadwaj U, Zhang R, Zhang S, Mu H, Fisher WE, Brunicardi FC, Chen C, Yao Q. Mesothelin is a malignant factor and therapeutic vaccine target for pancreatic cancer . *Mol Cancer Ther*. 2008; 7: 286-296.

[26] Sioud M, Sørensen D. Generation of an effective anti-tumor immunity after immunization with xenogeneic antigens. *Eur J Immunol*. 2003; 33: 38-45.

[27] Zhang W, Liu J, Wu Y, Xiao F, Wang Y, Wang R, Yang H, Wang G, Yang J, Deng H, Li J, Wen Y, Wei Y.. Immunotherapy of hepatocellular carcinoma with a vaccine based on xenogeneic homologous a fetoprotein in mice. *Biochem Biophys Res Commun*. 2008; 376: 10-14.

[28] Papewalis C, Wuttke M, Seissler J, Meyer Y, Kessler C, Jacobs B, Ullrich E, Willenberg HS, Schinner S, Baehring T, Scherbaum WA, Schott M. Dendritic cell vaccination with xenogenic polypeptide hormone induces tumor rejection in neuroendocrine cancer. *Clin Cancer Res*. 2008; 14: 4298-4305.

[29] Zheng S, Huang F, Zheng S, Wang W, Yin H, Wu R. Vaccination with a recombinant chicken FGFR-1 bypasses immunological tolerance against self-FGFR-1 in mice. *J Huazhong Univ Sci Technolog Med Sci*. 2006; 26: 389-391.

[30] Su JM, Wei YQ, Tian L, Zhao X, Yang L, He QM, Wang Y, Lu Y, Wu Y, Liu F, Liu JY, Yang JL, Lou YY, Hu B, Niu T, Wen YJ, Xiao F, Deng HX, Li J, Kan B. Active immunogene therapy of cancer with vaccine on the basis of chicken homologous matrix metalloproteinase-2. *Cancer Res*. 2003; 63 : 600-607.

[31] Yi T, Wei YQ, Tian L, Zhao X, Li J, Deng HX, Wen YJ, Zou CH, Tan GH, Kan B, Su JM, Jiang Y, Mao YQ, Chen P, Wang YS. Humoral and cellular immunity induced by tumor cell vaccine based on the chicken xenogeneic homologous matrix metalloproteinase-2. *Cancer Gene Ther*. 2007; 14: 158-164.

[32] Jiao JG, Zhang YD, Li YN. A DNA vaccine encoding the extracellular domain of porcine endoglin induces antitumor immunity in a mouse colon carcinoma model. *Ai Zheng*. 2005; 24: 1179-1183.

[33] Tan GH, Wei YQ, Tian L, Zhao X, Yang L, Li J, He QM, Wu Y, Wen YJ, Yi T, Ding ZY, Kan B, Mao YQ, Deng HX, Li HL, Zhou CH, Fu CH, Xiao F, Zhang XW.Active immunotherapy of tumors with a recombinant xenogeneic endoglin as a model antigen. *Eur J Immunol*. 2004; 34: 2012-2021.

[34] Tan GH, Li YN, Huang FY, Wang H, Bai RZ, Jang J. Combination of recombinant xenogeneic endoglin DNA and protein vaccination enhances anti-tumor effects. *Immunol Invest*. 2007; 36: 423-440.

[35] Jiao JG, Li YN, Wang H, Liu Q, Cao JX, Bai RZ, Huang FY. A plasmid DNA vaccine encoding the extracellular domain of porcine endoglin induces anti-tumour immune

response against self-endoglin-related angiogenesis in two liver cancer models. *Dig Liver Dis.* 2006; 38: 578-587.

[36] Luo Y, Wen YJ, Ding ZY, Fu CH, Wu Y, Liu JY, Li Q, He QM, Zhao X, Jiang Y, Li J, Deng HX, Kang B, Mao YQ, Wei YQ. Immunotherapy of tumors with protein vaccine based on chicken homologous Tie-2. *Clin Cancer Res* 2006; 12: 1813-1819.

[37] Wei YQ, Wang QR, Zhao X, Yang L, Tian L, Lu Y, Kang B, Lu CJ, Huang MJ, Lou YY,Xiao F, He QM, Shu JM, Xie XJ, Mao YQ, Lei S, Luo F, Zhou LQ, Liu CE, Zhou H, Jiang Y, Peng F, Yuan LP, Li Q, Wu Y, Liu JY. Immunotherapy of tumors with xenogeneic endothelial cells as a vaccine. *Nat Med.* 2000; 6: 1160-1166.

[38] Okaji Y, Tsuno NH, Kitayama J, Saito S, Takahashi T, Kawai K, Yazawa K, Asakage M, Hori N, Watanabe T, Shibata Y, Takahashi K, Nagawa H. Vaccination with autologous endothelium inhibits angiogenesis and metastasis of colon cancer through autoimmunity. *Cancer Sci.* 2004; 95: 85-90.

[39] Kamstock D, Elmslie R, Thamm D, Dow S. Evaluation of a xenogeneic VEGF vaccine in dogs with soft tissue sarcoma. *Cancer Immunol Immunother.* 2007; 56: 1299-1309.

[40] Felicetti P, Mennecozzi M, Barucca A, Montgomery S, Orlandi F, Manova K, Houghton AN, Gregor PD, Concetti A, Venanzi FM.Tumor endothelial marker 8 enhances tumor immunity in conjunction with immnization against differentiation Ag . *Cytotherapy* 2007; 9: 23-34.

[41] Fong L, Brockstedt D, Benike C, Breen JK, Strang G, Ruegg CL, Engleman EG. Dendritic cell-based xenoantigen vaccination for prostate cancer immunotherapy. *J Immunol.* 2001; 167: 7150-7156.

[42] Wolchok JD, Yuan J, Houghton AN, Gallardo HF, Rasalan TS, Wang J, Zhang Y,Ranganathan R, Chapman PB, Krown SE, Livingston PO, Heywood M, Riviere I, Panageas KS, Terzulli SL, Perales MA. Safety and immunogenicity of tyrosinase DNA vaccines in patients with melanoma. *Mol Ther.* 2007; 15: 2044-2050.

[43] HT, Restifo NP. Natural selection of tumor variants in the generation of "tumor escape" phenotypes. *Nat Immunol* 2002; 3: 999- 1005.

[44] Galili U. Interaction of the natural anti-Gal antibody with a-galactosyl epitopes: a major obstacle for xenotransplantation in humans. *Immunol Today* 1993; 14: 480-482.

[45] Galili U, Rachmilewitz EA, Peleg A, Flechner I. A unique natural human IgG antibody with anti-a-galactosyl specificity. *J Exp Med* 1984; 160: 1519-1531.

[46] Clynes R, Takechi Y, Moroi Y, Houghton A, Ravetch JV. Fc receptors are required in passive and active immunity to melanoma. *Proc Natl Acad Sci USA* 1998; 95: 652-656.

[47] Rossi GR, Unfer RC, Seregina T, Link CJ. Complete protection against melanoma in absence of autoimmune depigmentation after rejection of melanoma cells expressing alpha(1,3)galactosyl epitopes. *Cancer Immunol Immunother* 2005; 54: 999-1009.

[48] Felde MA, Samarin DM, Niza NA, Shishkov AA, K aschenko EA, Seledtsov VI, Seledtsova GV, Kozlov VA. Examination of cellular immunoreactivity in xenovaccine-treated patients with IV stage colorectal cancer. *Medical immunology(Russian)* 2006; № 1: 67-72.

[49] Seledtsov VI., Felde MA, Samarin DM, Seledtsova GV, Shishkov AA, Niza NA, Tyuryumin YaL, Kaschenko EA, Poveschenko OV, Kozlov VA. Immunological and clinical aspects of applying xenovaccinotherapy in treating melanoma. *Russian Oncological Journal (Russian).* 2006; № 4: 23-29.

[50] Seledtsov VI, Shishkov AA, Surovtseva MA, Samarin DM, Seledtsova GV, Niza NA, Seledtsov DV. Xenovaccinotherapy for melanoma. *Eur. J. Dermatol.* 2006; 16: 655-661.

[51] Seledtsov VI, Niza NA, Surovtseva M A, Shishkov AA, Samarin DM, Seledtsova GV, Seledtsov DV. Xenovaccinotherapy for colorectal cancer. *Biomed. Pharmacother.* 2007; 61: 125-130.

3

NKG2D-Based Cancer Immunotherapy

Jennifer Wu[1] and Xuanjun Wang[2]
[1]University of Washington
[2]Yunnan Agriculture University
[1]USA
[2]China

1. Introduction

NKG2D (nature killer group 2, member D) is a C-type lectin-like activating receptor expressed by all human nature killer (NK) cells, most NKT cells, subsets of γδ T cells, and CD8 T cells. In mouse, NKG2D is also expressed by all NK cells and subsets od splenic γδ T cells and NKT cells, but only expressed by activated mouse CD8 T cells and activated mouse macrophages. NKG2D is located on a syntanic region of human choromosome 12 and on mouse chromosome 6, clustered with other NKG2 family members (Glienke et al., 1998; Ho et al., 1998) (**Figure 1**). NKG2D serves as an invariant immune activating receptor upon engagement by ligands expressed on target cells, transformed or viral infected cells. Engagement of NKG2D by its ligands can activate NK cell and co-stimulate CD8 and γδ T cells (Bauer et al., 1999; Groh et al., 2001; Wu et al., 2002). The activation signals transmitted by NKG2D can override inhibitory signals transmitted by other NK receptors. NKG2D is therefore referred as the master activating receptor for NK cells to sense cells under abnormal physiological stress. The ligands for NKG2D are not commonly present in normal tissues but can be induced under abnormal physiological condition, such as cellular transformation or viral infection. The expression pattern of NKG2D ligands in tumor cells has been extensively studied. Emerging experimental evidence have indicated that NKG2D-mediated immunity can be very effective for tumor clerance by activating NK cells, and in some cases CD8 T cells. However, it is widely accepted that NKG2D function is subverted in cancer patients, due to mechanisms of tumor immunoediting and immune suppressive effect of tumor microenvironment (**Figure 2**). Thus, inventions are in need to overcome tumor immune evasion of NKG2D immunity as an effective cancer treatment. In this chapter, we will review the basic understandings of NKG2D function in anti-tumor immunity and the challenges and advances in NKG2D-based cancer treatment.

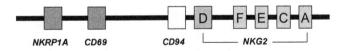

Fig. 1. The NKG2 family gene cluster. Except NKG2D, all other members of the NKG2 family form a heterodimeric complex with CD94. Different from other members, NKG2D forms a homodimer on cell surface.

2. NKG2D

2.1 Molecular structure and expression

NKG2D is a type II transmembering glycoprotein, containing C-type lectin-like domains, similar to other known NKG2 family (Eagle and Trowsdale, 2007). Although physically clustered with other NKG2 family members, NKG2D only displays 20-30% sequence homology with other members of the NKG2 family. NKG2D is highly conserved between species. For instance, human NKG2D and mouse NKG2D share 70% amino acid identity (Raulet, 2003). NKG2D was originally identified as a key activating receptor of NK cells. Subsequently NKG2D is identified on all human CD8 T cells, NKT cells, subsets of γδ T cells. In murine, NKG2D was expressed by activated and memory CD8 T cells, a proportion (25%) of splenic γδ T cells, and activated macrophages (Diefenbach et al., 2000; Mistry and O'Callaghan, 2007).

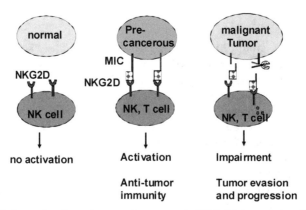

Fig. 2. Tumor cells have developed strategies to evade NKG2D immunity. The ligand of NKG2D is generally absent in normal tissues. In pre-cancerous tissues, NKG2D ligand is induced to stimulate NKG2D immunity in NK and T cells and prevents tumorigenesis. In malignant tissues, NKG2D function is impaired which allows tumor evade to immunity.

2.2 Signaling

The NKG2D molecule contains two β-sheets, two α-helices, four disulfate bonds, and a β-strand (Mistry and O'Callaghan, 2007). NKG2D forms homodimers on the cell membrane (Raulet, 2003). In both human and mouse lymphocytes, stable surface expression of NKG2D requires a complex formation of NKG2D homodimer with a Tyr-X-X-Met (YXXM) adaptor signaling molecule DAP10 at the cell membrane (Ogasawara and Lanier, 2005). Activated mouse NK cells also express a splice variant NKG2D-S, which is 13 aa shorter than normal NKG2D and signals through either DAP10 or the immunoreceptor tyrosine-based activation motif (ITAM)-containing adaptor molecule DAP12 (Long, 2002). Upon ligand engagement of NKG2D, DAP 10 is phosphorylated by src-family kinases (Figure 3), which permits the recruitment of the PI3K subunit p85 and the signaling intermediate Grb2-Vav 1 to fully activate NK cell cytotoxic pathways. In activated mouse NK cells, NKG2D-s may also independently signal through ITAM which, after phosphorylation, recruits ZAP70 (zeta-chain-associated protein kinase 70) and Syk (spleen tyrosine kinase). In NK cells, NKG2D-initiated activation signals can bypass signals transmitted through inhibitory receptors, presumably because SHP phosphotases which are usually recruited by activation of NK inhibitory receptors do not participate NKG2D signaling (Watzl, 2003). Because of this trait, NKG2D is also regarded as the "Master" activation receptor of NK cells. Activation signal provided by NKG2D can override inhibitory signals provided by NKG2D inhibitory receptors.

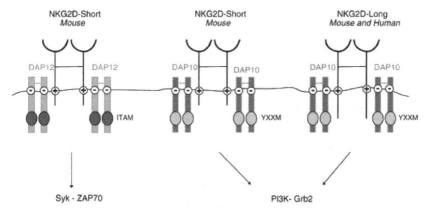

Fig. 3. NKG2D signalling pathways. Mouse NKG2D associates with both DAP10 and DAP12, whereas human NKG2D associates with DAP10 only. Adopted from Champsaur and Lanier, 2010.

3. NKG2D ligands

Multiple genes encode ligands for NKG2D have been identified in human and mice (Table 1). In human, expression of NKG2D is mostly restricted to tumor or certain viral infected cells and rarely identified in normal tissues. The expression pattern of NKG2D ligand in mouse tissues is not well understood. Nonetheless, the regulation of the NKG2D ligand expression is a delicate matter. Inappropriate expression of NKG2D ligands in normal tissues may induce autoimmune diseases, while failure to sustain surface ligand expression in transformed tissues would favor disease development and progression.

3.1 NKG2D ligands in human

Two families of NKG2D ligands are identified in humans: the MHC class I chain related family molecules A (MICA) and B (MICB) and the family of HCMV(human cytomegalovirus) UL16-binding proteins 1-6 (ULBPs 1-6) (Bahram et al., 2005). All these molecules are distant HLA class I homologues but not associated with β-2 microglobulin nor have roles in antigen presentation (Eagle and Trowsdale, 2007). Althogh highly conserved within each family, members of the MIC family share little sequence or structural similarity with those of the ULBP family. The expression pattern of the MIC and ULBPs are also dissimilar.

3.1.1 Tumor-associated expression of MIC family NKG2D ligand

MIC genes are located within the MHC class I region of chromosome 6 (Bahram et al., 2005). Seven MIC loci exist, but only two loci encode translated genes (MICA and MICB) (Eagle and Trowsdale, 2007). Although MICA and MICB transcripts are widely found in normal human tissues (Schrambach et al., 2007), MICA and MICB protein are predominantly found in epithelial originated tumors, rarely expressed in normal tissue with an exception to intestinal epithelium, possibly due to the contact of these cells with intestinal microbes. MICA and MICB share over 80% amino acid identity. Both MICA and MICB are highly plymorphic. There are 51 identified MICA alleles and 23 identified MICB alleles (Bahram et al., 2005; Viny et al., 2010). To some degree, this diversity may provide protection against rapidly evolving cancers (Eagle and Trowsdale, 2007). The MIC(A/B) molecule is consisted of three extracellular domains ($\alpha1$, $\alpha2$, and $\alpha3$), a trans-membrane region, and a cytoplasmic tail (Bahram et al., 1994; Bahram et al., 2005).

Name	Alternate Name	Cell Surface Attachment	NKG2D Affinity (K_D)
Human			
MICA	PERB11.1	Transmembrane	1 μM
MICB	PERB11.2	Transmembrane	0.8 μM
ULBP1	RAET1I	GPI anchor	1.1μM
ULBP2	RAET1H	GPI anchor or not	ND
ULBP3	RAET1N	GPI anchor	ND
ULBP4	RAET1E,LETAL	Transmembrane	ND
ULBP5	RAET1G	Transmembrane or GPI anchor	ND
ULBP6	RAET1L	GPI anchor	ND
Mice			
Rae-1α	Raet 1a	GPI anchor	690nM
Rae-1β	Raet 1b	GPI anchor	345nM
Rae-1γ	Raet 1c	GPI anchor	586nM
Rae-1δ	Raet 1d	GPI anchor	726nM
Rae-1ε	Raet e	GPI anchor	20n M
H60-a	n/a	Transmembrane	26nM
H60-b	n/a	Transmembrane	310nM
H60-c	n/a	GPI anchor	8.7μM
MULT1	n/a	Transmembrane	6 nM

Table 1. NKG2D ligands in human and mouse

3.1.2 Tumor-associated expression of ULBP family NKG2D ligand

The ULBPs were named for their ability to bind to the human cytomegalovirus UL16. protein Six members of human ULBP gene family are identified to encode functional proteins. ULBPs 1-3 and 6 are glycosylphosphatidylinositol (GPI)-linked proteins, whereas ULBPs 4 and 5 are type I transmembrane proteins (Mistry and O'Callaghan, 2007) (Figure 4). Unlike the MICs family, the ULBP family lack the $\alpha3$ domain and only have the MHC class I-like $\alpha1$ and $\alpha2$ domains (Mistry and O'Callaghan, 2007). The expression pattern of ULBP family members are not well defined. ULBP transcripts appear widely expressed in humans (Cosman et al., 2001; Radosavljevic et al., 2002), not restrcited to transformed tissues.

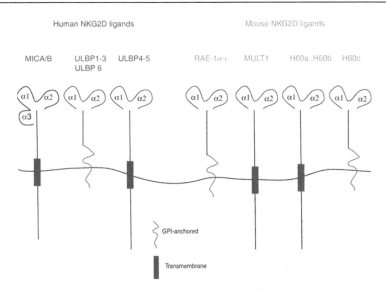

Fig. 4. Structure of NKG2D ligands in human and mice. MICA and MICB are the only known ligands containing three extracellular domains. All others (human and mouse) lack the α3 domain and are either transmembrane or GPI-anchored. Adopted from Champsaur and Lanier, 2010.

3.2 NKG2D ligands in mice

No homologue to human MIC protein was identified in mice. The identified mouse NKG2D ligands include family members of: the MHC I-related family members of retinoic acid early transcript RAE-1(α, β, γ, δ, and ε) and H60 (a, b, c), and the murine ULBP-like transcript 1 (MULT1) (Cerwenka et al., 2000; Diefenbach et al., 2003; O'Callaghan et al., 2001; Takada et al., 2008). All of these ligands only have the MHC class I-like α1 and α2 extracelluar domains. The prototype member of Rae-1 gene family was first discovered as retinoic acid (RA) early inducible cDNA clone-1 (Rae-1), which was rapidly induced on F9 teratocarcinoma cells in response to treatment with retinoic acid (Chalupny et al., 2003; Nomura et al., 1994). Presently, there are five known members of the Rae-1 family, named Rae-1α, Rae-1β, Rae-1γ, Rae-1δ, and Rae-1ε, which are differentially expressed in various mouse strains but highly related to each other (>85% identity). The H60 family comprises three members. H60a, the first ligand of the family was initially identified as a minor histocompatibility antigen by immunizing C57BL/6 mice with MHC-identical BALB.B cells (Malarkannan et al., 1998). Two novel members of H60 family were identified, and named as H60b and H60c (Takada et al., 2008). MULT1 is the unique member of the ULBP-like family of mouse NKG2D ligands and was found by database searching for mouse sequences with similarities to human ULBP (Carayannopoulos et al., 2002).

In mice, NKG2D ligand expression in primary tumorigenesis has not been extensively analyzed. Transcripts of mouse NKG2D ligand was found to be expressed in a broad range of normal tissues. H60a mRNA was found in multiple tissues, including the spleen, cardiac, skeletal muscle, thymus, and skin, whereas H60b mRNA is limited to cardiac and skeletal muscles (Zhang et al. 2010). The most recent addition to the H60 family, H60c, is transcribed largely in the skin (Takada et al., 2008; Whang et al., 2009). H60a is productively expressed in BALB/c mice but not in C57BL/6 mice, whereas H60b and H60c transcripts are detected in both C57BL/6 and BALB/c mouse. MULT1 mRNA is found in the heart, thymus, lung, and kidney across most mice strains (Carayannopoulos et al., 2002; Takada et al., 2008). However, the expression level of NKG2D ligand on normal tissues seem to be below the threshold of inducing activate immune response to cause tissue injury.

3.3 Regulation of the NKG2D ligand expression
As NKG2D serves as the master activating receptor on NK cells, expression of NKG2D ligand NKG2D be delicatedly regulated in a pathological condition to protect normal tissue intergrity and yet maintain the alertness to diseases. The regulation is acheived at multiple levels of regulatory mechanisms, each of which will be discussed below.

3.3.1 Transcriptional regulation
The known mechanisms which regulate the NKG2D ligand transcription are mainly cellular stress, DNA damage, TLR stimulation, and cytokine exposure. The promoter region of the MICA and MICB contains contain sequences that are highly homologous to the heat shock elements of HSP70 (Venkataraman et al., 2007), a stress induced gene. Viral oncoproteins, such as adenoviral E1A protein, or cellular stress-response related products can bind to the promoter region of MICA and/or MICB to induce or upregulate its expression (Venkataraman et al., 2007). Treatment of hepatocellular carcinoma cells with RA was shown to induce the expression of MICA and MICB (Jinushi et al., 2003b). The transcription factor AP-1, which is involved in tumorigenesis and cellular stress responses, was found to regulate Rae-1 transcription through the JunB subunit (Nausch et al., 2006).

The DNA damage response pathway is involved in maintaining the integrity of the genome. The PI3K-related protein kinases ATM (ataxia telangiectasia, mutated) and ATR (ATM and Rad3-related) sense DNA lesions, specifically double-strand breaks and stalled DNA replication, respectively. This sensing results in cell cycle arrest and DNA repair or cell apoptosis if the DNA damage is too extensive to be repaired. This pathway has been shown to be constitutively active in human cancer cells (Bartkova et al., 2005; Gasser and Raulet, 2006; Gorgoulis et al., 2005). Both mouse and human cells upregulate NKG2D ligands expression following treatment with DNA-damaging agents. This effect was dependent on ATR function, as inhibitors of ATR and ATM kinases can prevent ligand upregulation in a dose-dependent fashion.

TLR signaling also results in NKG2D ligand transcription in multiple mechanisms (Eissmann et al., 2010). Treatment of peritoneal macrophages with TLR agonists in vitro and injection of LPS in vivo both resulted in Rae-1 upregulation on peritoneal macrophages (Hamerman et al., 2004). TLR agonists increased the transcription of Raet1 genes, but not MULT1 or H60, in a Myd88-dependent fashion. TLR agonists have a similar effect on human cells (Kloss et al., 2008; Nedvetzki et al., 2007). TLR signaling also results in NKG2D ligand expression on DCs.

Cytokines can differentially affect NKG2D ligand expression in different cell types and environments. In humans, IFN-α leads to the expression of MICA on DCs (Jinushi et al., 2003a). IFN-α and IFN-γ treatment can down-regulate H60 expression on mouse sarcoma cells(Bui et al., 2006). Treatment of human melanoma cells with IFN-γ can decrease mRNA levels of MICA in STAT-1 dependent fashion (Schwinn *et al.*, 2009). Transforming growth factor-β (TGF-β) also decreases the transcription of MICA, ULBP2, and ULPB4 on human malignant gliomas (Friese *et al.*, 2004). Macrophages cultured in the presence of IL-10 show elevated expression of MICA and MICB and ULBPs 1-3 (Schulz *et al.*, 2010).

3.3.2 Post-transcriptional regulation

Various mechanisms are responsible for the post-transcriptional regulation of NKG2D ligands. The endogenous cellular microRNAs (miRNAs) that bound to the 3'-UTR (untranslated region) of MICA,MICB and ULBP1 can repress the translation of these ligands (Stern-Ginossar *et al.*, 2008; Himmelreich *et al.*, 2011). Four miRNAs that suppressed MICA expression have been identified (Yadav *et al.*, 2009). In these findings, silencing of Dicer, a key protein in the miRNA processing pathway, leads to the upregulation of MICA and MICB (Tang *et al.*, 2008). However, miRNA-induced upregulation of NKG2D ligands was found to be dependent on the DNA damage sensor ATM, thus suggesting that upregulation of NKG2D ligands in the absence of Dicer might be due to genotoxic stress in addition to the absence of regulatory miRNAs.

3.3.3 Post-translational regulation

Expression of NKG2D ligand can also be regulated post-translationally via various mechanisms. The ubiquitination on the lysines in cytoplasmic tail of MULT1 was shown to mediate its rapid degradation (Nice *et al.*, 2009). Ubiquitination can be reduced in response to heat shock or ultraviolet irradiation through the MARCH family of E3 ligases and thus allow upregulation of NKG2D ligand expression, such as MULT1 in mice and MIC (A/B) in humans (Nice *et al.*, 2010). The presence of multiple lysines in the cytoplasmic tail of H60a, H60b, MICA, MICB, and RAET-1G suggests that this translational control mechanism might be used by other NKG2D ligands. KSHV (Kaposi's sarcoma-associated herpesvirus)-encoded E3 ubiquitin ligase K5 can down-regulate cell surface expression of MICA and MICB (Thomas *et al.*, 2008). The ubiquitination may also redistribute MICA to the plasma membrane, rather than target to degradation as observed with MULT1. The sorting/internalization motif in H60a may confer the regulation mechanism (Samarakoon *et al.*, 2009). Lastly, one of the most commonly described mechanism to regulate surface NKG2D ligand expression in human cancer cells is protease-mediated shedding (Fernandez-Messina *et al.*, 2010; Liu *et al.*, 2010). This level of regulation will be discussed in details in section 6.1.

4. NKG2D in anti-tumor immunity

4.1 Evidence in experimental models

NKG2D-mediated tumor rejection has been demonstrated very effective in experimental animal models. The rejection was mediated primarily by NK cells or through a cooperation of NK cells with CD8 T cells. Overexpression of a high level of mouse NKG2D ligands Rae-1 or H60 in mouse tumor cells of various origin, including the thymoma cell line EL4, the T-cell lymphoma cell line RMA, and the poorly immunogenic and highly metastatic melanoma variant B16-BL6, induced *in vivo* rejection or retarded tumor growth when implanted into syngeneic mice (Cerwenka et al., 2001; Diefenbach et al., 2001). It was also found that the rejection of a small dose of Rae-1 or H60-expressing tumors (e.g. 1×10^4 cells) could be achieved by NK cells or CD8 T cells alone whereas inhibition the growth of large dose of Rae-1 or H60-expressing tumor cells (e.g. 1×10^6 cell) required a cooperation of NK cells and CD8 T cells (Diefenbach et al., 2001).

The significance of NKG2D in controlling tumor growth was further emphasized by *in vivo* NKG2D neutralization in experimental models. When mice (B6 or balb/c background) were injected with antibody to neutralize NKG2D, these animals showed increased susceptibility to carcinogen MCA-induced fibrosarcoma in comparison to control IgG-treated mice (Smyth et al., 2005). Perhaps the most direct genetic evidence to demonstrate the role of NKG2D in tumor immunity comes from the NKG2D-deficient mice. When TRAMP mice were crossed with NKG2D-deficient mice, the progeny had 4-time increased frequency of developing poorly-differentiated tumors than NKG2D^{WT} counterparts (Guerra et al., 2008).

4.2 Human cancer

Although NKG2D ligands are prevalently expressed in tumors of many types of human malignancies, there is so far no direct evidence to demonstrate the role of NKG2D in controlling tumor growth or progression. Understanding the significance of NKG2D in human cancer progression mainly comes from correlative observation in cancer patients. Massive clinical data demonstrating impaired NKG2D function in cancer patients was mediated by various mechanisms. A number of studies elegantly demonstrating the positive correlation of impaired NKG2D function with cancer disease stages. We are one of the first groups demonstrating that impaired NKG2D-mediated NK cell function correlated with cancer stages in prostate cancer patients (Wu et al., 2004). In this study, circulating NK cells were isolated from prostate cancer patients with various stages of diseases. NKG2D expression and NK cell function were analyzed *in vitro*. The result showed a gradually loss of NKG2D$^+$ NK population from patients with low grade to high grade of cancer, with complete loss of NKG2D expression on NK cells from patients with advanced diseases. As an obvious consequence, NKG2D-mediated cytotoxicity of these NK cells against tumor cells was severely subverted. Similar observations were demonstrated in the progression of other types of cancers, such as multiple myeloma and colon cancer (Doubrovina et al., 2003; Jinushi et al., 2008). In gliomas patients, tumor burden was found to be associated with deficiency of NKG2D expression on NK and CD8 T cells (Crane et al. 2010). A number of studies have also described that dysfunction of NKG2D on CD3$^+$CD56$^+$ NK-like T cells and subsets of γδ T cells was associated with poor prognosis of certain cancers (Bilgi et al., 2008; Marten et al., 2006; Wang et al., 2008).

5. Tumor immune evasion of NKG2D immunity

5.1 Tumor shedding of NKG2D ligand as the immune evasion mechanism

Expression of NKG2D ligand on tumors should effectively trigger immune response, at least NK cell innate response at the early stage of tumorigenesis, to eradicate tumors in human. However, in many types of established tumors of human malignancy, the NKG2D ligand MIC was highly expressed (Groh et al., 1999). The very paradoxical question is: how can human epithelial tumors develop and persist while the surface MIC molecule should identify them as abnormal and flag them for immune destruction? Clinical studies demonstrated that most of the human malignancies have developed mechanisms to evade NKG2D-mediated anti-tumor immunity. One of the common mechanisms by which human cancers evade NKG2D immunity is shedding of the NKG2D ligand MIC from tumor cell surface to release a stable soluble form of MIC (sMIC) to the circulation (Groh et al., 2002). This mechanism has been identified in an array of human malignancies, including carcinomas of prostate, breast, lung, colon, Kidney, and ovarian, gliomas, neuroblasttomas, and melanoma (Groh et al., 2002). Elevated serum levels of sMIC has been shown to be correlative with advanced cancer stages (Doubrovina et al., 2003; Holdenrieder et al., 2006a, b; Jinushi et al., 2008; Rebmann et al., 2007; Tamaki et al., 2010; Tamaki et al., 2009; Tamaki et al., 2008; Wu et al., 2004). Some studies have suggested that serum levels of sMIC may be used as a valid prognosis factor for cancer progression (Tamaki et al.,2010 ; Tamaki et al., 2009). Tumor-derived sMIC can impose several negative imprints on host immune system. First, shedding can reduce the density of membrane-bound NKG2D lgand, namely MIC on tumor cells and thus reduce the visibility of tumor cells by the immune surveillance. Second, sMIC in the circulation can not only mask NKG2D on effector NK, NKT and T cells, but also induce NKG2D internalization (Champsaur and Lanier, 2010). Third, sMIC may induce the expansion of immune suppressive NKG2D+CD4 T cells in the tumor microenvironment (Groh et al., 2003).

5.2 The alternative hypothesis

The hypothesis that tumor-derived sMIC is immune suppressive in cancer patients is widely accepted. Currently, an alternative hypothesis that chronic exposure to membrane-bound ligands also impairs NKG2D function was also proposed, based on several *in vitro* and *in vivo* studies. This alternative hypothesis raised a concern on the effectiveness and stratege on NKG2D-based immune therapy. The *in vitro* study was conducted by co-culturing purified mouse splenic NK cells with RAE-1-overexpressing tumor cells. The investigator found that NKG2D expression was down-regulated (Coudert et al., 2005). It was not clear in this study whether the down-regulation of prolonged in vitro culture is due to soluble RAE-1 or membrane-bound RAE-1, as RAE-1 was recently shown to be shed by mouse tumor cells (Champsaur and Lanier, 2010). With a different aspect of limitations, the existing evidence from *in vivo* studies was based on enforced ectopic constitutive expression of NKG2D ligand on normal mouse, not in the context of tissue-specific expression without resembling the feature of NKG2D ligand expression in cancer patients. For example, one transgenic mouse model that was created by expressing human MICA under the constitutive and ubiquitous mouse MHC class I H-2K^b promoter on a C57BL/6 background showed impaired ability of NK cells to reject MICA-transfected RMA tumors in comparison to the wild-type counterparts (Wiemann et al., 2005). In other models, NKG2D ligand RAE-1ε was expressed in normal mice under the constitutive involucrin promoter (inducing squamous epithelium expression) or the ubiquitous chicken β-actin promoter; local and systemic NKG2D downregulation was noted in these mice in comparison to the wild-type counterparts (Oppenheim et al., 2005). Notably, in these transgenic mouse models, NKG2D ligand expression was "ectopic" under the direction of a constitutive or ubiquitous promoter in somatic cells. Given the magnitude of ligand-induced NKG2D signaling on activating NK cell cytoxicity, down-regulation of NKG2D function may be expected in these transgenic mice in compare to an otherwise wild type counterpart. This would be a self-regulatory mechanism in response to "a suicide machinery" to allow normal embryonic development. Thus, whether the sustained systemic ligand-induced downregulation of NKG2D in these mouse models truly represents the real situation in cancer patients should be carefully evaluated.

5.3 Does chronic exposure to membrane-bound ligand impair NKG2D function?

The alternative hypothesis raised a fatal therapeutic concern whether sustaining NKG2D ligand on tumor cell surface would be beneficial or detrimental for host anti-tumor immunity. To resolve the controversial, we constructed a mutant shedding resistant membrane-restricted NKG2D ligand MICB.A2. We overexpressed the native shedding-sensitive MICB and the mutant MICB.A2 both of which can be recognized by mouse NKG2D (Wu et al., 2009) respectively in a highly tumorigenic mouse prostate tumor cell line TRAMP-C2 and implanted these cell lines into SCID mice. Interestingly, expression of the membrane-restricted MICB.A2 prevented TRAMP-C2 to form tumors *in vivo* whereas expression of native shedding-sensitive MICB did not (Wu et al., 2009). When the mice were injected with purified sMICB prior to tumor inoculation to imitate the expression of shedding-sensitive MICB, expression of MICB.A2 could not prevent TRAMP-C2 tumor formation. This study provided a proof-of-principle that tumor-specific membrane-bound ligand does not impair NKG2D function *in vivo* and that only the soluble ligand derived from the membrane-bound ligand as a result of shedding induces NKG2D dysfunction to promote tumorigenesis. To provide further evidence supporting this notion, we have created double transgenic TRAMP-MICB and TRAMP-MICB.A2 mice where MICB and MICB.A2 was concurrently expressed with the SV40T oncoprotein in the mouse prostate epithelium directed by the prostate-specific probasin promoter. Sustained immunity was generated by enforced expression of membrane-restricted MICB.A2 to allow long-term tumor-free survival of animals; conversely, enforced expression of shedding-sensitive MICB facilitated bound MIC, is immune suppressive to facilitate tumor progression and metastasis (Wu, unpublished). Together, these studies have suggested that stabilizing membrane-bound NKG2D ligand expression may become valuable avenue for tumor immune therapy.

5.4 Modulation of NKG2D function by tumor microenvironment

Other soluble components than soluble NKG2D ligands in the tumor microenvironment have also been described to facilitate tumors evading NKG2D immunity. One of the widely described factors is TGF-β, which can be secreted by regulatory T cells or tumor cells. TGF-β was well demonstrated to down-regulate of NKG2D expression in Glioma patients (Castriconi et al., 2003; Crane et al., ; Friese et al., 2004). In some cases, TGF-β was also found to inhibit the expression of tumor cell surface NKG2D ligand expression at the transcriptional level (Friese et al., 2004). Indoleamine 2,3-dioxygenase (IDO), a tryptophan (Trp) catabolite, is another well studied component in the tumor microenvironment that may negatively regulate NKG2D function. IDO is generally absent or inactive in cells of the immune system, but it can be induced or activated in macrophages and subsets of dendritic-cell (DC) by specific cytokines, in particular IFN-γ. IDO has also been found in various tumors of different histotypes. Elevated IDO activity was found to be correlated with cancer, such as lung, ovarian, breast cancers, and many other types of malignancies (Ino, 2010; Prendergast et al.). There is evidence that IDO can directly down-regulate NKG2D expression *in vitro* in a time and dose-dependent manner (Song et al. 2010).

6. Interventions to harness NKG2D immunity for cancer treatment

Ample evidence demonstrating that NKG2D function is impaired in cancer patients and that NKG2D dysfunction can facilitate cancer progression to advanced diseases. With the understanding of the mechanisms by which NKG2D function was compromised, in this section, rationales and optimal strategies to harness NKG2D immunity for potential cancer therapy will be discussed.

6.1 Mechanisms of MIC shedding

Studies have been done in many investigators to understand the mechanisms that regulate MIC shedding for potential therapeutic interventions. A diverse group of enzymes have recently been shown to be involved in MIC shedding. Studies from several groups have shown that inhibition of cellular metalloproteinase activity by GM6001 markedly interferes with MIC shedding. Specific metalloproteinases, such as ADAM (a disintegrin and metalloproteinase)-10 and ADAM-17, were found contributing to MICA shedding (Waldhauer et al., 2008) and ADAM-17 protease was found contributing to MICB shedding (Boutet et al., 2009). The type I membrane MMP (MT1-MMP, also called MMP14) also directly regulates MICA shedding independent of ADAMS (Liu et al., 2010). The thiol isomerase ERp5, which catalyzes disulfide bond formation, reduction, and isomerization, was shown to be required for MIC shedding (Kaiser et al., 2007). This was presumably accomplished by chaperoning conformational alterations of surface MIC through disulphide-bond exchange that render MIC susceptible for proteolytic cleavage.

6.2 Targeting proteases to inhibit MIC shedding

ADAM-10 and -17 and the thioreductase ERp5 have been proposed to be potential cancer therapeutic targets for inhibiting MIC shedding. However, these enzymes are not only involved in pathology of diseases, but also involved in many normal physiological functions. For instance, ADAM-17 is required for generation of the active forms of Epidermal Growth Factor Receptor (EGFR) ligands that is essential for the development of epithelial tissues. In addition, although there are many examples of expression or upregulation of ADAMs in both tumor tissues and cell lines, the precise pattern of their expression within tumors is not always clear (Edwards et al., 2008). Furthermore, targeting ADAM-17 has been in clinical trials with a spectrum of inhibitors for over a decade. However, no single ADAM-17 inhibitor has passed a Phase II clinical trial because of high toxicity and non-specific targeting (DasGupta et al., 2009). As to the possibility of targeting ERp5, it has been suggested that disulfide bond exchange with cell surface molecule to enable the shedding may be a general mechanism by which ERp5 modulates cell signaling (Jordan and Gibbins, 2006). In addition, a wide role of ERp5 in cellular function has been implicated, such as in normal platelet activation (Jordan et al., 2005). These studies suggest that there are many facets of these enzymes that need to be understood before embarking with confidence on targeting them for cancer therapy. Therefore, a more specific and feasible target is needed for inhibiting MIC shedding for cancer therapy.

6.3 Targeting MIC shedding regulatory sequences

By Mass-spectrometry analyses, we and others have shown that MIC is cleaved at multiple sites in the near transmembrane region aa 253-289 in tumor cell lines (Kaiser et al., 2007; Waldhauer et al., 2008; Wang et al., 2009), suggesting that targeting the cleavage site(s) for inhibiting MIC shedding is not therapeutically feasible. Using genetic approach, a dispensable six-aa motif in the α3 ectodomain of MIC (A and B) was identified to be critical for regulating MIC shedding (Wang et al., 2009). Mutation in the six-aa motif completely prevented MIC shedding but did not interfere with MIC to be recognized by NKG2D.

Further study revealed that the six-aa motif is required for MIC to form a physical complex with ERp5, a presumable requirement for MIC to be shed. Due to the "non-invasive" feature of the six-aa motif, molecules or antibodies targeting this six-aa shedding regulatory motif to prevent MIC to interact with ERp5 may be a more feasible therapy.

6.4 Neutralizing sMIC

In a clinical trial with a anti-CTLA-4 antibody blockade or vaccines for melanoma therapy, patients who generated anti-MICA antibodies during the therapy showed significantly better clinical outcome than those who did not (Jinushi et al., 2006). The beneficial effect was shown to act through antibody antagonizing sMICA-induced suppression of NK and CD8 T cell anti-tumor responses. Although not being discussed in this study, the effect of anti-MICA antibody in this particular clinical setting may also be due to elimination of sMIC in the serum and thus elimination of immune suppressive NKG2D+ CD4 T cells. More, anti-MIC antibody has also been shown to sensitive tumor cells to antigen-specific T cells by enhancing DC cross-priming (Groh et al., 2005). Based on these observations, using anti-MIC monoclonal antibody (mAb) to neutralize circulating sMIC and concomitantly to enhance DC cross-priming has been proposed as a cancer therapy. However, clinical implication using anti-MIC antibody must take into consideration that the antibody will also block the interaction of tumor-cell surface MIC with NKG2D and thus block NKG2D-mediated NK cell anti-tumor function. Thus, when applying this approach, it is critical to understand whether NK cell or T cell play a critical role in a particular stage of a specific cancer type. As an alternative approach, phase I clinical trial using adoptively transferred haploidentical NK cells to scavenge plasma sMIC has shown some effect in neuropblastoma patients (Kloess et al. 2010). If donor NK cells are obtainable, this approach may become an effective therapy for many type of cancers.

6.5 Engineering T cells with chimeric NKG2D

A new and very interesting mechanism to utilize the NKG2D-mediated immunity in tumor therapy is expressing chimeric NKG2D-CD3ζ (chNKG2D) in T cells for adoptive cell therapy. By fusing NKG2D with the cytoplasmic signaling domain of CD3ζ chain, NKG2D may induce the anti-tumor activation of T cells independent of TCR signaling, when NKG2D ligand is present on tumor cells. The chNKG2D expressed on NK cells and T cells does not seem to be down-regulated by soluble NKG2D ligand (Zhang et al., 2006; Zhang et al., 2005). This approach had been demonstrated to be very effective in controlling tumor growth in several experimental animal models (Barber et al., 2011; Barber et al., 2008a; Barber et al., 2008b; Zhang et al., 2007). Treatment of mice bearing established ovarian and multiple myeloma with T cells expressing the chNKG2D receptor can lead to long-term, tumor-free survival and induce host memory responses to tumor antigens. This protection is not restricted to the direct effect of chNKG2D-induced activation of T cells upon ligand engagement. Sustained long-term protection against tumors in animal models was found to be achieved through cytokines secreted by the chNKG2D-engineered T cells to induce a proinflammatory environment and re-activate host NK, CD4 and CD8 T cell anti-tumor responses. In ovarian mouse models, adoptive transfer of chNKG2D T cells was found to not only to induce systemic increase in IFNγ, GM-CSF, and perforin but also to eliminate immunosuppressive regulatory CD4 T cells in the tumor microenvironment (Barber and Sentman, 2009; Barber et al., 2008a). Adoptive transferring chNKG2D engineered T cells has also been shown effective in our tumor models. However, due to the systemic immunoactivation induced by chNKG2D T cells, the long-term safety in clinical application has to be evaluated. chNKG2D-engineered autologous T cells is currently in phase I clinical trial for treating ovarian cancer patients.

7. Conclusion

As emerging evidence demonstrating the significance of sustained NKG2D-NKG2D ligand interaction in anti-tumor responses, in particular solid tumors, it is time to develop therapeutic interventions to harness the NKG2D immunity for anti-tumor therapy. As soluble NKG2D ligands are the culprit for tumor evading NKG2D immunity, interventions to enforce NKG2D-mediated anti-tumor response should be focused on preventing tumor shedding, removal of soluble NKG2D ligand or counteracting the effect of soluble ligand on NKG2D function. More, in the development of tumor vaccines, one should also take into the consideration that across-priming by NKG2D ligand may boost the clinical efficiency of vaccine-induced immune responses. Last but not least, as tumor microenvironment can negatively regulate NKG2D function, co-targeting tumor microenvironment may be necessarily in stratifying NKG2D anti-tumor immunity.

8. Acknowledgment

We thank grant support by National Institute of Health (NIH) Temin Award 1K01CA116002, and NIH 1R01CA149405 to J.W

9. References

Bahram, S., Bresnahan, M., Geraghty, D.E., and Spies, T. (1994). A second lineage of mammalian major histocompatibility complex class I genes. Proc Natl Acad Sci U S A 91, 6259-6263.

Bahram, S., Inoko, H., Shiina, T., and Radosavljevic, M. (2005). MIC and other NKG2D ligands: from none to too many. Curr Opin Immunol 17, 505-509.

Barber, A., Meehan, K.R., and Sentman, C.L. Treatment of multiple myeloma with adoptively transferred chimeric NKG2D receptor-expressing T cells. Gene Ther.

Barber, A., and Sentman, C.L. (2009). Chimeric NKG2D T cells require both T cell- and host-derived cytokine secretion and perforin expression to increase tumor antigen presentation and systemic immunity. J Immunol 183, 2365-2372.

Barber, A., Zhang, T., Megli, C.J., Wu, J., Meehan, K.R., and Sentman, C.L. (2008a). Chimeric NKG2D receptor-expressing T cells as an immunotherapy for multiple myeloma. Exp Hematol 36, 1318-1328.

Barber, A., Zhang, T., and Sentman, C.L. (2008b). Immunotherapy with chimeric NKG2D receptors leads to long-term tumor-free survival and development of host antitumor immunity in murine ovarian cancer. J Immunol 180, 72-78.

Bartkova, J., Horejsi, Z., Koed, K., Kramer, A., Tort, F., Zieger, K., Guldberg, P., Sehested, M., Nesland, J.M., Lukas, C., et al. (2005). DNA damage response as a candidate anti-cancer barrier in early human tumorigenesis. Nature 434, 864-870.

Bauer, S., Groh, V., Wu, J., Steinle, A., Phillips, J.H., Lanier, L.L., and Spies, T. (1999). Activation of NK cells and T cells by NKG2D, a receptor for stress-inducible MICA. Science 285, 727-729.

Bilgi, O., Karagoz, B., Turken, O., Kandemir, E.G., Ozturk, A., Gumus, M., and Yaylaci, M. (2008). Peripheral blood gamma-delta T cells in advanced-stage cancer patients. Adv Ther 25, 218-224.

Boutet, P., Aguera-Gonzalez, S., Atkinson, S., Pennington, C.J., Edwards, D.R., Murphy, G., Reyburn, H.T., and Vales-Gomez, M. (2009). Cutting edge: The metalloproteinase ADAM17/TNF-alpha-converting enzyme regulates proteolytic shedding of the MHC class I-related chain B protein. J Immunol 182, 49-53.

Bui, J.D., Carayannopoulos, L.N., Lanier, L.L., Yokoyama, W.M., and Schreiber, R.D. (2006). IFN-dependent down-regulation of the NKG2D ligand H60 on tumors. J Immunol 176, 905-913.

Carayannopoulos, L.N., Naidenko, O.V., Fremont, D.H., and Yokoyama, W.M. (2002). Cutting edge: murine UL16-binding protein-like transcript 1: a newly described transcript encoding a high-affinity ligand for murine NKG2D. J Immunol 169, 4079-4083.

Castriconi, R., Cantoni, C., Della Chiesa, M., Vitale, M., Marcenaro, E., Conte, R., Biassoni, R., Bottino, C., Moretta, L., and Moretta, A. (2003). Transforming growth factor beta 1 inhibits expression of NKp30 and NKG2D receptors: consequences for the NK-mediated killing of dendritic cells. Proc Natl Acad Sci U S A 100, 4120-4125.

Cerwenka, A., Bakker, A.B., McClanahan, T., Wagner, J., Wu, J., Phillips, J.H., and Lanier, L.L. (2000). Retinoic acid early inducible genes define a ligand family for the activating NKG2D receptor in mice. Immunity 12, 721-727.

Cerwenka, A., Baron, J.L., and Lanier, L.L. (2001). Ectopic expression of retinoic acid early inducible-1 gene (RAE-1) permits natural killer cell-mediated rejection of a MHC class I-bearing tumor in vivo. Proc Natl Acad Sci U S A 98, 11521-11526.

Chalupny, N.J., Sutherland, C.L., Lawrence, W.A., Rein-Weston, A., and Cosman, D. (2003). ULBP4 is a novel ligand for human NKG2D. Biochem Biophys Res Commun 305, 129-135.

Champsaur, M., and Lanier, L.L. (2010). Effect of NKG2D ligand expression on host immune responses. Immunol Rev 235, 267-285.

Cosman, D., Mullberg, J., Sutherland, C.L., Chin, W., Armitage, R., Fanslow, W., Kubin, M., and Chalupny, N.J. (2001). ULBPs, novel MHC class I-related molecules, bind to CMV glycoprotein UL16 and stimulate NK cytotoxicity through the NKG2D receptor. Immunity 14, 123-133.

Coudert, J.D., Zimmer, J., Tomasello, E., Cebecauer, M., Colonna, M., Vivier, E., and Held, W. (2005). Altered NKG2D function in NK cells induced by chronic exposure to NKG2D ligand-expressing tumor cells. Blood 106, 1711-1717.

Crane, C.A., Han, S.J., Barry, J.J., Ahn, B.J., Lanier, L.L., and Parsa, A.T. TGF-beta downregulates the activating receptor NKG2D on NK cells and CD8+ T cells in glioma patients. Neuro Oncol 12, 7-13.

DasGupta, S., Murumkar, P.R., Giridhar, R., and Yadav, M.R. (2009). Current perspective of TACE inhibitors: a review. Bioorg Med Chem 17, 444-459.

Diefenbach, A., Hsia, J.K., Hsiung, M.Y., and Raulet, D.H. (2003). A novel ligand for the NKG2D receptor activates NK cells and macrophages and induces tumor immunity. Eur J Immunol 33, 381-391.

Diefenbach, A., Jamieson, A.M., Liu, S.D., Shastri, N., and Raulet, D.H. (2000). Ligands for the murine NKG2D receptor: expression by tumor cells and activation of NK cells and macrophages. Nat Immunol 1, 119-126.

Diefenbach, A., Jensen, E.R., Jamieson, A.M., and Raulet, D.H. (2001). Rae1 and H60 ligands of the NKG2D receptor stimulate tumour immunity. Nature 413, 165-171.

Doubrovina, E.S., Doubrovin, M.M., Vider, E., Sisson, R.B., O'Reilly, R.J., Dupont, B., and Vyas, Y.M. (2003). Evasion from NK cell immunity by MHC class I chain-related molecules expressing colon adenocarcinoma. J Immunol 171, 6891-6899.

Eagle, R.A., and Trowsdale, J. (2007). Promiscuity and the single receptor: NKG2D. Nat Rev Immunol 7, 737-744.

Edwards, D.R., Handsley, M.M., and Pennington, C.J. (2008). The ADAM metalloproteinases. Mol Aspects Med 29, 258-289.

Eissmann, P., Evans, J.H., Mehrabi, M., Rose, E.L., Nedvetzki, S., and Davis, D.M. (2010). Multiple mechanisms downstream of TLR-4 stimulation allow expression of NKG2D ligands to facilitate macrophage/NK cell crosstalk. J Immunol 184, 6901-6909.

Fernandez-Messina, L., Ashiru, O., Boutet, P., Aguera-Gonzalez, S., Skepper, J.N., Reyburn, H.T., and Vales-Gomez, M. (2010). Differential mechanisms of shedding of the glycosylphosphatidylinositol (GPI)-anchored NKG2D ligands. J Biol Chem 285, 8543-8551.

Friese, M.A., Wischhusen, J., Wick, W., Weiler, M., Eisele, G., Steinle, A., and Weller, M. (2004). RNA interference targeting transforming growth factor-beta enhances NKG2D-mediated antiglioma immune response, inhibits glioma cell migration and invasiveness, and abrogates tumorigenicity in vivo. Cancer Res 64, 7596-7603.

Gasser, S., and Raulet, D.H. (2006). Activation and self-tolerance of natural killer cells. Immunol Rev 214, 130-142.

Glienke, J., Sobanov, Y., Brostjan, C., Steffens, C., Nguyen, C., Lehrach, H., Hofer, E., and Francis, F. (1998). The genomic organization of NKG2C, E, F, and D receptor genes in the human natural killer gene complex. Immunogenetics 48, 163-173.

Gorgoulis, V.G., Vassiliou, L.V., Karakaidos, P., Zacharatos, P., Kotsinas, A., Liloglou, T., Venere, M., Ditullio, R.A., Jr., Kastrinakis, N.G., Levy, B., et al. (2005). Activation of the DNA damage checkpoint and genomic instability in human precancerous lesions. Nature 434, 907-913.

Groh, V., Bruhl, A., El-Gabalawy, H., Nelson, J.L., and Spies, T. (2003). Stimulation of T cell autoreactivity by anomalous expression of NKG2D and its MIC ligands in rheumatoid arthritis. Proc Natl Acad Sci U S A 100, 9452-9457.

Groh, V., Li, Y.Q., Cioca, D., Hunder, N.N., Wang, W., Riddell, S.R., Yee, C., and Spies, T. (2005). Efficient cross-priming of tumor antigen-specific T cells by dendritic cells sensitized with diverse anti-MICA opsonized tumor cells. Proc Natl Acad Sci U S A 102, 6461-6466.

Groh, V., Rhinehart, R., Randolph-Habecker, J., Topp, M.S., Riddell, S.R., and Spies, T. (2001). Costimulation of CD8alphabeta T cells by NKG2D via engagement by MIC induced on virus-infected cells. Nat Immunol 2, 255-260.

Groh, V., Rhinehart, R., Secrist, H., Bauer, S., Grabstein, K.H., and Spies, T. (1999). Broad tumor-associated expression and recognition by tumor-derived gamma delta T cells of MICA and MICB. Proc Natl Acad Sci U S A *96*, 6879-6884.

Groh, V., Wu, J., Yee, C., and Spies, T. (2002). Tumour-derived soluble MIC ligands impair expression of NKG2D and T-cell activation. Nature *419*, 734-738.

Guerra, N., Tan, Y.X., Joncker, N.T., Choy, A., Gallardo, F., Xiong, N., Knoblaugh, S., Cado, D., Greenberg, N.M., and Raulet, D.H. (2008). NKG2D-deficient mice are defective in tumor surveillance in models of spontaneous malignancy. Immunity *28*, 571-580.

Hamerman, J.A., Ogasawara, K., and Lanier, L.L. (2004). Cutting edge: Toll-like receptor signaling in macrophages induces ligands for the NKG2D receptor. J Immunol *172*, 2001-2005.

Ho, E.L., Heusel, J.W., Brown, M.G., Matsumoto, K., Scalzo, A.A., and Yokoyama, W.M. (1998). Murine Nkg2d and Cd94 are clustered within the natural killer complex and are expressed independently in natural killer cells. Proc Natl Acad Sci U S A *95*, 6320-6325.

Holdenrieder, S., Stieber, P., Peterfi, A., Nagel, D., Steinle, A., and Salih, H.R. (2006a). Soluble MICA in malignant diseases. Int J Cancer *118*, 684-687.

Holdenrieder, S., Stieber, P., Peterfi, A., Nagel, D., Steinle, A., and Salih, H.R. (2006b). Soluble MICB in malignant diseases: analysis of diagnostic significance and correlation with soluble MICA. Cancer Immunol Immunother *55*, 1584-1589.

Ino, K. Indoleamine 2,3-dioxygenase and immune tolerance in ovarian cancer. Curr Opin Obstet Gynecol *23*, 13-18.

Jinushi, M., Hodi, F.S., and Dranoff, G. (2006). Therapy-induced antibodies to MHC class I chain-related protein A antagonize immune suppression and stimulate antitumor cytotoxicity. Proc Natl Acad Sci U S A *103*, 9190-9195.

Jinushi, M., Takehara, T., Kanto, T., Tatsumi, T., Groh, V., Spies, T., Miyagi, T., Suzuki, T., Sasaki, Y., and Hayashi, N. (2003a). Critical role of MHC class I-related chain A and B expression on IFN-alpha-stimulated dendritic cells in NK cell activation: impairment in chronic hepatitis C virus infection. J Immunol *170*, 1249-1256.

Jinushi, M., Takehara, T., Tatsumi, T., Kanto, T., Groh, V., Spies, T., Kimura, R., Miyagi, T., Mochizuki, K., Sasaki, Y., and Hayashi, N. (2003b). Expression and role of MICA and MICB in human hepatocellular carcinomas and their regulation by retinoic acid. Int J Cancer *104*, 354-361.

Jinushi, M., Vanneman, M., Munshi, N.C., Tai, Y.T., Prabhala, R.H., Ritz, J., Neuberg, D., Anderson, K.C., Carrasco, D.R., and Dranoff, G. (2008). MHC class I chain-related protein A antibodies and shedding are associated with the progression of multiple myeloma. Proc Natl Acad Sci U S A *105*, 1285-1290.

Jordan, P.A., and Gibbins, J.M. (2006). Extracellular disulfide exchange and the regulation of cellular function. Antioxid Redox Signal *8*, 312-324.

Jordan, P.A., Stevens, J.M., Hubbard, G.P., Barrett, N.E., Sage, T., Authi, K.S., and Gibbins, J.M. (2005). A role for the thiol isomerase protein ERP5 in platelet function. Blood *105*, 1500-1507.

Kaiser, B.K., Yim, D., Chow, I.T., Gonzalez, S., Dai, Z., Mann, H.H., Strong, R.K., Groh, V., and Spies, T. (2007). Disulphide-isomerase-enabled shedding of tumour-associated NKG2D ligands. Nature *447*, 482-486.

Kloess, S., Huenecke, S., Piechulek, D., Esser, R., Koch, J., Brehm, C., Soerensen, J., Gardlowski, T., Brinkmann, A., Bader, P., et al. IL-2-activated haploidentical NK cells restore NKG2D-mediated NK-cell cytotoxicity in neuroblastoma patients by scavenging of plasma MICA. Eur J Immunol 40, 3255-3267.

Kloss, M., Decker, P., Baltz, K.M., Baessler, T., Jung, G., Rammensee, H.G., Steinle, A., Krusch, M., and Salih, H.R. (2008). Interaction of monocytes with NK cells upon Toll-like receptor-induced expression of the NKG2D ligand MICA. J Immunol 181, 6711-6719.

Liu, G., Atteridge, C.L., Wang, X., Lundgren, A.D., and Wu, J.D. (2010). The membrane type matrix metalloproteinase MMP14 mediates constitutive shedding of MHC class I chain-related molecule A independent of A disintegrin and metalloproteinases. J Immunol 184, 3346-3350.

Long, E.O. (2002). Versatile signaling through NKG2D. Nat Immunol 3, 1119-1120.

Malarkannan, S., Shih, P.P., Eden, P.A., Horng, T., Zuberi, A.R., Christianson, G., Roopenian, D., and Shastri, N. (1998). The molecular and functional characterization of a dominant minor H antigen, H60. J Immunol 161, 3501-3509.

Marten, A., von Lilienfeld-Toal, M., Buchler, M.W., and Schmidt, J. (2006). Soluble MIC is elevated in the serum of patients with pancreatic carcinoma diminishing gammadelta T cell cytotoxicity. Int J Cancer 119, 2359-2365.

Mistry, A.R., and O'Callaghan, C.A. (2007). Regulation of ligands for the activating receptor NKG2D. Immunology 121, 439-447.

Nausch, N., Florin, L., Hartenstein, B., Angel, P., Schorpp-Kistner, M., and Cerwenka, A. (2006). Cutting edge: the AP-1 subunit JunB determines NK cell-mediated target cell killing by regulation of the NKG2D-ligand RAE-1epsilon. J Immunol 176, 7-11.

Nedvetzki, S., Sowinski, S., Eagle, R.A., Harris, J., Vely, F., Pende, D., Trowsdale, J., Vivier, E., Gordon, S., and Davis, D.M. (2007). Reciprocal regulation of human natural killer cells and macrophages associated with distinct immune synapses. Blood 109, 3776-3785.

Nice, T.J., Coscoy, L., and Raulet, D.H. (2009). Posttranslational regulation of the NKG2D ligand Mult1 in response to cell stress. J Exp Med 206, 287-298.

Nice, T.J., Deng, W., Coscoy, L., and Raulet, D.H. (2010). Stress-regulated targeting of the NKG2D ligand Mult1 by a membrane-associated RING-CH family E3 ligase. J Immunol 185, 5369-5376.

Nomura, M., Takihara, Y., and Shimada, K. (1994). Isolation and characterization of retinoic acid-inducible cDNA clones in F9 cells: one of the early inducible clones encodes a novel protein sharing several highly homologous regions with a Drosophila polyhomeotic protein. Differentiation 57, 39-50.

O'Callaghan, C.A., Cerwenka, A., Willcox, B.E., Lanier, L.L., and Bjorkman, P.J. (2001). Molecular competition for NKG2D: H60 and RAE1 compete unequally for NKG2D with dominance of H60. Immunity 15, 201-211.

Ogasawara, K., and Lanier, L.L. (2005). NKG2D in NK and T cell-mediated immunity. J Clin Immunol 25, 534-540.

Oppenheim, D.E., Roberts, S.J., Clarke, S.L., Filler, R., Lewis, J.M., Tigelaar, R.E., Girardi, M., and Hayday, A.C. (2005). Sustained localized expression of ligand for the activating NKG2D receptor impairs natural cytotoxicity in vivo and reduces tumor immunosurveillance. Nat Immunol 6, 928-937.

Prendergast, G.C., Metz, R., and Muller, A.J. Towards a genetic definition of cancer-associated inflammation: role of the IDO pathway. Am J Pathol 176, 2082-2087.

Radosavljevic, M., Cuillerier, B., Wilson, M.J., Clement, O., Wicker, S., Gilfillan, S., Beck, S., Trowsdale, J., and Bahram, S. (2002). A cluster of ten novel MHC class I related genes on human chromosome 6q24.2-q25.3. Genomics 79, 114-123.

Raulet, D.H. (2003). Roles of the NKG2D immunoreceptor and its ligands. Nat Rev Immunol 3, 781-790.

Rebmann, V., Schutt, P., Brandhorst, D., Opalka, B., Moritz, T., Nowrousian, M.R., and Grosse-Wilde, H. (2007). Soluble MICA as an independent prognostic factor for the overall survival and progression-free survival of multiple myeloma patients. Clin Immunol 123, 114-120.

Samarakoon, A., Chu, H., and Malarkannan, S. (2009). Murine NKG2D ligands: "double, double toil and trouble". Mol Immunol 46, 1011-1019.

Schrambach, S., Ardizzone, M., Leymarie, V., Sibilia, J., and Bahram, S. (2007). In vivo expression pattern of MICA and MICB and its relevance to auto-immunity and cancer. PLoS One 2, e518.

Schulz, U., Kreutz, M., Multhoff, G., Stoelcker, B., Kohler, M., Andreesen, R., and Holler, E. (2010). Interleukin-10 promotes NK cell killing of autologous macrophages by stimulating expression of NKG2D ligands. Scand J Immunol 72, 319-331.

Schwinn, N., Vokhminova, D., Sucker, A., Textor, S., Striegel, S., Moll, I., Nausch, N., Tuettenberg, J., Steinle, A., Cerwenka, A., et al. (2009). Interferon-gamma down-regulates NKG2D ligand expression and impairs the NKG2D-mediated cytolysis of MHC class I-deficient melanoma by natural killer cells. Int J Cancer 124, 1594-1604.

Smyth, M.J., Swann, J., Cretney, E., Zerafa, N., Yokoyama, W.M., and Hayakawa, Y. (2005). NKG2D function protects the host from tumor initiation. J Exp Med 202, 583-588.

Song, H., Park, H., Kim, J., Park, G., Kim, Y.S., Kim, S.M., Kim, D., Seo, S.K., Lee, H.K., Cho, D., and Hur, D. IDO metabolite produced by EBV-transformed B cells inhibits surface expression of NKG2D in NK cells via the c-Jun N-terminal kinase (JNK) pathway. Immunol Lett 136, 187-193.

Takada, A., Yoshida, S., Kajikawa, M., Miyatake, Y., Tomaru, U., Sakai, M., Chiba, H., Maenaka, K., Kohda, D., Fugo, K., and Kasahara, M. (2008). Two novel NKG2D ligands of the mouse H60 family with differential expression patterns and binding affinities to NKG2D. J Immunol 180, 1678-1685.

Tamaki, S., Kawakami, M., Ishitani, A., Kawashima, W., Kasuda, S., Yamanaka, Y., Shimomura, H., Imai, Y., Nakagawa, Y., Hatake, K., and Kirita, T. Soluble MICB serum levels correlate with disease stage and survival rate in patients with oral squamous cell carcinoma. Anticancer Res 30, 4097-4101.

Tamaki, S., Kawakami, M., Ishitani, A., Kawashima, W., Kasuda, S., Yamanaka, Y., Shimomura, H., Imai, Y., Nakagawa, Y., Hatake, K., and Kirita, T. (2010). Soluble MICB serum levels correlate with disease stage and survival rate in patients with oral squamous cell carcinoma. Anticancer Res 30, 4097-4101.

Tamaki, S., Kawakami, M., Yamanaka, Y., Shimomura, H., Imai, Y., Ishida, J., Yamamoto, K., Ishitani, A., Hatake, K., and Kirita, T. (2009). Relationship between soluble MICA and the MICA A5.1 homozygous genotype in patients with oral squamous cell carcinoma. Clin Immunol 130, 331-337.

Tamaki, S., Sanefuzi, N., Kawakami, M., Aoki, K., Imai, Y., Yamanaka, Y., Yamamoto, K., Ishitani, A., Hatake, K., and Kirita, T. (2008). Association between soluble MICA levels and disease stage IV oral squamous cell carcinoma in Japanese patients. Hum Immunol 69, 88-93.

Tang, K.F., Ren, H., Cao, J., Zeng, G.L., Xie, J., Chen, M., Wang, L., and He, C.X. (2008). Decreased Dicer expression elicits DNA damage and up-regulation of MICA and MICB. J Cell Biol 182, 233-239.

Thomas, M., Wills, M., and Lehner, P.J. (2008). Natural killer cell evasion by an E3 ubiquitin ligase from Kaposi's sarcoma-associated herpesvirus. Biochem Soc Trans 36, 459-463.

Venkataraman, G.M., Suciu, D., Groh, V., Boss, J.M., and Spies, T. (2007). Promoter region architecture and transcriptional regulation of the genes for the MHC class I-related chain A and B ligands of NKG2D. J Immunol 178, 961-969.

Viny, A.D., Clemente, M.J., Jasek, M., Askar, M., Ishwaran, H., Nowacki, A., Zhang, A., and Maciejewski, J.P. MICA polymorphism identified by whole genome array associated with NKG2D-mediated cytotoxicity in T-cell large granular lymphocyte leukemia. Haematologica 95, 1713-1721.

Viny, A.D., Clemente, M.J., Jasek, M., Askar, M., Ishwaran, H., Nowacki, A., Zhang, A., and Maciejewski, J.P. (2010). MICA polymorphism identified by whole genome array associated with NKG2D-mediated cytotoxicity in T-cell large granular lymphocyte leukemia. Haematologica 95, 1713-1721.

Waldhauer, I., Goehlsdorf, D., Gieseke, F., Weinschenk, T., Wittenbrink, M., Ludwig, A., Stevanovic, S., Rammensee, H.G., and Steinle, A. (2008). Tumor-associated MICA is shed by ADAM proteases. Cancer Res 68, 6368-6376.

Wang, H., Yang, D., Xu, W., Wang, Y., Ruan, Z., Zhao, T., Han, J., and Wu, Y. (2008). Tumor-derived soluble MICs impair CD3(+)CD56(+) NKT-like cell cytotoxicity in cancer patients. Immunol Lett 120, 65-71.

Wang, X., Lundgren, A.D., Singh, P., Goodlett, D.R., Plymate, S.R., and Wu, J.D. (2009). An six-amino acid motif in the alpha3 domain of MICA is the cancer therapeutic target to inhibit shedding. Biochem Biophys Res Commun 387, 476-481.

Watzl, C. (2003). The NKG2D receptor and its ligands-recognition beyond the "missing self"? Microbes Infect 5, 31-37.

Whang, M.I., Guerra, N., and Raulet, D.H. (2009). Costimulation of dendritic epidermal gammadelta T cells by a new NKG2D ligand expressed specifically in the skin. J Immunol 182, 4557-4564.

Wiemann, K., Mittrucker, H.W., Feger, U., Welte, S.A., Yokoyama, W.M., Spies, T., Rammensee, H.G., and Steinle, A. (2005). Systemic NKG2D down-regulation impairs NK and CD8 T cell responses in vivo. J Immunol 175, 720-729.

Wu, J., Groh, V., and Spies, T. (2002). T cell antigen receptor engagement and specificity in the recognition of stress-inducible MHC class I-related chains by human epithelial gamma delta T cells. J Immunol 169, 1236-1240.

Wu, J.D., Atteridge, C.L., Wang, X., Seya, T., and Plymate, S.R. (2009). Obstructing shedding of the immunostimulatory MHC class I chain-related gene B prevents tumor formation. Clin Cancer Res 15, 632-640.

Wu, J.D., Higgins, L.M., Steinle, A., Cosman, D., Haugk, K., and Plymate, S.R. (2004). Prevalent expression of the immunostimulatory MHC class I chain-related molecule is counteracted by shedding in prostate cancer. J Clin Invest 114, 560-568.

Yadav, D., Ngolab, J., Lim, R.S., Krishnamurthy, S., and Bui, J.D. (2009). Cutting edge: down-regulation of MHC class I-related chain A on tumor cells by IFN-gamma-induced microRNA. J Immunol 182, 39-43.

Zhang, H., Hardamon, C., Sagoe, B., Ngolab, J., and Bui, J.D. Studies of the H60a locus in C57BL/6 and 129/Sv mouse strains identify the H60a 3'UTR as a regulator of H60a expression. Mol Immunol 48, 539-545.

Zhang, T., Barber, A., and Sentman, C.L. (2006). Generation of antitumor responses by genetic modification of primary human T cells with a chimeric NKG2D receptor. Cancer Res 66, 5927-5933.

Zhang, T., Barber, A., and Sentman, C.L. (2007). Chimeric NKG2D modified T cells inhibit systemic T-cell lymphoma growth in a manner involving multiple cytokines and cytotoxic pathways. Cancer Res 67, 11029-11036.

Zhang, T., Lemoi, B.A., and Sentman, C.L. (2005). Chimeric NK-receptor-bearing T cells mediate antitumor immunotherapy. Blood 106, 1544-1551.

4

Cancer Vaccine

Shinichiro Akiyama and Hiroyuki Abe
Kudan Clinic Immune Cell Therapy Center
Japan

1. Introduction

According to the GLOBOCAN 2008 estimates, about 12.7 million cancer cases and 7.6 million cancer deaths are estimated to have occurred in 2008; of these, 56% of the cases and 64% of the deaths occurred in the economically developing world (Jemal et al., 2011). It is now 51 years since Macfarlane Burnet and Peter Medawar won the Nobel Prize in Physiology or Medicine for the discovery of acquired immunological tolerance, and Burnet's 'hypothesis that called for experiment' has driven an enormous amount of progress. A recent advance in anti-cancer therapies has been the use of cancer antigen to develop vaccines. However, immunization with cancer cell-based vaccines has not resulted in significant long-term therapeutic benefits. The search for human tumor antigens as potential targets for cancer immunotherapy has led to the discovery of several molecules expressed mainly or selectively on cancer cells.

Vaccination is an effective medical procedure of clinical oncology setting based on the induction of a long-lasting immunologic memory characterized by mechanisms endowed with high destructive potential and specificity. In the last few decades, identification of tumor-associated antigens (TAA) has prompted the development of different strategies for antitumor vaccination, aimed at inducing specific recognition of TAA in order to elicit a persistent immune memory that may eliminate residual tumor cells and protect recipients from relapses. Current data from trials with cancer vaccine for patients with advanced cancer are however not uniform. Because enormous problems arise from the variability of protocols in the preparation of vaccine, such as dendritic cell-based or peptide vaccine, and the vaccination itself.

Widely occurring, over-expressed TAAs have been detected in different types of tumors as well as in many normal tissues, and their over-expression in tumor cells can reach the threshold for T cell recognition, breaking the immunological tolerance and triggering an anticancer response. Many antigens have been identified and studied as potential targets for vaccine therapy, and several vaccine methods have been investigated to target them. The most well-studied and promising vaccines for the treatment of cancer can be subdivided into three main groups: antigen-specific vaccines, tumor cell vaccines, and dendritic cell vaccines.

Active immunotherapy is aimed either at eliciting a specific host immune response against selected cancer antigens by employing cancer vaccines or at amplifying the existing antitumor immune response by administering nonspecific proinflammatory molecules or adjuvants. Dendritic cells (DCs) are the most potent antigen-presenting cells in vitro and in vivo. DCs have a central function in the activation of specific effector T cells. On this basis, vaccination strategies with DC were regarded as a promising therapeutic approach even in advanced tumor diseases. DC have always been described as having two distinct functional stages: 1) immature, with high antigen uptake and processing ability, and poor T-cell stimulatory function; 2) mature, with high stimulatory function and poor antigen uptake and processing ability. DC internalize cancer antigens and process their proteins then display them as short peptides on the extracellular surface, in conjunction with major histocompatibility complex (MHC) class I and II molecules. DC then migrates into the corresponding lymph nodes, where it matures and present antigen to naïve T lymphocytes. Helper T cells (CD4$^+$) recognize their cognate antigens (MHC class II molecules) located on DCs, whereas CD8$^+$ cytotoxic T lymphocytes (CTLs) recognize affected foreign or cancer cells which display the complementary peptide-MHC class I molecule on their cell surfaces. Targeted cell death occurs by perforin/granzyme-induced apoptosis or FAS-L/Fas interaction. Activation of CD4$^+$ T cells leads to the secretion of cytokines such as IFN-γ and IL-12, which in turn augment the stimulation of active CD8$^+$ T cells. Cancer vaccine aimed at inducing specific recognition of TAA as well as eliciting persistent immune memory T lymphocytes. Programmed death-1 (PD-1) and anti-cytotoxic T lymphocyte-associated protein 4 (CTLA-4) are induced on T cells after a TCR signal, and result in cell cycle arrest and termination of T-cell activation. Blocking by either CTLA-4 or PD-1 monoclonal antibodies can sustain the activation and proliferation of tumor-specific T cells (Hirano et al., 2005; Hodi et al., 2008). Although, to date, no autologous cellular immunotherapy has gained wide use in clinical practice, the first such therapy to show clinical efficacy in a phase 3 study recently gained U.S. Food and Drug Administration (FDA) approval for the treatment of prostate cancer. Sipuleucel-T consists of autologous PBMCs loaded with recombinant human prostatic acid phosphatase (PAP) linked to granulocyte-macrophage colony stimulating factor (PAP-GM-CSF), which has proven to be effective in phase III clinical trials. DC based Vaccine are typically prepared by harvesting large numbers of autologous peripheral blood mononuclear cells (PBMCs) by leukapheresis, then culturing these cells and loading them with antigens ex vivo and injecting them back into the patient. Three general methods have been described concerning DC based vaccine: (1)differentiating DCs from non-proliferating monocyte precursors (so-called "monocyte-derived DCs"; (2)differentiating DCs from proliferating CD34$^+$ hematopoietic progenitor cells; or (3)directly isolating DCs or mixed APCs from periphereal blood. Autologous DC can be loaded with a wide assortment of antigen types, including whole tumor cells or cell lysates, or TAA in the form of synthetic peptides, purified or recombinant proteins, RNA, plasmid DNA or non-replicating recombinant viral vectors (Mayordomo et al., 1995; Thurner et al., 1999). Immunogenicity may be enhanced by using antigens combined or fused with other more immunogenic molecules, including xenogeneic proteins such as Keyhole Limped Hemocyanin (KLH) or IL-2, TNF-α, IFN-γ or Toll-like receptor agonist. Adapting single peptide for vaccine is not preferable, because after complete objective response to NY-ESO-1 peptide vaccine, but later recurred with a NY-ESO-1–negative tumor, proving that single-target immunization can result in immune escape tumor variants after initial response (Odunsi et al., 2007). A desirable alternative to vaccines are multiepitope or whole tumor antigen vaccines created using autologous tumor lysate or tumor-derived RNA, which may have universal applicability (Chianese-Bullock et al., 2008; Tsuda et al., 2007).

However, the immune responses are often weak, and data on clinical efficacy are limited, as most of these have been small, single arm studies designed only to evaluate safety and immunogenicity. An enormous problem arises from the variability of protocols in the preparation of DC and in the vaccination itself. A meta-analysis of 56 published peer-reviewed immunotherapy trials of melanoma that used either molecular defined synthetic antigens or whole tumor antigen (4,375 patients) found that only 25.3% of patients vaccinated had objective clinical control (Chi & Dudek , 2011).

A number of studies have found that development of tumor and an unfavorable prognosis for cancer patients were accompanied by accumulation of natural $CD4^+CD25^+Foxp3^+$ T regulatory cells (Tregs) in peripheral blood, as well as of peripherally induced Tregs in the tumor itself (Wilczynski et al., 2008). Furthermore, depletion of Treg is a critical maneuver to enhance vaccine therapy. Different therapeutic immune strategies have been tested preclinically and are currently in evaluation in early phase I and II trials. DC based vaccine is usually given to peripheral site, whereas Natural Killer (NK)-T cell and LAK are either delivered systematically or into the tumor site. Results from these trials vary, but the overall increased survival and/or clinical efficient benefit obtained so far has been limited. In addition, MHC expression level vary cancer type and stage, it seems difficult to eradicate cancer just administrating vaccine. Because CTL induced by vaccine targets MHC expressed cancer cell, whereas NK cell attacks MHC non-expressed cancer cell.

Only three randomized phase 3 clinical trials of DC/APC vaccines for the treatment of cancer have been published. The first study compared subcutaneously administered cytokine-matured, Mo-DCs loaded with a mixture of MHC class II and II-restricted peptide antigens to conventional chemotherapy in patients with stage IV melanoma. Designed to compare clinical response rates as measured by tumor regression, the study showed no statistically significant difference in clinical outcomes between the two treatments. With the FDA-approval of sipuleucel-T, cancer vaccine has become an accepted approach for the treatment of cancer. However, it is not known if the use of dendritic cells or mixed APCs for the active immunotherapy of cancer has an advantage over more conventional vaccine approaches, which are simpler and much less expensive. We usually propose WT1, MUC1, CEA, CA125, HER-2/neu, and PSA as cancer antigens for DC based therapy according to the patient's primary lesion and elevated tumor marker (Sugiyama, 2005; Mukherjee et al., 2000; Nair et al., 1999; Larbcurrentet et al., 2007). It been reported that WT1 and MUC1 is antigens with high immunogenicity and their-targeted immunotherapy have confirmed its safety and clinical efficacy, although there is few description concerning cancer vaccine adapting WT1 and MUC1 simultaneously to cancer antigen (Ramanathan et al., 2005). Dr Okamoto and his colleagues have already reported that OK-432 generates mature DCs via Toll-like receptor 4 signaling and that OK-432-activated DCs stimulates $CD8^+$ T cells to induce antigen-specific CTLs (Ahmed et al., 2004, Itoh et al., 2003; Nakahara et al., 2003; Okamoto et al., 2003, 2004, 2006; Oshikawa et al., 2006). In this analysis efficacy of cancer vaccine, different potential means of DC based vaccination in experimental settings and preliminary data from clinical trial have been examined.

2. Material and method

2.1 Patients, treatment and sampling

This retrospective study was carried out in accordance with the standards of our Institutional Committee for the Protection of Human Subjects. Eligible patients must be those who have failed standard treatment. Informed written consent according to the Declaration of Helsinki was obtained from all patients before giving this therapy, and the collection of the samples was approved by the Institutional Review Board. From 2007 to 2010, 127 patients with advanced cancer refractory to standard treatment were treated with DC-based immunotherapy (DC vaccine alone or DC vaccine plus NK-T cell therapy) at Kudan Clinic Immune Cell Therapy Center.

Initial patient evaluations included a medical history and physical examination; measurement of performance status, hemoglobin, WBC count, platelet count, blood urea nitrogen, creatinine, alkaline phosphatase, lactate dehydrogenase, AST, ALT, bilirubin, and tumor marker levels; HbA1c; Computed Tomography (CT) scans or Magnetic Resonance Imaging (MRI) of whole body. Patients with evidence of operable tumor were ineligible. To be eligible, patients were required to have an ECOG performance status of less than 3.

Eligible Adequate hematologic, hepatic, and renal function, within the following parameters: WBC count of 2,500/µl or greater; platelet count of 100,000/µl or greater; hemoglobin value of 10 g/dl or greater; blood urea nitrogen value less than 50 mg/dl; serum bilirubin level less than 5.0 mg/dl; AST level lower than 500 IU.

Autologous DCs (1×10^7 cells) were administered intradermally at 14-day intervals. Tolerable 1 to 5 KE of OK-432 (Chugai Pharmaceutical Co., Ltd., Tokyo, Japan), a streptococcal immunological adjuvant, was administered together with DC vaccine. NK-T cells were simultaneously injected in as many patients at 14-day intervals.

The clinical response was evaluated on the basis of the Response Evaluation Criteria in Solid Tumors (RECIST) Ver1.0 as follows: complete remission (CR), partial remission (PR), stable disease (SD), and progressive disease (PD). Adverse events were evaluated by grading the toxicity according to the National Cancer Institute (NCI) Common Terminology Criteria for Adverse Events (CTCAE) Version 4.0.

2.2 Preparation of DCs and NK-T cells

PBMCs-rich fraction was obtained from leukapheresis (400 ml x 13 cycles) using COM.TEC (Fresenius Kabi, Homburg, Germany). The PBMCs were isolated from the heparinized leukapheresis products by Ficoll-Hypaque gradient density centrifugation (Böyum, 1967). These PBMCs were placed into 100 mm plastic tissue-culture plates (Becton Dickinson Labware, Franklin Lakes, NJ) in AIM-V medium (Gibco, Gaithersburg, Md). After 30 min of incubation at 37°C, nonadherent cells were removed, and the adherent cells were cultured in AIM-V containing granulocyte-macrophage colony stimulating factor (GM-CSF, 500 ng/ml; Primmune Inc., Kobe, Japan), and IL-4 (250 ng/ml; R&D Systems Inc., Minneapolis, MN) to generate immature DCs (Okamoto et al., 2004). The population of the adherent cells remaining in the wells was composed of 95.6 ± 3.3% CD14+. After 5 days of the cultivation, the immature DCs were stimulated to be matured with OK-432 (10 µg/ml) and Prostaglandin E2 (50 ng/ml; Daiichi Fine Chemical Co. LTD., Toyama, Japan) for 24 hrs. It has been reported that Prostaglandin E2 acquires the ability to migrate to the lymph node to DCs (Sato et al., 2003). Peptides (20 µg/ml) for WT1, Her2 and CEA were pulsed into the DCs at 24 hrs after the treatment with OK-432 and with Prostaglandin E2, while MUC1 long peptide (30 mer) (20 µg /ml), CA125 protein (500 U/ml) and autologous tumor lysates (50 µg/ml) were added into the DC culture media at the same time as adding OK-432 and Prostaglandin E2, then incubated for 24 hrs (Kontani et al., 2002; Cannon et al., 2004). To prepare the autologous tumor lysates, tumor masses were obtained by surgical resection exclusion, and were then homogenized. Aliquots of the isolated tumor cells were then lysed by putting them through 10 freeze (in liquid nitrogen) and thaw (in a 37 °C water bath) cycles. The lysed cells were centrifuged at 14000 g for 5 min, and the supernatants were passed through a 0.22 µm filter (Millipore Corporation, Bedford, MA). The protein contents of the resultant cell-free lysates were determined using DC protein assay kits (Bio-Rad Laboratories, Hercules Aliquots (500 µg/tube) were then cryopreserved at -135 °C until use (Nagayama et al., 2003). Surface molecules expressed in the DCs were determined using flow cytometry. The cells defined as the mature DCs were CD14-, HLA-DR+, HLA-ABC+, CD80+, CD83+, CD86+, CD40+, and CCR7+.

For preparation of NK-T cells, PBMCs were cultured with an immobilized monoclonal anti-CD3 antibody (5 µg/mL OKT3; Jansen Pharmaceutical K.K., Tokyo, Japan) in the presence of recombinant human IL-2 (175 U/mL; CHIRON, Benelux B.V., Amsterdam, Netherlands) and autologous plasma for 14 days. Fresh NK-T cells were prepared every injection as described above; it was composed of more than 85% of αβ-T cells and about 10% of NK/NKT cells.

2.3 Vaccine quality control

All vaccines were subjected to a quality-control evaluation, which were assessed the total number of live dendritic cell, monocyte-derived dendritic cell characteristics, and percentage of viable cells. For a vaccine to be deemed "adequate," there must have been 4 x 10^7 viable dendritic cells.

2.4 FACS analysis

The frozen cells were allowed to thaw in a 37 °C water bath quickly and retrieved from the cryopreservation tubes by rinsing with 0.02% albumin containing Cell Wash™ (eBioscience, San Jose, CA) (FACS buffer). The FACS analysis was performed for cell surface antigen staining. FITC-labeled anti-human CD14, CD40, CD80, HLA-A, B, C, PE-labeled anti-human CD11c, CD83, CD197 (CCR7+), HLA-DR and FACS Calibur Flowcytometer were purchased from BD Bioscience, and used for the FACS analysis.

3. Results

3.1 Clinical outcome of patients with DC-based vaccine

Computed tomography scans or MRI was done before and at the end of dendritic cell therapy. Of 127 patients who received DC vaccine, complete responses (n = 4; 3.1%), partial responses (n = 26; 20.5%), or stable disease were observed in 34 (26.8%) (Table 1.).

Although the study was not designed or powered to detect differences between other vaccine treatment groups, it was of interest to compare the response and survival of patients treated with other vaccines.

Most patients received NK-T therapy in combination with the DC vaccination as to induce Th (helper T cell) 1-dominant state for improved CTL response and to attack non-MHC expressed carcinoma cells. The NK-T cells generated according to the methods described in the "Materials and Methods" section secrete IFN-γ and IL-2, and induce helper T cell (Th) 1-dominant state in the cytokine balance of the patients (Chong et al., 1994).

3.2 Adverse events

Therapy was well-tolerated during the treatment and 3 months after last administration. None of the patients experienced adverse events of grade 3 or higher during the treatment period, grade 1 to 2 fevers, grade 1 injected-site reaction consisting of erythema, induration

Cancer type	patient No.	CR (%)	PR (%)	SD (%)	PD (%)	total (%)
esophagus	10	0	20.0	10.0	70.0	100
gastric	24	0	16.7	20.8	62.5	100
colorectal	9	0	22.2	44.4	33.3	100
hapetocellular	8	12.5	25.0	12.5	50.0	100
pancreas	18	5.6	27.8	38.9	27.8	100
lung	14	7.1	21.4	42.9	28.6	100
breast	21	0	9.6	33.3	57.1	100
gynecological	3	0	0	33.3	66.6	100
malignant lymphoma	3	33.3	0	0	66.6	100
prostate	10	0	60.0	20.0	20.0	100
thyroid	3	0	0	0	100	100
malignant melanoma	4	0	0	0	100	100
total (No.)	127	4	26	34	63	100
total (%)		3.1	20.5	26.8	49.6	100

Table 1. Clinical Outcome of Patients treated with DC based vaccine

and tenderness, lasting 24 to 48 hours after injection in 8 patients and resulted in no dose modifications or delays. No signs or symptoms of auto-immune phenomena (eg, arthritis, colitis, inflammation of skin) were observed either during or after therapy.

4. Discussion

Interest in antitumor vaccination arose around 1900 when a series of microbial vaccines by Dr William B. Coley proved to be effective. Boon T and others provided an unambiguous definition of TAA, an important finding the genetic and molecular identification of a large series of TAA (Coulie, 1997; Robbins & Kawakami, 1996).

In many cases, TAA are peptides presented by class I and class II glycoproteins of the MHC. A similar picture is emerging from phase I studies on vaccination of cancer patients. However, clinical responses to the immunotherapy with DC vaccination have only been observed in a minority of patients with solid cancer. Initiation of immune responses requires that professional APC deliver a first signal to T-lymphocytes through the binding of the T-cell receptor by the peptide enclosed in the HLA molecule, that is responsible for the specificity of the immune response, and a second or co-stimulatory signal that is not antigen-specific but it is required for T-cell activation mainly through CD80 (B7-1) and CD86 (B7-2) binding to CD28 receptor, or the CD40:CD40L pathway (Janeway & Bottomly, 1994). Moreover, the capacity of DC to activate NK cells by ligation of the CD40 molecule with its counter-receptor has recently been demonstrated (Cayeux et al., 1999; Kitamura et al., 1999).

Therefore, given the complex network of regulatory signals by professional APC and naïve and memory T lymphocytes occurring in antigen-specific immune responses, it is not surprising that tumor cells may fail to induce efficient immune reactions even when a well known TAA is present. From among the professional APC, DC are the most potent stimulators of T cell responses and play a crucial role in the initiation of primary immune responses (Banchereau & Steinman, 1998). DC have always been described as having two distinct functional stages: 1) immature, with high antigen uptake and processing ability, and poor T-cell stimulatory function; 2) mature, with high stimulatory function and poor antigen uptake and processing ability. Despite several immunotherapeutic approaches having been tested for colon cancer patients, only one study has reported clinical results in a prospective randomized study (Vermorken et al., 1999). Experimental data and clinical evidence suggest that antitumor vaccines will be a new form of tumor treatment that will be able to be adopted for the management of defined stages of carcinoma, in sequential association with conventional treatments (Sadanaga et al., 2001). Prediction of when the efficacy of antitumor vaccination will be assessed and will become a routine procedure is beyond a simple scientific evaluation. While pre-clinical research has identified several possible targets and strategies for tumor vaccination, the clinical scenario is far more complex. The main cell populations taking part in immunoregulation of tumor growth are presented in Fig. 1.

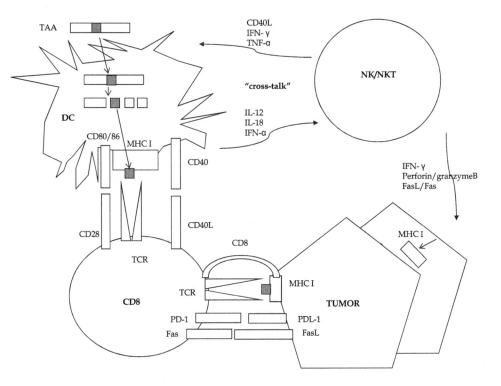

Fig. 1. The main anti-tumor immune cell responses by DC and NK/NKT cell

Most peptide-based vaccines have considered HLA class I restricted peptides only, whereas there is increasing evidence that tumor-specific CD4+ T-cells may be important in inducing an effective antitumor immunity. The addition of peptides that bind class II HLA glycoproteins to peptide vaccines could lead to an amplification of the immune response as well as to better clinical effect. The possibility of effectively monitoring the immune response induced acquires critical importance since it may provide a much earlier surrogate end-point, predictive of the clinical outcome. An ideal TAA is a protein that is essential for sustaining the malignant phenotype, and that is not stripped or down modulated by the immune reaction. TAAs were sorted by their anti-tumor potential such as therapeutic function, immunogenicity, oncogenicity, specificity, expression level and % positive cells, and cancer stem cell expression. Among the 75 peptides evaluated by Dr Martin A. Cheever, WT1 was the 1st and MUC1 was the 2nd anti-tumor effect (Cheever et al., 2009). WT1 was originally identified as tumor suppressor gene for Wilm's tumor. WT1 over-expression has been detected in different malignant cell types including gastroenterological carcinoma, gynecological carcinoma, lung carcinoma, prostate, breast carcinoma and hematological malignancy. MUC1 is expressed at high levels over the entire surface of diverse types of carcinoma cells such as gastroenterological carcinoma, gynecological carcinoma, NSCLC, prostate and breast carcinoma. MUC1 transmembrane receptor has revealed a function for this subunit as an oncoprotein that is targeted to the nucleus and regulates gene expression. MUC1-C accelerates the malignant potential by regulating gene transcription, blocking stress-induced apoptosis and necrosis, and attenuating activation of death receptor pathways.

When compared with conventional cancer management, vaccination is a *soft*, non-invasive treatment free from particular distress and iatrogenic side effects. Antitumor vaccines can be expected to have a considerable social impact, but a few large clinical trials enrolling the appropriate patients are now necessary to assess their efficacy. In conclusion, even if cancer vaccines are an old dream, only recently has their design become a rational enterprise (Ehrlich, 1909). There are now many ways of constructing vaccines able to elicit a strong protective immunity. This progress is offering ground for optimism.

Here, we demonstrate that WT1 and/or MUC1 pulsed DC vaccination is feasible, safe, and sufficiently powerful to induce objective clinical and immune responses even in patients with significant tumor burden. Several studies of ex vivo, custom-manufactured cancer vaccines using patient-specific idiotype, idiotype-pulsed dendritic cells, and tumor lysate–pulsed dendritic cells have also demonstrated objective clinical responses and these prior results prompted our pursuit of the practicable in situ approach.

This approach-by its nature-must be studied in patients with clinically evident disease, in contrast to the described randomized studies (Flowers, 2007; Freedman et al., 2009). As compared with other comparably practical vaccines current vaccination has the potential advantage of using more potential TAA encompassing each individuals' relevant tumor antigens. In addition, several recent immune-response studies showing that vaccine-induced T cells peak at day 14 and decline sharply thereafter, have prompted earlier immune-response measurements in an ongoing follow-up study (Deng et al., 2004; Kim et al., 2007; Treanor et al., 2006). There is little or no controversy that patients with Treg-inducing tumors had poorer clinical outcomes after vaccination. This biomarker could be either a specific predictor of response to in situ vaccination or a general prognosticator of poor outcomes regardless of therapy. Interestingly, patients with highly Treg-infiltrated tumors have shown favorable clinical outcomes after standard therapy (Carreras et al., 2006; Tzankov et al., 2008). If Treg induction predicts good response to standard therapy, but a poor response to the in situ vaccine, then it would be a powerful clinical tool for selecting appropriate patients for vaccination. This interesting finding is still preliminary and is being evaluated prospectively in an ongoing follow study (ClinicalTrials.gov-ID: NCT00880581). That the vaccine preparation in current study was optimal was evident from quality-control assessments, because in the study presented here, all vaccines didn't fail to meet quality-control specifications. As prognosis of most advanced carcinoma who failed standard therapy is poor, establishment of effective therapeutic modality for advanced carcinoma is an urgent issue.

Immunotherapy would be implied as one of the important therapeutic modalities against advanced carcinoma and even adjuvant settings because WT1 and MUC1, highly immunogenic target molecules for adaptive anti-tumor immune response, were frequently expressed in most carcinoma tissue (Cheever et al., 2009; Oka et al., 2006). DC-based vaccination has several advantageous aspects for induction and activation of tumor antigen-specific CTLs compared with CTL-epitope peptide-based vaccination (Melief & van der Burg, 2008). Patients with advanced carcinoma who failed standard therapy and met eligible criteria enrolled in current study. Response rate was 23.6%, whereas control ratio was 50.4%. It is a significant tumor control ratio compared with other historical modalities much less no severe adverse event. Is the strongest result from this trial the apparent increase in control ratio? It would be important to understand the mechanisms of immune system underlying the significant increase in cancer control ratio. These results indicate that WT1 and/or MUC1 pulsed DC-based vaccination can elicit significant clinical benefit even for the advanced cancer patients refractory to the standard therapies. Although there was a trend toward treatment being superior to standard treatment only, there was no statistical consideration. However, the study demonstrated that successful active specific immunotherapy with WT1 and/or MUC1 pulsed DC-based vaccine may be dependent on the quality of the vaccine as well as TAAs. These encouraging preliminary results suggest that WT1 and/or MUC1 pulsed DC-based vaccination warrants further study as a novel therapy for patients with advanced carcinoma. The combination of cytotoxic therapy and intratumoral immune stimulation has been studied preclinically for a variety of common tumor types and might also be directly translated to the clinic (Meng et al., 2005; Najar et al., 2008; VanOosten & Griffith, 2007). This trial clearly supports the idea that to be immunologically effective, control of the vaccine preparation and the quality assurance that the vaccine meets specifications are of the highest priority and must be considerations in any future tumor cell vaccine study. A key element in these novel strategies is the identification of suitable patients, the selection being based on detailed immunological and molecular characterization. The most promising finding that emerges from this study is that WT1 and/or MUC1 pulsed DC-based vaccine together with NK-T cell therapy elicit strong anti-tumor response. Progress in the formulation of cancer vaccines will be brought by a more precise knowledge of the requirements for the potent generation of efficient CTL induction and NK cell expansion as well as discovering potent TAA, together with the current ability to closely monitor molecular immune response prediction markers in, will likely provide powerful, individualized vaccines in the near future.

5. Acknowledgements

The authors express their appreciation to tella, Inc. for technical assistance.

6. References

Ahmed, S.U., Okamoto, M., Oshikawa, T., Tano, T., Sasai, A., Kan, S., Hiroshima, T., Ohue, H., Moriya, Y., Ryoma, Y., Saito, M., Sato, M. (2004). Anti-tumor effect of an intratumoral administration of dendritic cells in combination with TS-1, an oral fluoropyrimidine anti-cancer drug, and OK-432, a streptococcal immunopotentiator: Involvement of Toll-like receptor 4. *Journal of immunotherapy*, Vol.27, No.6, pp. 432-41, ISSN 1524-9557

Banchereau, J., Steinman, R.M. (1998). Dendritic cells and the control of immunity. *Nature*, Vol.392, No.2, pp. 245-52, ISSN 0028-0836

Böyum, A. (1967). Isolation of mononuclear cells and granulocytes from human blood. *Scandinavian journal of clinical and laboratory investigation*, Vol.21, pp. 77-89, ISSN 0085-591X

Cannon, M.J., Santin, A.D., O'Brien, T.J. (2004). Immunological treatment of ovarian cancer. *Current opinion in obstetrics & gynecology*, Vol.16, No.1, pp. 87-92, ISSN 1040-872X

Carreras, J., Lopez-Guillermo, A., Fox, B.C., Colomo, L., Martinez, A., Roncador, G., Montserrat, E., Campo, E., Banham, A.H. (2006). High numbers of tumor-infiltrating FOXP3-positive regulatory T cells are associated with improved overall survival in follicular lymphoma. *Blood*, Vol.1, No.108, pp. 2957-64, ISSN 0006-4971

Cayeux, S., Richter, G., Becker, C., Pezzutto, A., Dörken, B., Blankenstein, T. (1999). Direct and indirect T cell priming by dendritic cell vaccines. *European journal of immunology*, Vol.29, No.1, pp. 225-34, ISSN 0014-2980

Cheever, M.A., Allison, J.P., Ferris, A.S., Finn, O.J., Hastings, B.M., Hecht, T.T., Mellman, I., Prindiville, S.A., Viner, J.L., Weiner, L.M., Matrisian, L.M. (2009). The prioritization of cancer antigens: a national cancer institute pilot project for the acceleration of translational research. *Clinical cancer research*, Vol.1, No.15, pp. 5323-37, ISSN 1078-0432

Chianese-Bullock, K.A., Irvin, W.P. Jr., Petroni, G.R., Murphy, C., Smolkin, M., Olson, W.C., Coleman, E., Boerner, S.A., Nail, C.J., Neese, P.Y., Yuan, A., Hogan, K.T., Slingluff, C.L. Jr. (2008). A multipeptide vaccine is safe and elicits T-cell responses in participants with advanced stage ovarian cancer. *Journal of immunotherapy*, Vol.31, no.4, pp. 420-430, ISSN 1524-9557

Chi, M., Dudek, A.Z. (2011). Vaccine therapy for metastatic melanoma: systematic review and meta-analysis of clinical trials. *Melanoma research*, Vol.21. No.3, pp.165-74, ISSN 0960-8931

Chong, A.S., Jiang, X.L., Scuderi, P., Lamas, M., Graf, L.H. Jr. (1994). ICAM-1 and LFA-3 enhance the ability of anti-CD3 mAb to stimulate interferon gamma production in interleukin-2-activated T cells. *Cancer immunology, immunotherapy*, Vol.39, No.2, pp. 127-34, ISSN 0340-7004

Coulie, P.G. (1997). Human tumour antigens recognized by T cells: new perspectives for anti-cancer vaccines? *Molecular medicine today*, Vol.3, No.6, pp. 261-8, ISSN 1357-4310

Deng, Y., Jing, Y., Campbell, A.E., Gravenstein, S. (2004). Age-related impaired type 1 T cell responses to influenza: reduced activation ex vivo, decreased expansion in CTL culture in vitro, and blunted response to influenza vaccination in vivo in the elderly. *Journal of immunology*, Vol.15, No.172, pp. 3437-46, ISSN 0022-1767

Ehrlich, P. (1909). Ueber den jetzigen Stand der Karzinomforschung. *Ned Tijdschr Geneeskd*, Vol.i, pp. 273-90, ID 30308001160

Flowers, C.R. (2007). BiovaxID idiotype vaccination: active immunotherapy for follicular lymphoma. *Expert review of vaccines*, Vol. 6, No.3, pp. 307-17, ISSN 1476-0584

Freedman, A., Neelapu, S.S., Nichols, C., Robertson, M.J., Djulbegovic, B., Winter, J.N., Bender, J.F., Gold, D.P., Ghalie, R.G., Stewart, M.E., Esquibel, V., Hamlin, P. (2009). Placebo-controlled phase III trial of patient-specific immunotherapy with mitumprotimut-T and granulocytemacrophage colony-stimulating factor after rituximab in patients with follicular lymphoma. *Journal of clinical oncology*, Vol.20, No.27, pp. 3036-3043, ISSN 0277-3732

Hirano, F., Kaneko, K., Tamura, H., Dong, H., Wang, S., Ichikawa, M., Rietz, C., Flies, D.B., Lau, J.S., Zhu, G., Tamada, K., Chen, L. (2005). Blockade of B7-H1 and PD-1 by monoclonal antibodies potentiates cancer therapeutic immunity. *Cancer research*, Vol.1, No.65, pp. 1089-96, ISSN 0008-5472

Hodi, F.S., Butler, M., Oble, D.A., Seiden, M.V., Haluska, F.G., Kruse, A., Macrae, S., Nelson, M., Canning, C., Lowy, I., Korman, A., Lautz, D., Russell, S., Jaklitsch, M.T., Ramaiya, N., Chen, T.C., Neuberg, D., Allison, J.P., Mihm, M.C., Dranoff, G. Immunologic and clinical effects of antibody blockade of cytotoxic T lymphocyte-associated antigen 4 in previously vaccinated cancer patients. (2008). *Proceedings of the National Academy of Sciences of the United States of America*, Vol. 26, No. 105, pp. 3005-10. ISSN 0027-8424

Itoh, T., Ueda, Y., Okugawa, K., Fujiwara, H., Fuji, N., Yamashita, T., Fujiki, H., Yamagishi, H. (2003). Streptococcal preparation OK432 promotes functional maturation of human monocyte-derived dendritic cells. *Cancer immunology, immunotherapy*, Vol.52, No.4, pp. 207-214, ISSN 0340-7004

Janeway, C.A. Jr., Bottomly, K. (1994). Signals and signs for lymphocyte responses. *Cell*, Vol.28, No.76, pp. 275-85, ISSN 0092-8674

Jemal, A., Bray, F., Center, M.M., Ferlay, J., Ward, E., Forman, D. (2011). Global cancer statistics. *CA: a cancer journal for clinicians*, Vol.61, No.2, pp. 69-90, ISSN 0007-9235

Kim, S.H., Choi, S.J., Park, W.B., Kim, H.B., Kim, N.J., Oh, M.D., Choe, K.W. (2007). Detailed kinetics of immune responses to a new cell culture-derived smallpox vaccine in vaccinia-naïve adults. *Vaccine*, Vol. 14, No. 25, pp. 6287-91, ISSN 0264-410X

Kitamura, H., Iwakabe, K., Yahata, T., Nishimura, S., Ohta, A., Ohmi, Y., Sato, M., Takeda, K., Okumura, K., Van Kaer, L., Kawano, T., Taniguchi, M., Nishimura, T. (1999). The natural killer T (NKT) cell ligand alpha-galactosylceramide demonstrates its immunopotentiating effect by inducing interleukin (IL)-12 production by dendritic cells and IL-12 receptor expression on NKT cells. *The Journal of experimental medicine*, Vol.5, No. 189, pp. 1121-8, ISSN 0022-1007

Kontani, K., Taguchi, O., Ozaki, Y., Hanaoka, J., Tezuka, N., Sawai, S., Inoue, S., Fujino, S., Maeda, T., Itoh, Y., Ogasawara, K., Sato, H., Ohkubo, I., Kudo, T. (2002). Novel vaccination protocol consisting of injecting MUC1 DNA and nonprimed dendritic cells at the same region greatly enhancedMUC1-specific antitumor immunity in a murine model. *Cancer gene therapy*, Vol. 9, No.4, pp. 330-7, ISSN 0929-1903

Larbcurrentet, C., Robert, B., Navarro-Teulon, I., Thèzenas, S., Ladjemi, M.Z., Morisseau, S., Campigna, E., Bibeau, F., Mach, J.P., Pèlegrin, A., Azria, D. (2007). In vivo therapeutic synergism of anti-epidermal growth factor receptor and anti-HER2 monoclonal antibodies against pancreatic carcinomas. *Clinical cancer research*, Vol.1, No. 13, pp. 3356-62, ISSN 1078-0432

Mayordomo, J.I, Zorina, T., Storkus, W.J., Zitvogel, L., Celluzzi, C., Falo, L.D., Melief, C.J., Ildstad, S.T., Kast, W.M., Deleo, A.B. (1995). Bone marrow-derived dendritic cells pulsed with synthetic tumour peptides elicit protective and therapeutic antitumour immunity. *Nature medicine*, Vol.1, No. 12, pp. 1297-302, ISSN 1078-8956

Melief, C.J., van der Burg, S.H. (2008). Immunotherapy of established (pre)malignant disease by synthetic long peptide vaccines. *Nature reviews. Cancer*, Vol.8, No.5, pp. 351-360, ISSN 1474-175X

Meng, Y., Carpentier, A.F., Chen, L., Boisserie, G., Simon, J.M., Mazeron, J.J., Delattre, J.Y. (2005). Successful combination of local CpG-ODN and radiotherapy in malignant glioma. *International journal of cancer*, Vol.10, No.116, pp. 992-997, ISSN 0020-7136

Mukherjee, P., Ginardi, A.R., Madsen, C.S., Sterner, C.J., Adriance, M.C., Tevethia, M.J., Gendler, S.J. (2000). Mice with spontaneous pancreatic cancer naturally develop MUC1-specific CTLs that erradicate tumors when adoptively transferred. *Journal of immunology*, Vol.15, No.165, pp. 3451-60, ISSN 0022-1767

Nagayama, H., Sato, K., Morishita, M., Uchimaru, K., Oyaizu, N., Inazawa, T., Yamasaki, T., Enomoto, M., Nakaoka, T., Nakamura, T., Maekawa, T., Yamamoto, A., Shimada, S., Saida, T., Kawakami, Y., Asano, S., Tani, K., Takahashi, T.A., Yamashita, N. (2003). Results of a phase I clinical study using autologous tumour lysate-pulsed monocyte-derived mature dendritic cell vaccinations for stage IV malignant melanoma patients combined with low dose interleukin-2. *Melanoma research*, Vol.13, No.5, pp. 521-30, ISSN 0960-8931

Nair, S.K., Hull, S., Coleman, D., Gilboa, E., Lyerly, H.K., Morse, M.A. (1999). Induction of carcinoembryonic antigen (CEA)-specific cytotoxic T-lymphocyte responses in vitro using autologous dendritic cells loaded with CEA peptide or CEA RNA in patients with metastatic malignancies expressing CEA. *International journal of cancer*, Vol.2, No.82, pp. 121-4, ISSN 0020-7136

Najar, H.M., Dutz, J.P. (2008). Topical CpG enhances the response of murine malignant melanoma to dacarbazine. *The Journal of investigative dermatology*, Vol.128, No.9, pp. 2204-2210, ISSN 0022-202X

Nakahara, S., Tsunoda, T., Baba, T., Asabe, S., Tahara, H. (2003). Dendritic cells stimulated with a bacterial product, OK-432, efficiently induce cytotoxic T lymphocytes specific to tumor rejection peptide. *Cancer research*, Vol.15, No.63, pp. 4112-4118, ISSN 0008-5472

Odunsi, K., Qian, F., Matsuzaki, J., Mhawech-Fauceglia, P., Andrews, C., Hoffman, E.W., Pan, L., Ritter, G., Villella, J., Thomas, B., Rodabaugh, K., Lele, S., Shrikant, P., Old, L.J., Gnjatic, S. (2007). Vaccination with an NY-ESO-1 peptide of HLA class I/II specificities induces integrated humoral and T cell responses in ovarian cancer. *Proceedings of the National Academy of Sciences of the United States of America*, Vol.31, No.104, pp. 12837-12842, ISSN 0027-8424

Oka, Y., Tsuboi, A., Kawakami, M., Elisseeva, O.A., Nakajima, H., Udaka, K., Kawase, I., Oji, Y., Sugiyama, H. (2006). Development of WT1 peptide cancer vaccine against hematopoietic malignancies and solid cancers. *Current medicinal chemistry*, Vol.13, No.20, pp. 2345-52, ISSN 0929-8673

Okamoto, M., Oshikawa, T., Tano, T., Ohe, G., Furuichi, S., Nishikawa, H., Ahmed, S.U., Akashi, S., Miyake, K., Takeuchi, O., Akira, S., Moriya, Y., Matsubara, S., Ryoma, Y., Saito, M., Sato, M. (2003). Involvement of Toll-like receptor 4 signaling in interferon-γ production and anti-tumor effect by a streptococcal agent OK-432. *Journal of the National Cancer Institute*, Vol.19, No. 95, pp. 316-26, ISSN 0027-8874

Okamoto, M., Furuichi, S., Nishioka, Y., Oshikawa, T., Tano, T., Ahmed, S.U., Takeda, K., Akira, S., Ryoma, Y., Moriya, Y., Saito, M., Sone, S., Sato, M. (2004). Expression of toll-like receptor 4 on dendritic cells is significant for anticancer effect of dendritic cell-based immunotherapy in combination with an active component of OK-432, a streptococcal preparation. *Cancer research*, Vol. 1, No.64, pp. 5461-70, ISSN 0008-5472

Okamoto, M., Oshikawa, T., Tano, T., Ahmed, S.U., Kan, S., Sasai, A., Akashi, S., Miyake, K., Moriya, Y., Ryoma, Y., Saito, M., Sato, M. (2006). Mechanism of anti-cancer host response induced by OK-432, a streptococcal preparation, mediated by phagocytosis and Toll-like receptor 4 signaling. *Journal of immunotherapy*, Vol.29, No.1, pp. 78-86, ISSN 1524-9557

Oshikawa, T., Okamoto, M., Tano, T., Sasai, A., Kan, S., Moriya, Y., Ryoma, Y., Saito, M., Akira, S., Sato, M. (2006). Anti-tumor effect of OK-432-derived DNA: One of the active constituents of OK-432, a streptococcal immunotherapeutic agent. *Journal of immunotherapy*, Vol.29, No.2, pp. 143-150, ISSN 1524-9557

Ramanathan, R.K., Lee, K.M., McKolanis, J., et al. Ramanathan RK, Lee KM, McKolanis J, Hitbold E, Schraut W, Moser AJ, Warnick E, Whiteside T, Osborne J, Kim H, Day R, Troetschel M, Finn OJ. (2005). Phase I study of a MUC1 vaccine composed of different doses of MUC1 peptide with SB-AS2 adjuvant in resected and locally advanced pancreatic cancer. *Cancer immunology, immunotherapy*, Vol.54, No.3, pp. 254-64, ISSN 0340-7004

Robbins, P.F., Kawakami, Y. (1996). Human tumor antigens recognized by T cells. *Current opinion in immunology*, Vol.8, No.5, pp. 628-36, ISSN 0952-7915

Sadanaga, N., Nagashima, H., Mashino, K., Tahara, K., Yamaguchi, H., Ohta, M., Fujie, T., Tanaka, F., Inoue, H., Takesako, K., Akiyoshi, T., Mori, M. (2001). Dendritic cell vaccination with MAGE peptide is a novel therapeutic approach for gastrointestinal carcinomas. *Clinical cancer research*, Vol. 7, No.8, pp. 2277-84, ISSN 1078-0432

Sato, M., Takayama, T., Tanaka, H., Konishi, J., Suzuki, T., Kaiga, T., Tahara, H. (2003). Generation of mature dendritic cells fully capable of T helper type 1 polarization using OK-432 combined with prostaglandin E (2). *Cancer science*, Vol.94, No.12, pp.1091-8, ISSN 1347-9032

Sugiyama, H. (2005). Cancer immunotherapy targeting Wilms' tumor gene WT1 product. *Expert review of vaccines*, Vol. 4, No.4, pp. 503-512, ISSN1476-0584

Thurner, B., Haendle, I., Röder, C., Dieckmann, D., Keikavoussi, P., Jonuleit, H., Bender, A., Maczek, C., Schreiner, D., von den Driesch, P., Bröcker, E.B., Steinman, R.M., Enk, A., Kämpgen, E., Schuler, G. (1999). Vaccination with mage-3A1 peptide-pulsed mature, monocyte-derived dendritic cells expands specific cytotoxic T cells and induces regression of some metastases in advanced stage IV melanoma. *The Journal of experimental medicine*, Vol.6, No. 190, pp. 1669-78, ISSN 0022-1007

Treanor, J., Wu, H., Liang, H., Topham, D.J. (2006). Immune responses to vaccinia and influenza elicited during primary versus recent or distant secondary smallpox vaccination of adults. *Vaccine*, Vol.17, No.24, pp. 6913-23, ISSN 0264-410X

Tsuda N, Mochizuki K, Harada M, Sukehiro, A., Kawano, K., Yamada, A., Ushijima, K., Sugiyama, T., Nishida, T., Yamana, H., Itoh, K., Kamura, T. Vaccination with predesignated or evidence-based peptides for patients with recurrent gynecologic cancers. *Journal of immunotherapy*, (2004). Vol.27, No.1, pp. 60-72, ISSN 1524-9557

Tzankov, A., Meier, C., Hirschmann, P., Went, P., Pileri, S.A., Dirnhofer, S. (2008). Correlation of high numbers of intratumoral FOXP3+ regulatory T cells with improved survival in germinal center-like diffuse large B-cell lymphoma, follicular lymphoma and classical Hodgkin's lymphoma. *Haematologica*, Vol.93, No.2, pp. 193-200. ISSN 0390-6078

VanOosten, R.L., Griffith, T.S. (2007). Activation of tumor-specific CD8+ T cells after intratumoral Ad5-TRAIL/CpG oligodeoxynucleotide combination therapy. *Cancer research*, Vol.15, No.67, pp. 11980-11990, ISSN 0008-5472

Vermorken, J.B., Claessen, A.M., van Tinteren, H., Gall, H.E., Ezinga, R., Meijer, S., Scheper, R.J., Meijer, C.J., Bloemena, E., Ransom, J.H., Hanna, M.G. Jr., Pinedo, H.M. (1999). Active specific immunotherapy for stage II and stage III human colon cancer: a randomised trial. *Lancet*, Vol.30, No. 353, pp. 345-50, ISSN 0140-6736

Wilczynski, J.R., Kalinka, J., Radwan, M. (2008). The role of T-regulatorycells in pregnancy and cancer. *Frontiers in bioscience*, Vol.1, No.13, pp. 2275–2289, ISSN 1945-0494

5

Antiangiogenic Treatment Concepts in Gynecologic Oncology

M. Eichbaum, C. Mayer, E. Bischofs, J. Reinhardt, J. Thum and C. Sohn
Departments of Obstetrics and Gynecology, University of Heidelberg, Heidelberg, Germany

1. Introduction

Gynecologic malignancies count for about 80,000 of all new cancer diagnoses in women in the United States (Jemal et al., 2010). In the US almost 20,000 patients a year are diagnosed with epithelial ovarian cancer, 11,000 with cervical cancer and 42,000 with endometrial cancer (Jemal et al., 2010). A relevant part of these tumor situations are found in an early-stage disease setting, for instance most of all newly diagnosed endometrial cancers. But frequently there is no possibility for an early-stage diagnosis and the tumor is already advanced when primarily detected, like in the majority of all cases with epithelial ovarian cancer (EOC).

Though tumor biology and standard treatment concepts are different for all three entities, there is a common need for new therapeutic approaches to improve the patients' outcome. Many preclinical studies have suggested that antiangiogenic strategies are beneficial against these cancers (Delli Carpini, 2010). One reason may be the fact that these tumors are able to form large single tumor nodulations during intraabdominal spread or local progression with hypoxic cores triggering tumor-associated neo-angiogenesis (Bryant et al., 2010). Furthermore, the frequently seen phenomenon of peritoneal carcinosis, closely related to gynecologic malignancies, induces angiogenesis to preserve nutritive supply to all metastatic tumor nodes (Fagotti et al., 2010, Figure 1).

Since Folkman first proposed the strategy of targeting the tumor vasculature as a novel therapeutic strategy, considerable progress has been made to understand the underlying mechanisms of angiogenesis (Folkman, 1971). The control of angiogenesis is under the influence of both pro- and anti-angiogenesis factors. Of these, vascular endothelial growth factor (VEGF) and its family of receptors play a key role in the regulation of angiogenesis. The VEGF gene family consists of several members including placenta growth factor (PlGF), VEGF-A, VEGF-B, VEGF-C and VEGF-D, but VEGF-A (often referred to as VEGF) is the dominant protein (Ferrara, 2003). The VEGF receptor family consists of three members including VEGFR-1(Flt-1), VEGFR-2 (KDR or Flk-1), and VEGFR-3 (Flt-4). Given the key role of VEGF and its family of receptors in regulating angiogenesis, inhibitors of both VEGF and its receptors are actively being developed as anti-cancer therapies. To inhibit the VEGF pathway two different options are used:

1. VEGF ligand inhibition by antibodies or soluble receptors
2. VEGF receptor inhibition by tyrosine kinase inhibitor (TKIs) or receptor antibodies

Several further antiangiogenic targets beside the VEGF pathway are identified and explored (Figure 2).

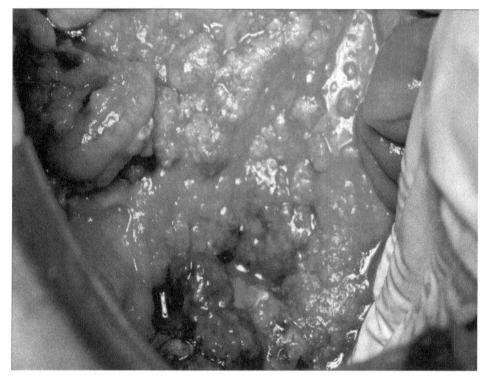

Fig. 1. Peritoneal carcinosis and Angiogenesis.

The clinical evaluation of antiangiogenic drugs revealed new, unique toxicity profiles and potential side-effects, such as hypertension, proteinuria and GI-toxicities that have so far not been in the focus of the oncologist and need to be understood and closely considered during therapy. However, under careful and responsible advise most of the established and documented treatment concepts can be performed without difficulties.

In summary, antiangiogenic drugs are reasonable and promising new therapeutic strategies under clinical investigation. Subsequently, current antiangiogenic treatment strategies against the three main gynecologic malignancies ovarian cancer, cervical cancer and endometrial cancer will be presented and discussed.

2. Ovarian cancer

2.1 Background
In the US about 21,880 women a year develop a malignant tumour of the ovary. The incidence of ovarian carcinoma has remained unchanged in the last few decades. With more than 13,850 deaths, it is the fifth highest cause of cancer-related mortality in women. Symptoms of the disease usually develop at a very late stage. For this reason about 70% of patients are already in an advanced stage of the tumor at the time of diagnosis (FIGO III or

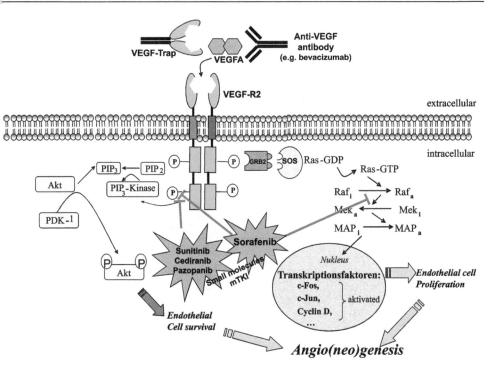

Fig. 2. Molecular mechanisms in tumor-associated angiogenesis and main targets of current investigations.

IV). Surgical tumor removal is the primary treatment. Whether and to what extent residual tumour formation is present postoperatively is the deciding factor in the subsequent prognosis for the patient. After surgery, chemotherapy involving paclitaxel plus carboplatin is generally indicated in the event of an initially advanced tumour stage (McGuire et al., 1999; McGuire et al., 2001; Parmar et al., 2003). Despite improved surgical procedures and a high primary response to chemotherapy, about 70% of patients with advanced ovarian carcinoma develop a tumor relapse and die from the disease.

Angiogenesis is a critical pathway in the development and progression of ovarian cancer. Therefore, identification and development of novel agents with limited toxicity that target mechanisms of tumor progression such as angiogenesis are of high priority. Data from numerous preclinical and clinical trials support the assumption of VEGF/VEGFR, PDGFR as well as FDGF as target molecules for the treatment of ovarian cancer (Burger, 2010). Beyond these currently intensively investigated targets, further antiagiogenic pathways are explored, such as angiopoetin or vascular disrupting agents (VDA) (Theo et al., 2010; Zweifel et al., 2011).

Anti-angiogenic agents in investigational clinical trials

Several anti-angiogenic agents are evaluated in investigational clinical trials to improve the therapy of recurrent and also primary ovarian cancer. Results from a number of phase I and phase II trials are available and also phase III trials have been performed and have led to first reported data, in particular the GOG 218 as well as the ICON-7-trial.

Author	patients	Treatment	ORR [%]	Median OS [months]	Median PFS [months]	
Micha 2007	n=20 (first line, advanced EOC, PPC, FTC)	Paclitaxel i.v. (175 mg/m²) and carboplatin i.v. (AUC %) q3w for 6 cycles and bevacizumab (15 mg/kg) at cycles 2-6.	80	NR	NR	48,3 % neutropenia of 116 cycles 10% hypertension
Burger 2007	n=62 persistent/recurrent EOC/PPC	bevacizumab 15 mg/kg i.v. q3w	21	17	4,7	9,4% hypertension 6,4% GI events (nausea,emesis) 4,8% pain 3,2% allergic
Cannistra 2007	n=44 platinum-resistant EOC/PPC	bevacizumab 15 mg/kg i.v. q3w	16	10,7	4,4	9,1% hypertension 15,9 % proteinuria 2,3% bleeding 2,3 % wound-healing complications 11,4% GI perforation
Garcia 2008	n=70 recurrent EOC/PPC	bevacizumab 10 mg/kg i.v. q2 w and cyclophosphamide 50 mg/d p.o.	24	16,9	Median TTP: 7,2	19,4 % lymphopenia 18,6% pain 8,6% fatigue Bevacizumab-related: 15,7% hypertension 5,7% GI-Perforation or fistula 4,3 proteinuria
Tillmanns[a] 2010	n=48	bevacizumab 10 mg/kg i.v. q2 w and nab-paclitaxel 100 mg/m²	46	16,5	8,3	3,8% nausea 3,8% nosebleed 3,8% bowel obstruction 2,8% neuropathy 2,6% neutropenia 2,4% anemia 1,6% infection
Penson 2010	n=62 newly diagnosed	Carboplatin i.v. (AUC5), paclitaxel i.v.(175 mg/m²) and bevacizumab 15 mg/kg i.v. for 6-8 cycles on day 1 every 21 days. Bevacizumab was omitted in the first cycle and continued as a single agent for 1	76	Not reached	29,8	Chemotherapy phase: 22,6% neutropenia 12,9% metabolic 9,7% hypertension 6,5% thrombocytopenia,

Table 1. Antiangiogenic drugs currently under investigation in EOC.

Bevacizumab

The most clinical experiences have been collected targeting VEGF with the recombinant humanized monoclonal anti-VEGF antibody (bevacizumab, avastin®).

Several phase II studies showed efficacy and tolerability as well in the palliative as in the adjuvant setting. Recently, bevacizumab in combination with the standard chemotherapy of carbolatin/paclitaxel was evaluated in two phase III trials demonstrating a significant improvement in PFS compared to the standard chemotherapy treatment (GOG 218 and ICON 7). Table 1 provides an overview of all published phase II and III studies (Table 1).

Treating ovarian cancer patients with bevacizumab single agent regimens demonstrated very promising reponse rates (Table 1), furthermore some combined therapies including cytotoxic drugs seemed to enhance not only direct antitumoral efficacy but also antiangiogenic potentials. This is in particular the case for so called metronomic treatment strategies, where chemotherapeutic agents are administered in low dosages in regular, short time intervals, for example, cyclophosphamide in daily oral application (Sanchez-Munoz et al., 2010).

The main toxic effects of bevacizumab as documented in the available trials are hypertension, headache, proteinuria, thrombosis and hemoptysis (Table 1). A particular attention has been drawn on GI perforations that have been observed and seem to be a specific phenomenon on bevacizumab-therapies in patients with EOC. The exact pathomechanism of this potentially fatal complication is not fully understood though there are several explaining theories (Richardson et al., 2010). Currently, the average risk of developing a GI perforation during bevacizumab-therapy can be estimated at 7-8 % for patients with EOC (Richardson et al., 2010, Tanyi et al., 2011).

VEGF trap

VEGF trap (aflibercept®), a molecular fusion protein, inhibits VEGF-mediated events as a high affinity VEGF decoy. It is also able to bind to other VEGF familiy members e.g. PlGF. Tew et al. published a multicenter phase II study in women with recurrent ovarian cancer who were treated with 2mg/kg or 4mg/kg aflibercept, but the study only showed a moderate response rate (ORR 7 %, Moroney et al., 2009)

Toxic effects of aflibercept are hypertension, headache, fatigue and GI –perforations (1,8%). Colombo et al. could show that aflibercept reduces ascites in patients with advanced ovarian cancer. They achieved a response in terms of less often repeated paracenteses.

Ramucirumab

Ramucirumab (IMC-1121B) is a novel fully human antibody targeting VEGFR2. It showed significant antitumor activity in several mouse tumors and human tumor xenografts by inhibiting angiogenesis mediated by reduction of microvessel density, tumor cell apoptosis and necrosis, as well as a decreased tumor cell proliferation (Prewett et al., 1999; Spratlin, 2011).

Ramucirumab is currently being explored in phase III trials in hepatocellular carcinomas (ImCLON HCC-Ramucirumab), NSCLC (Lilly study I4T-MC-JVB(a)), in previously untreated patients with HER2-negative, unresectable, locally recurrent or metastatic breast cancer (Trio-012) and in patients with metastatic colorectal carcinoma. A phase III study is designed in patients with metastatic adenocarcinoma of the stomach. The safety and efficacy of Ramucirumab is also evaluated in a randomized phase II trial in patients with metastatic melanoma with or without dacarbazine (Carvajal et al., 2010), as second-line therapy in patients with locally advanced or metastatic transitional cell carcinoma of the bladder, urethra, ureter, or renal pelvis and metastatic androgen-independent prostate cancer with or without mitoxantrone and prednisone.

At the time of publication, ramucirumab was undergoing assessment in a non-randomized, open-label, multicenter phase II study as a monotherapy in the treatment of persistent or recurrent EOC, FTC, or PPC. Ramucirumab is given at 8mg/kg q2w. The results of these trials will tell whether ramucirumab is a useful addition to current antiangiogenic therapies and an option in the treatment of patients with ovarian cancer.

Tyrosine kinase inhibitors

Tyrosine kinase inhibitors repress the VEGF pathway by binding directly to the VEGFRs.

Sorafenib

Sorafenib is an oral tyrosine kinase inhibitor which not only targets VEGFR2 and 3 and PDGFR-beta but also the Ras/Raf/Mek/ERK pathways. In the GOG 170 trial Matei et al. evaluated Sorafenib as a single agent treatment in patients with recurrent ovarian cancer. In this phase II trial preliminary results showed a progression free survival for at least six months in 12 of 59 patients, partial response in 2 patients and stable disease in 20 patients. Progressive disease was determined in 30 patients (Matei et al., 2010).

Siu et al. tested Sorafenib in combination with gemcitabine in a phase I trial in solid tumors and could show that the combination was well tolerated (Siu et al., 2006). In contrast to this and in line with Matei et al. Pölcher and colleagues pointed out that sorafenib showed markable toxicity in ovarian cancer study protocols, thus this drug needs to be further evaluated in clinical trials (Pölcher et al., 2010).

Sunitinib

Sunitinib (Sutent®) is also an oral tyrosine kinase inhibitor that binds to VEGFR 1-3 as well as PDGFR-alpha and beta. Sunitinib is approved for the treatment of advanced or metastatic renal cell carcinoma as first line therapy, of nonresectable gastrointestinal stromal tumours and for the treatment of patients with unresectable, locally advanced, or metastatic pancreatic neuroendocrine tumors (pNET). There a lots of clinical trials to determine the efficacy and safety of sunitinib in several tumor entities e.g glioblastoma, colon cancer and breast cancer. [http://clinicaltrialsfeeds.org/clinical-trials/results/term=sunitinib]

In a preclinical study sunitinib inhibited tumor growth and reduced peritoneal metastasis of human ovarian cancer in xenografted mice. (Bauerschlag et al., 2010). The following phase II study of sunitinib (initial dose 50mg/d p.o) in 30 patients with recurrent EOC or PPC showed only a partial response (3,3%). Hand-foot-syndrome, hypertension, fatigue and gastrointestinal symptoms but no gastrointestinal perforation were the main toxicities. (Biagi et al., 2011).

Pazopanib

Pazopanib is an investigational, oral, angiogenesis inhibitor targeting VEGFR, PDGFR and c-kit. Pazopanib is currently being studied in a number of different tumour types; clinical trials are currently underway in renal cell carcinoma (Phase III), breast cancer (Phase III in inflammatory breast cancer), ovarian cancer, STS, NSCLC, cervical cancer and other solid tumours. It is being evaluated as a monotherapy, in combination with targeted therapies and in combination with cytotoxic chemotherapy.

Author	patients	Treatment	ORR [%]	Median OS [months]	Median PFS [months]	
Welch 2010	n=33 recurrent EOC	Gemcitabine 1000mg/m² i.v. weekly for 7 of 8 weeks in the first cycle, then weekly for 3 weeks of each subsequent 4-week cycle. Sorafenib 400 mg p.o.	4,7	13	Median TTP: 5,4	hand-foot syndrome, fatigue, hypokalemia, diarrhea
2010	n=102 (was planned),4 were enrolled neoadjuvant advanced EOC	Carboplatin AUC5 and Paclitaxel 175 mg/m² preoperatively and concomitant sorafenib 400 mg twice daily. (After four cycles of postoperative chemotherapy, a maintenance phase of single agent oral Sorafenib through 1 year was planned)	-	-	-	3 patients had life threatening events (cardiac output failure, myocardial infarction, anastomotic leak): **The study was interrupted!**
Matei 2011	n=71 recurrent/persistent EOC/PPC	Sorafenib 400 mg twice daily.	2,8	NR	At 6 months (n=12)	14% metabolic 12,6% hand-foot syndrome 9,9 % rash
Biagi 2011	n=30	Sunitinib 50 mg daily, 4 of 6 weeks	3,3	NR	4,1	fatigue, gastrointestinal symptoms, hand-foot syndrome and hypertension.
Matulonis 2009	n=46 recurrent EOC/FTC/PPC	Cediranib 45 mg daily (Because of toxicities the dose was lowered to 30 mg)	17,4	Not yet reached	5,2	46% hypertension 24%fatigue 13% diarrhea
Friedlander 2010	n=31 recurrent EOC/FTC/PPC	pazopanib 800 mg once daily	18			

Table 2. Overview of published phase II and phase III trials on bevacizumab in patients with ovarian cancer.

VEG104450 is a Phase II study to assess the biochemical response rate (determined by CA-125 response) to pazopanib monotherapy in subjects with epithelial ovarian, fallopian tube, or primary peritoneal carcinoma that have responded to standard treatment and who have a high risk of recurrence due to a rising CA-125. Data reported recently (Friedlander, 2008) showed that, in 36 ovarian subjects with biochemical (i.e. CA-125) recurrence after < 2 treatment regimens, the most frequent AEs (reported by more than 20% of subjects) are diarrhoea, fatigue, nausea (all 47%), hypertension and abdominal pain (31%), AST and ALT increase (25%), anorexia and vomiting (22%). These were primarily Grade 1 and 2, with only one Grade 4 event reported in the study (of peripheral oedema, considered unrelated to the study drug); there were no Grade 5 events and no bowel perforations reported in this study. Currently, the German PACOVAR-trial analysis in a phase I/II setting evaluates activity and tolerability of pazopanib combined with orally administered metronomic cyclophosphamide in patients with recurrent, intensively pretreated ovarian cancer. First results of the phase I are expected in 2012.

Endometrial cancer

Endometrial cancer is the most common gynecologic malignancy with a peak incidence between the ages of 55 and 65. Worldwide about 142.000 women are affected by endometrial cancer every year (Jemal et al., 2010). It is frequently diagnosed at an early stage as women affected often present by abnormal vaginal bleeding. At an early stage endometrial cancer can be treated surgically with curable intention (van Wijk et al., 2009). In patients with high-risk endometrial cancer postoperative pelvic radiotherapy, adjuvant radiation therapy or adjuvant chemotherapy have shown to improve outcome (Ray et al., 2009).

However, about 13% of all patients with endometrial cancer develop recurrent disease. (Van Wijk et al., 2009). In the treatment of recurrent endometrial cancer different therapeutic modalities consisting of radiotherapy, surgery and systemic therapies as chemotherapy and hormone therapy are in use (Ray et al., 2009). Clinical trials evaluating chemotherapeutic regimen for patients with endometrial cancer include combinations of doxorubicin and cisplatin, cyclophosphamide or paclitaxel and carboplatin, most of them administered in palliative situation (Ray et al., 2009).

Due to promising results of antiangiogenic treatment concepts in many solid tumors, some efforts have already been made to elucidate the role of VEGF in endometrial cancer. Kamat et al. examined serum samples of endometrial cancer patients and established an endometrioid orthotopic mouse model to approach the role of VEGF in endometrial cancer. The authors found significantly increased levels of VEGF in approximately half of the tumors. These high levels were independently associated with a poor outcome of the affected patients, as an overexpression of VEGF enhances tumor growth. Moreover, in a published mouse model study the combination of docetaxel and bevacizumab has proven a greater therapeutic efficacy than docetaxel or bevacizumab alone (Kamat et al., 2005).

Recently, Aghajanian et al published data of a phase II GOG trial of bevacizumab in patients with recurrent or advanced endometrial cancer. In a series of n=56 patients the authors could demonstrate that a treatment regimen consisting of 15mg/kg bevacizumab i.v. every three weeks led to an ORR of 13.5% and a PFS at 6 months of 40.4% (Aghajanian et al., 2010). Furthermore, it could be shown that high VEGF-A immunohistochemical staining in archival tumors was associated with a reduced risk of death but that high circulating VEGF-A levels were associated with poor outcome. For possible explanation authors suggested that VEGF staining in tumor did not reflect the state of the tumor before treatment when

VEGF-levels in plasma where measured. Finally, in 2011, Reinhardt and colleagues published a case report presenting the successful remission in a patient with recurrent, heavily pretreated endometrial cancer using a combination regimen with bevacizumab and metronomic cyclophosphamide (Reinhardt et al., 2011). Adverse events of bevacizumab therapies in endometrial cancer patients include GI-hemorrhage, proteinuria, hypertension, thrombosis and pulmonary embolism. So far no GI-perforations or fistulae have been reported (Aganajian et al., 2010)

Beside bevacizumab as antiangiogenic treatment concept the oral tyrosine kinase inhibitors of multiple VEGF receptors sunitinib and sorafenib have been evaluated in clinical studies for the treatment of endometrial cancer.

Sorafenib showed minimal activity with PFS at 6 months of 29% and median overall survival of 11.4 months. As adverse events hypertension, hand-foot-syndrome, anemia, thrombosis, fatigue and bleeding were found (Nimeiri et al., 2008).

Accordingly, in a phase II study in recurrent or metastatic endometrial cancer sunitinib demonstrated activity with an ORR of 15% and median overall survival of 19 months. Adverse events were fatigue and hypertension. (Correa et al., 2010)

Cervical cancer

Cervical cancer is the second most cause of female cancer mortality worldwide with 288 000 deaths every year. About 510.000 cases of cervical cancer are reported each year with nearly 80% in developing countries. Cervical cancer is preventable and generally curable if diagnosed at early stage (Wright et al., 2006). Surgery is the goldstandard in early lesions, whereas locally advanced lesions are managed with concurrent cisplatin chemotherapy and pelvic radiation (Monk et al., 2009). Metastatic disease or recurrent lesions not amenable to radical local excision or regional radiation are treated with palliative chemotherapy (Tewari et al., 2009). Patients diagnosed with locally advanced or metastatic cancer of the cervix have a very poor prognosis with a 5-year survival between 5 and 15 % (patients with stage IV disease) (Takano et al., 2009).

Recurrent tumors within the irradiated and therefore devascularized fields likely have microenvironment changes that make chemotherapy delivery far from optimal. For these reasons, this patient population is not one that is ideally suited to receive multiple lines of chemotherapy. Biologic therapies offer another therapeutic strategy that has demonstrated effectiveness in tumors resistant to chemotherapy (Monk et al., 2010).

Angiogenesis seems to play an important role in the development and progression of cervical cancer. Evidence that angiogenesis plays an important role in locally advanced cervical cancer has been shown in recent years (Mackay et al., 2010; Carpini et al., 2010). In one study of 111 patients with cervical cancer, Cooper et al identified tumor angiogenesis (as reflected by the tumor microvessel density) as a significant prognostic factor within a Cox multivariate analysis, where it was associated with poor locoregional control and overall survival. Data from prospective studies in women with advanced cervical cancer, treated with anti-angiogenic therapy, are limited to a few small studies.

Bevacizumab

Corresponding to other solid tumors, most experiences are also reported in targeting VEGF with bevacizumab.

Wright et al first evaluated the effect of the VEGF-Inhibitor bevacizumab in a retrospective trial in women with recurrent cervical cancer (Wright et al., 2006). Five patients were treated with bevacizumab and 5-fluoruracil, one patient with bevacizumab and capecitabine, respectively. The median age of these patients was 43 years, the stage distribution was IB2, IIB and IIIB at 2 patients a throw. All of the patients had received prior platinum-based chemotherapy. Bevacizumab was given intravenously every other week to five of the six patients with a starting dose of either 5 mg/kg or 10 mg/kg. One patient was given bevacizumab at a dose of 15 mg/kg every three weeks. A total of 30 doses of bevacizumab was given. The regimen was well tolerated. There was a grade 4 neutropenic sepsis encountered in one patient after 2 cycles of bevacizumab and one extremity thrombosis in another subject. The overall response rate (ORR) was 33 % (2 of the 6 patients). One of these patients showed a complete response, the other one a partial response. There was a stable disease in two patients (33 %). The median time to progression for the four patients with clinical benefit (CR, PR, SD) was 4.3 months. None of the patients demonstrated a progression free intervall > 6 months. Though only a small number of patients was observed, this study indicated that the combination of bevacizumab and 5-fluoruracil-based chemotherapy seems to be feasible and associated with significant activity in patients with recurrent cervical cancer.

In 2009 Monk published a phase II-trial of bevacizumab in the treatment of persistent in recurrent squamous cell carcinoma of the cervix (GOG protocol 227C) (Monk et al., 2009).

46 patients were randomized to the trial and received bevacizumab in a dose of 15 mg/kg intravenously every 3 weeks. Primary endpoints of the study were PFS for at least 6 months and evaluation of adverse events. A total of 254 cycles of bevacizumab as a single agent therapy were administered with a median of 4 cycles per patient. Eleven patients (23.9 %) experienced a progression free survival of > 6 months, whereas five patients (10.9 %) showed partial responses. Median overall survival for all patients was 7.29 months. There were several grade 3/ 4 adverse events demonstrated in this trial, including hypertension (n = 7), thromboembolism (n = 5), gastrointestinal complaints (n = 4), anemia (n = 2), vaginal bleeding (n = 1), neutropenia (n = 1) and fistula (n = 1) No unusual toxicities were noted. This trial provided that bevacizumab as a single agent therapy was relatively well tolerated, safe and demonstrated remarkable activity. Importantly, the results of this protocol constitute the first prospective clinical trial of a biologic agent that shows clinical activity in cervical cancer (Tewari et al., 2009). Exploratory analyses suggested an increased risk of progression (or death) for those who are African- American, are young, and have a poor performance status. Additional analyses also suggested an increased risk of death for those who have more prior chemotherapy regimens.

Takano et al (Takano et al., 2009) reported of two cases of patients with cervical cancer treated with bevacizumab (2 mg/kg), paclitaxel (80 mg/m2) and carboplatin (AUC = 2.0). Therapy consisted of carboplatin/paclitaxel weekly on days 1, 8, 15 and bevacizumab weekly on days 1, 8, 15, 21, q28d. In both patients full remission was notified and there was no evidence of disease for > 10 months as well as no adverse events higher than grade 3.

Based on the findings in the studies described, a phase III trial with bevacizumab for treatment of cervical cancer is planned by the GOG. In GOG 240, patients will be randomized to one of four regimens: paclitaxel/cisplatin, paclitaxel/cisplatin plus bevacizumab, paclitaxel/topotecan and paclitaxel/topotecan plus bevacizumab.

Also, other anti-angiogenesis compounds will soon be investigated by the GOG. For example, brivanib, a highly potent dual inhibitor of VEGFR and fibroblast growth factor receptor (FGFR) will be under study (Monk et al., 2010).

Sunitinib

There is one phase II study published in 2010 by Mackay et al. that evaluates the activity of sunitinib, a tyrosine kinase inhibitor in the treatment of locally advanced or metastatic cervical cancer (Mackay et al., 2010) (NCIC CTG Trial IND.184). Sunitinib is an oral, multi-targeted tyrosine kinase inhibitor, that inhibits receptors for VEGF, c-Kit and platelet-derived growth factor. 19 patients received sunitinib at a dose of 50 mg/day in 6-week cycles (4 weeks, followed by 2 weeks off treatment). 16 patients (84 %) showed stable disease, but there was no objective response noted in any of the patients. However, 4 patients developed fistulae during treatment and one patient had an enterocutaneous fistula 3.5 months post-study. All of the fistulae occured within the previous radiation fields. Although SD-rate was 84 %, the overall progression free survival was only 3.5 months in this study, which compares with the progression free survival in the phase II trial published by Monk and described before. But the observation of five cases of fistulae (26 %) was of particular concern, so that sunitinib as a single agent therapy does not have enough sufficient activity in women with advanced cervical cancer to recommend further study.

3. Conclusion and future perspectives

There is consensus that angiogenesis is a crucial phenomenon in the progression of gynecologic tumors. Many promising efforts have been made so far demonstrating that ovarian cancer as well as uterine cancers can be targeted by antiangiogenic treatment strategies.

As gynecologic tumors still often respond very differently to antiangiogenic therapies future studies will have to work on identifying patients that will likely respond to specific antiangiogenic regimens. Existing and already proven active therapies will have to be confirmed in further long-term experiences, in particular regarding their potential long-terms toxicity or side-effects and finally new, additional targets beyond the VEGF/ VEGFR-mechanism have to be evaluated. Finally, a new attention should be paid to the concept of maintenance treatments, in particular in EOC, as antiangiogenic treatment concepts, might be especially useful in keeping a major cytotoxic therapeutic success. A particular role may be attributed in the future to combined antiangiogenic and metronomic cytotoxic regimens.

4. References

Aghanjanian C, Sill MW, Darcy KM, Greer B, McMeekin DS, Rose PG, et al: Phase II Trial of Bevacizumab in Recurrent or Persistent Endometrial Cancer: A Gynecologic Oncology Group Study.J ClinOncol, 2010.

Bauerschlag DO, Schem C, Tiwari S, Egberts JH, Weigel MT, Kalthoff H, Jonat W, Maass N, Meinhold-Heerlein I.Sunitinib (SU11248) inhibits growth of human ovarian cancer in xenografted mice. Anticancer Res. 2010 Sep;30(9):3355-60.

Biagi JJ, Oza AM, Chalchal HI, Grimshaw R, Ellard SL, Lee U, Hirte H, Sederias J, Ivy SP, Eisenhauer EA. A phase II study of sunitinib in patients with recurrent epithelial ovarian and primary peritoneal carcinoma: an NCIC Clinical Trials Group Study.Ann Oncol. 2011 Feb;22(2):335-40. Epub 2010 Aug 12.

Bryant CS, Munkarah AR, Kumar S, Batchu RB, Shah JP, Berman J, Morris RT, Jiang ZL, Saed GM. Reduction of hypoxia-induced angiogenesis in ovarian cancer cells by inhibition of HIF-1 alpha gene expression.Arch Gynecol Obstet. 2010 Dec;282(6):677-83. Epub 2010 Feb 7.

Burger RA. Overview of anti-angiogenic agents in development for ovarian cancer.Gynecol Oncol. 2011 Apr;121(1):230-8. Epub 2011 Jan 8. Review.

Carvajal et al. J Clin Oncol 28:15s, 2010 (suppl; abstr 8519 Carpini, J.D., A.K. Karam, and L. Montgomery, Vascular endothelial growth factor and its relationship to the prognosis and treatment of breast, ovarian, and cervical cancer.Angiogenesis, 2010.13(1): p. 43-58.

Correa R, Mackay H, Hirte HW, et al: A phase II study of sunitinib in recurrent or metastatic endometrial carcinoma: A trial of the princess MargaretHospital, The University of Chicago, and California Cancer Phase II Consortia.J ClinOncol 28:399s, 2010 (suppl; abstr 5038)

Delli Carpini J, Karam AK, Montgomery L.Vascular endothelial growth factor and its relationship to the prognosis and treatment of breast, ovarian, and cervical cancer.Angiogenesis. 2010 Mar;13(1):43-58. Epub 2010 Mar 14. Review. Erratum in: Angiogenesis. 2010 Sep;13(3):279. Carpini, Jennifer Delli [corrected to Delli Carpini, Jennifer].

Fagotti A, Gallotta V, Romano F, Fanfani F, Rossitto C, Naldini A, Vigliotta M, Scambia G. Peritoneal carcinosis of ovarian origin. World J Gastrointest Oncol. 2010 Feb 15;2(2):102-8.

Ferrara N, Gerber HP, LeCouter J. The biology of VEGF and its receptors. Nat Med. 2003 Jun;9(6):669-76. Review.

Folkman J. The biology of VEGF and its receptors. Tumor angiogenesis: therapeutic implications. N Engl J Med. 1971 Nov 18;285(21):1182-6. Review.

Friedlander M, Hancock KC, Rischin D, Messing MJ, Stringer CA, Matthys GM, Ma B, Hodge JP, Lager JJ. A Phase II, open-label study evaluating pazopanib in patients with recurrent ovarian cancer.

Gynecol Oncol. 2010 Oct;119(1):32-7. Epub 2010 Jun 27. Jemal A, Siegel R, Xu J, Ward E Cancer Stratistics CA Cancer J Clin. 2010 Sep-Oct;60(5):277-300. Epub 2010 Jul 7. Erratum in: CA Cancer J Clin. 2011 Mar-Apr;61(2):133-4.

Kamat AA, Merrit WM, Coffey D, Lin YG, Patel PR, et al: Clinical and Biological Significance of Vascular Endothelial Growth Factor in Endometrial Cancer.ClinCancer Res 2007; 13(24)

Mackay, H.J., Tinker, A., Winquist, E., Thomas, G., Swenerton, K., Oza, A., Sederias, J., Ivy, P. and Eisenhauer, E.A. A phase II study of sunitinib in patients with locally advanced or metastatic cervical carcinoma: NCIC CTG Trial IND. 184.Gynecologic oncology, 2010.116(2): p. 163-167.

Matei D, Sill MW, Lankes HA, DeGeest K, Bristow RE, Mutch D, Yamada SD, Cohn D, Calvert V, Farley J, Petricoin EF, Birrer MJ. Activity of sorafenib in recurrent ovarian cancer and primary peritoneal carcinomatosis: a gynecologic oncology group trial. J Clin Oncol. 2011 Jan 1;29(1):69-75. Epub 2010 Nov 22.

McGuire WP, Brady MF, and Ozols RF: The Gynecologic Oncology Group experience in ovarian cancer. Ann Oncol (1999)10: S29-34.

McGuire WP: Primary therapy of epithelial ovarian cancer. Amer Soc Clin Oncol Educational Book (Spring 2001) 477-480.

Monk, B.J., Sill, M.W., Burger, R.A., Gray, H.J., Buekers, T.E. and Roman, L.D. Phase II trial of bevacizumab in the treatment of persistent or recurrent squamous cell carcinoma of the cervix: a gynecologic oncology group study.Journal of Clinical Oncology, 2009.27(7): p. 1069.

Monk, B.J., L.J. Willmott, and D.A. Sumner, Anti-angiogenesis agents in metastatic or recurrent cervical cancer.Gynecologic oncology, 2010.116(2): p. 181-186.

Moroney JW, Sood AK, Coleman RL. Aflibercept in epithelial ovarian carcinoma. Future Oncol. 2009 Jun;5(5):591-600. Review.

Nimeiri HS, Oza AM, Morgan RJ, et al :Sorafenib in patients with advanced/recurrent uterine carcinoma or carcinosarcoma: A phase II trial of the university of chicago, PMH, and California Phase II Consortia.J ClinOncol. 26:313s, 2008 (suppl; abstr 5585)

Parmar MK, Ledermann JA, Colombo N, du Bois A, Delaloye JF, Kristensen GB, Wheeler S, Swart AM, Qian W, Torri V, Floriani I, Jayson G, Lamont A, Tropé C; ICON and AGO Collaborators.

Paclitaxel plus platinum-based chemotherapy versus conventional platinum-based chemotherapy in women with relapsed ovarian cancer: the ICON4/AGO-OVAR-2.2 trial. Tumor angiogenesis: therapeutic implications.

Pölcher M, Eckhardt M, Coch C, Wolfgarten M, Kübler K, Hartmann G, Kuhn W, Rudlowski C. Sorafenib in combination with carboplatin and paclitaxel as neoadjuvant chemotherapy in patients with advanced ovarian cancer. Cancer Chemother Pharmacol. 2010 May;66(1):203-7. Epub 2010 Mar 5.

Prewett M, Huber J, Li Y, Santiago A, O'Connor W, King K, Overholser J, Hooper A, Pytowski B, Witte L, Bohlen P, Hicklin DJ. Antivascular endothelial growth factor receptor (fetal liver kinase 1) monoclonal antibody inhibits tumor angiogenesis and growth of several mouse and human tumors. Cancer Res. 1999 Oct 15;59(20):5209-18

Ray M. and Fleming G, Management of advanced-stage and recurrent endometrial cancer.SeminOncol, 2009. 36(2): p. 145-54.

Reinhardt J, Schott S, Mayer C, Sohn C, Eichbaum M Long-term remission of an advanced recurrent endometrial cancer in a heavily pretreated patient using a combined regimen with bevacizumab and metronomic cyclophosphamide. Anticancer Drugs. 2011 Mar 2. [Epub ahead of print]

Richardson DL, Backes FJ, Hurt JD, Seamon LG, Copeland LJ, Fowler JM, Cohn DE, O'Malley DM. Which factors predict bowel complications in patients with recurrent epithelial ovarian cancer being treated with bevacizumab? Gynecol Oncol. 2010 Jul;118(1):47-51. Epub 2010 Apr 10 Spratlin J.

Ramucirumab (IMC-1121B): Monoclonal antibody inhibition of vascular endothelial growth factor receptor-2. Curr Oncol Rep. 2011 Apr;13(2):97-102.

Sánchez-Muñoz A, Mendiola C, Pérez-Ruiz E, Rodríguez-Sánchez CA, Jurado JM, Alonso-Carrión L, Ghanem I, de Velasco G, Quero-Blanco C, Alba E. Bevacizumab plus low-dose metronomic oral cyclophosphamide in heavily pretreated patients with recurrent ovarian cancer. Oncology. 2010;79(1-2):98-104. Epub 2010 Nov 15.

Siu LL, Awada A, Takimoto CH, Piccart M, Schwartz B, Giannaris T, Lathia C, Petrenciuc O, Moore MJ. Phase I trial of sorafenib and gemcitabine in advanced solid tumors with an expanded cohort in advanced pancreatic cancer. Clin Cancer Res. 2006 Jan 1;12(1):144-51.

Takano, M., Kikuchi, Y., Kita, T., Goto, T., Yoshikawa, T., Kato, M., Watanabe, A., Sasaki, N., Miyamoto, M. and Inoue, H. Complete remission of metastatic and relapsed uterine cervical cancers using weekly administration of bevacizumab and paclitaxel/carboplatin.Onkologie, 2009.32(10): p. 595-597.

Tanyi JL, McCann G, Hagemann AR, Coukos G, Rubin SC, Liao JB, Chu CS. Clinical predictors of bevacizumab-associated gastrointestinal perforation. Gynecol Oncol. 2011 Mar;120(3):464-9. Epub 2010 Dec 17.

Tew WP, Gordon M, Murren J, Dupont J, Pezzulli S, Aghajanian C, Sabbatini P, Mendelson D, Schwartz L, Gettinger S, Psyrri A, Cedarbaum JM, Spriggs DR.Phase 1 study of aflibercept administered subcutaneously to patients with advanced solid tumors. Clin Cancer Res. 2010 Jan 1;16(1):358-66. Epub 2009 Dec 22.

Tewari, K.S. and B.J. Monk. Recent achievements and future developments in advanced and recurrent cervical cancer: trials of the Gynecologic Oncology Group. inSeminars in Oncology. 2009: Elsevier.

Teoh DG, Secord AA. Antiangiogenic therapies in epithelial ovarian cancer. Cancer Control. 2011 Jan;18(1):31-43. Review.

Van Wijk FH, van der Burg MEL, Burger CW, Vergote I, van Doorn HC., Management of recurrent endometrioid endometrial cancer: an overview.Int J Gynecol Cancer, 2009. 19(3): p. 314-20.

Wright, J.D., Viviano, D., Powell, M.A., Gibb, R.K., Mutch, D.G., Grigsby, P.W. and Rader, J.S Bevacizumab combination therapy in heavily pretreated, recurrent cervical cancer.Gynecologic oncology, 2006.103(2): p. 489-493.

Zweifel M, Jayson GC, Reed NS, Osborne R, Hassan B, Ledermann J, Shreeves G, Poupard L, Lu SP, Balkissoon J, Chaplin DJ, Rustin GJ. Phase II trial of combretastatin A4 phosphate, carboplatin, and paclitaxel in patients with platinum-resistant ovarian cancer. Ann Oncol. 2011 Jan 27. [Epub ahead of print]

6

The Management of Small Renal Tumours by Ablative Therapies

Seshadri Sriprasad[1] and Howard Marsh[2]
[1]Consultant Urological Surgeon - Darent Valley Hospital, Dartford, Kent,
[2]Consultant Urological Surgeon- Medway Maritime Hospital, Gillingham, Kent,
UK

1. Introduction

Renal cell carcinoma (RCC) was the 9th commonest malignancy in Europe in 2008 [1] with an estimated 88400 new cases and 39300 deaths [2] making it the most lethal urological malignancy. Over the last 2 decades there has been a significant increase in the incidence of small renal masses (SRMs) at diagnosis often as an incidental finding as a result of abdominal imaging for the investigation of pain or other abdominal symptoms [3]. This has resulted in a stage migration to smaller and lower stage lesions in asymptomatic patients [4]. Many of these SRMs are slow growing and of low malignant potential although the precise natural history remains unclear [5]. The rate of radiographic growth in most series which have followed renal masses usually for 3 years is between 0 and 0.86 cm/yr with a meta-analysis by Chawla et al reporting an overall median growth rate of 0.28cm/year [6]. Some tumours however will behave more aggressively and at present it is not possible to determine in advance which tumours these are. Nephron sparing surgery (NSS) represents the gold standard for the small renal mass and radical surgery for the T2 and larger tumours.

Although laparoscopic nephron sparing surgery has been demonstrated to be both feasible and oncologically equivalent to open nephron sparing surgery it is widely acknowledged to be technically demanding with a steep learning curve and associated morbidity. This particularly relates to keeping warm ischaemia time to a minimum. In one of the largest series Gill et al reported a median surgical time of 3 hours and a median warm ischemia time of 27.8 minutes [7]. Although robotically assisted partial nephrectomy is gaining acceptance, active surveillance and minimally invasive alternatives including ablative techniques have emerged as alternatives to nephron sparing surgery or radical nephrectomy.

The main ablative techniques in clinical use are cryotherapy and radiofrequency ablation. Cryotherapy is more frequently applied laparoscopically and radiofrequency ablation percutaneously. In some institutions including the Cleveland Clinic selected tumours are preferentially treated with minimally ablative techniques rather than with partial nephrectomy [8]. In addition other emerging techniques that have been described include High Intensity Focused Ultrasound, Microwave thermotherapy, Interstitial Laser ablation and CyberKnife. Whilst there is increasing evidence in support of radiofrequency ablation and cryotherapy, there is less clear evidence in support of the other minimally invasive techniques at present.

2. Cryotherapy

Tissue destruction by freezing and thawing has been used in a variety of medical problems for over 150 years with minimal clinical significance. However, with the development of vacuum-insulated liquid nitrogen and argon cooled probes, a real breakthrough was made and targeted cryoablation of renal tumours became a reality. Currently cryoablation is performed using an argon gas based system which operates on the Joule- Thompson principle (i.e., rapid cooling of the tip of a probe by highly compressed liquid nitrogen or argon expanding through a restricted orifice to the gaseous state). Using this principle, very low temperatures of - 175^0C to - 190^0C can be focused on to kidney tissue to freeze tumours. Based on the same principle helium gas can be used for thawing [9]. Cryoprobes of varying diameters are now available and they produce ice balls of varying shapes [10].

3. Mechanism of cryoablation

Although the exact mechanism of tissue injury resulting from freezing is not completely understood, experimental studies have provided us with a fair knowledge of the mode of action of cryotherapy. The physiological changes of freezing are described as acute and delayed. When the tissues are exposed to temperature of -5^0C, ice is formed in the extracellular space. This changes the osmotic gradient and draws water from the intracellular to the extracellular compartment, leading to changes, in the intracellular solute composition, pH and eventually leads to protein denaturation [11,12]. When the temperature reaches to -20^0C, ice forms both intra and extracellularly. It is believed that the intracellular ice shears the cell membrane with irreversible cell damage. Complete destruction of normal renal parenchyma occurs at temperatures below -19.4 ^{0}C [13, 14]. Delayed tissue injury also occurs after cryoablation. This is due to damage to the microvasculature of the target tissue and formation of microthrombi. This phenomenon leads to delayed cell death and is believed to be the significant mechanism of action of cryotherapy [15]. Tissue destruction is achieved better by the combination of freezing and thawing processes. Double freezing, as compared to a single- freeze approach, has been shown to produce large areas of necrosis in animal models with significantly increased cell death [16].

4. Indications and contraindications for renal cryotherapy

The indications for cryotherapy are the same as that for partial nephrectomy. A peripherally situated, enhancing, well- circumscribed tumour which is less than 4cm is the ideal lesion for cryotherapy. In general younger patients are offered partial nephrectomy. In older patients or those with comorbidities such as diabetes, hypertension, congestive cardiac failure cryotherapy is considered. In certain special situations such as tumour less than 4cms in solitary or transplant kidney; hereditary conditions such as Von Hippel- Lindau disease and tuberous sclerosis, cryotherapy may be ideal [17].

The relative contraindications for cryotherapy are young age, tumours greater than 4cms, hilar tumours, intrarenal tumours, and cystic tumours. The only absolute contraindication is untreatable or irreversible coagulopathy [18].

5. Technique of cryotherapy

Most patients are treated with laparoscopic or percutaneous image guided minimally invasive techniques. Open cryotherapy may occasionally be necessary and is also described.

6. Laparoscopic cryotherapy

Tumours that are situated in the anterior aspect of kidney and in the polar region are ideally treated by a transperitoneal laparoscopic technique and the posterior tumours by the retroperitoneal approach. The transperitoneal technique that we use is as follows:

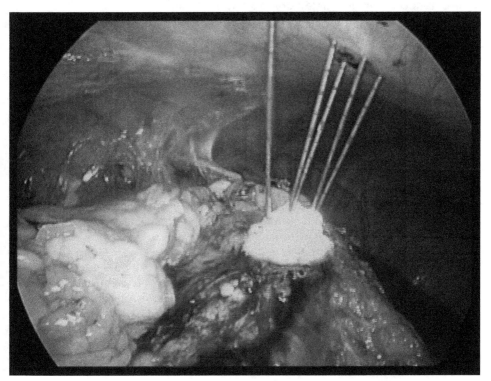

Fig. 1. Showing kidney tumour treated with argon gas cryotherapy- note the spectacular freezing of the tumour.

After placing the ports, the kidney is well mobilised. Gerota's fascia is incised and the perirenal fat is dissected from the surface of the kidney. The exophytic tumour is well seen at this stage and is defined. The position and the depth of the tumour are confirmed and measured using a laparoscopic ultrasound probe. Two to three good core biopsies are taken for histology. Cryoprobes are then placed perpendicularly into the tumour with the tip extending about 5mm beyond. The number of probes placed is determined by the size of the tumour. Two thermosensors are placed one in the centre of the lesion and the other beyond the margin of the tumour to monitor the temperature during cryoablation. The cryoablation starts with a freeze cycle with delivery of the argon gas through the probes. The cryolesion is readily visible as an ice ball and visible in the ultrasound. Typically the first freeze cycle is for 10 minutes. The target temperature in the centre of the lesion is -40⁰C and below. This is followed by a thaw cycle with helium gas. Like many other centres we follow a two freeze and two thaw cycle protocol. At the end of the procedure, a passive and an active thaw are performed and then the probes are removed slowly, after the ice has fully melted. Retrieval of the probes should not be attempted if any resistance is noted as it may lead to fracture of the tumour. In this situation continuing passive thaw for some time allows easy removal of the probes (Fig 1)

7. Percutaneous image-guided cryoablation

Most cryoablations are performed under CT and MRI guidance. Tumours situated in the posterior and inferior aspect of the kidneys are ideal for image guided cryoablation. The upper pole tumours are difficult to reach. The procedure of cryotherapy is essentially similar to laparoscopic techniques. The advantages of percutaneous techniques are short hospital stay, ice ball monitoring by cross- sectional imaging, decreased analgesic requirement and lower cost compared to laparoscopy. Currently however, only 25% of tumours are treated by percutaneous image guided cryoablation and the techniques are still evolving [19].

8. Success and follow up

The absence of enhancement in a post contrast CT-scan at three months following cryoablation is considered as a successful procedure. Although no algorithm exists the patients are closely followed with contrast CT- scans at six, nine and twelve months and ideally the tumour should show regression. Periodic long- term follow up should continue till the tumour is regressed completely and then annual surveillance to ensure that there is no recurrence from the margin. The presence of enhancement would indicate incomplete treatment. Rim enhancement only with no increase in size seems to occur commonly in the first few months after cryoablation and this usually settles. This usually is not an indication for biopsies as it is difficult to take and the yield is low [20]. A recent study from the Cleveland clinic concluded that biopsies did not provide sufficient additional information to contrast enhanced MRI or CT findings in the six months post treatment period and hence did not recommend biopsies [21].

9. Results

The accumulating medium and long term data suggests that cryoablation is associated with high efficacy and low morbidity. The oncological control seems to be promising. The recent review by Berger and associates indicated a five and 10- year cancer specific survival of 93% and 81% respectively [22]. A meta-analysis showed that local recurrence (treatment failure) ranges from 4.6% to 5.2% and metastatic progression ranged from 1% to 1.2% [23].

10. Complications

Cryotherapy is a minimally invasive treatment modality which ablates the renal tumour *in situ*. Although, it is reasonably safe it has a few complications. Minor renal laceration and bleeding from the needle site is common but settles with pressure. Renal fracture and haemorrhage can be avoided by perpendicular placement of the cryoprobes and waiting for complete thawing before removing the probes. The area of skin surrounding the cryoprobes needs to be protected, by warm gauze, to prevent cold injury to the skin. The adjacent internal organs also need protection from cryo injury. Pancreatic injury and ureteropelvic junction stricture has been reported [24]. Data from a retrospective multi centre study for 139 patients revealed that the major and minor complication rates associated with cryoablation were 1.8% and 9.2% respectively. The five major complications were ileus, haemorrhage, conversion to open surgery, scarring with ureteropelvic junction obstruction and urinary leakage. Overall, the most common complication as well as the most common minor complication was pain or paraesthesia at the probe insertion site [25].

11. Conclusions

Renal cryotherapy has proven its safety with good oncological control at medium term with some long term data. Currently the main application of cryotherapy in kidney tumours is for peripheral lesions less than 4cm in patients who would benefit from or require nephron sparing surgery but are not candidates because of comorbidity. Laparoscopic cryotherapy is also on the rise in patients with normal kidneys and relatively normal fitness. The percutaneous approach is constantly evolving and the field is very promising. We have to wait for the long term oncological data but it appears that cryotherapy is here to stay.

12. Radiofrequency ablation

First used in the targeted destruction of hepatic lesions radiofrequency ablation (RFA) has been used since the 1990s. It was first used in the kidney in 1997 [26]. Many of the treatment protocols in RFA are derived from the liver experience.

Although, it can be deployed laparoscopically it is most commonly applied percutaneously by interventional radiologists. The technique involves the insertion of 2 electrodes into the target tissue, in this case a renal tumour and conversion of electrical current between the two electrodes to ultrahigh (radio) frequency. This in turn ablates the intervening tissue with a margin of surrounding normal tissue. The mechanism of tissue destruction is immediate cellular damage and delayed microvascular impairment with the denaturation of proteins and the coagulation of tissue and the disruption of lipid cell membranes. The tissue needs to be heated to a temperature range of 50 to 100′C [27,28]. Over 105′C, the heat distribution and so tissue destruction becomes patchy and unreliable.

Real time imaging of RFA with intra operative USS CT or MRI has proved to be unreliable because of the similarity between normal and ablated tissue and because of the formation of gas bubble artefact. As a result imaging is usually confined to assisting initial probe placement with the RFA being monitored by temperature and or impedance changes.

The advantages of this minimally invasive technique include the ability to apply the energy percutaneously under light sedation, avoiding a general anaesthetic and allowing a more rapid recovery with low morbidity.

The disadvantages of the technique include a lower success rate compared to cryotherapy or nephron sparing surgery. In addition there are only short to medium term results available and the long term efficacy is not established. Also a significant proportion of the reported studies did not establish histological confirmation of a tumour before treatment and so histological confirmation of successful ablation or cure is problematic. It is difficult to interpret the results if it is not certain that the original lesion was malignant. Furthermore as the natural history of the small renal mass is still not completely clear it may be that a significant proportion of the lesions that are tumours would have followed an indolent course without treatment and that the application of an ablative technique is an over treatment. As with cryotherapy, proximity to large vessels may lead to the draining of ablative energy by conduction that in turn reduces efficacy of the procedure. Another challenge is confirmation of successful ablation or cure. Most series report biopsy of the lesion at 6 months together with serial imaging with CT, usually at 6 monthly intervals. A successful outcome is taken as a lack of contrast enhancement of the lesion on CT. In addition the lesion should show progressive shrinking on subsequent imaging.

13. Results

Early experience has shown promising short and medium term tumour control [29]. McDougal et al [30] have reported on patients with over 4 years follow-up and showed successful ablation of exophytic masses smaller than 5cm in diameter. 13 masses in 11 patients with a mean tumour size 3.2cm were followed over a mean of 4.6 years. 12 (92.3%) of the 13 masses treated showed compete ablation.

Zagoria et al [31] reported a retrospective series of 125 treated tumours in which 116 (93%) were completely ablated with a mean follow up of 13.8 months. All 95 tumours smaller than 3.7cm were completely ablated and 21 (70%) of 30 larger tumours were completely ablated with 9 showing evidence of residual viable tumour on follow-up scans. They reported that with each 1cm increase in tumour diameter over 3.6cm the likelihood of tumour free survival decreased by a factor of 2.19 (p<0.001). There were 8 (8%) complications none of which resulted in long-term morbidity.

Stern reported with a mean follow up of 30 months that RFA had the same outcome as partial nephrectomy for T1a lesions with a disease specific survival of 93.4% [32]. Levinson described over a period of at least 40 months a recurrence free survival of 90.3% in patients undergoing RFA for SRM in a single kidney [33].

There are concerns regarding the reliability of imaging to assess treatment response. Lack of enhancement of an ablated mass on CT does not always correlate with histological confirmation of no viable tumour tissue on biopsy. Weight reported that over 45% of renal tumours that showed no enhancement following RFA demonstrated viable tumour on biopsy at 6 months [34]. Others however have suggested that the presence of tumour on biopsy less than 12 months post treatment may be unreliable and have shown no viable tumour in 20 lesions that were biopsied over 12 months following treatment [35]. Where recurrences or cases of persistent disease do occur they tend to be demonstrated within 12 months of treatment. In one study from several institutions 92.1% of renal tumour recurrences were detectable 12 months or fewer after ablation [36].

One study reported the presence of pathological skip areas where tissue remains that has not been ablated. In this study this was found in seven of nine treated renal tumours [37].

A meta-analysis examining 47 studies comparing RFA and cryoablation for SRM has been published [38]. No differences were detected between the modalities in patient age, tumour size or follow-up. Pre-treatment biopsy was performed more often for lesions treated with cryoablation (82.3%) than with RFA (62.2%) (p<0.0001). There was a significantly higher rate of unknown pathology in lesions treated with RFA (40.4%) compared to those treated with cryoablation (24.5%) (p<0.0001). Repeat ablation was more frequently performed after RFA (8.5%) than after cryoablation (1.3%) (p<0.0001) and the rate of local tumour progression was significantly higher for RFA (12.9%) than for cryoablation (5.2%) (p<0.0001). Metastasis was reported more frequently for RFA (2.5%) than for cryoablation (1%) (p=0.06).

The authors of this large meta-analysis concluded that ablation of SRMs is a viable strategy based on short term oncological outcomes and that cryoablation results in fewer retreatments and improved local tumour control and may be associated with a lower risk of metastatic progression compared with RFA.

A further meta-analysis by the same authors looked at all studies reporting on the management of SRMs whether by open or laparoscopic partial nephrectomy, RFA, cryoablation or observation [39]. The analysis included 99 studies involving 6471 renal masses. Local recurrence was reported in 2.6% of masses treated with partial nephrectomy, 4.6% of cases treated with cryotherapy and 11.7% of masses treated with RFA.

Morbidity although low includes perinephric haematomas, bile and urinary fistulae, pancreatic pseudocysts and a ureteric stricture [40, 41].

14. Conclusions

Tumours most suitable for RFA are the same as those most suitable for nephron sparing surgery, that is those <3.5cm in diameter, peripheral, solid, exophytic lesions and away from the renal hilum and collecting system.

In addition RFA may be recommended for patients with conditions predisposing them to repeated development of renal tumours requiring multiple treatments such as Von Hippel Lindau disease.

A number of series have been reported with short and medium term follow up. The results appear to depend upon the position of the tumour with small exophytic peripheral tumours responding better than central lesions.

Although the majority of incomplete ablations are apparent by 12 months ongoing surveillance imaging much the same as following partial nephrectomy is recommended.

What remains to be seen is whether focal ablation actually alters the natural history of the small renal mass or whether the encouraging short and intermediate results are a function of the favourable nature of the lesion.

15. High Intensity Focused Ultrasound (HIFU)

HIFU is very attractive as a completely non-invasive treatment option. The focused ultrasound beam has a thermal and a cavitational effect. The thermal effect is caused by the absorption of ultrasonic sound waves by the tissues resulting in protein denaturation and coagulative necrosis [42]. The cavitation effect is caused by bubble implosion leading to mechanical disruption.

The first feasibility study was reported by Vallencien in 1993 [43] who found evidence of ablation in 8 patients with renal tumours. The limitations of the technique include difficulty in lesion localisation and targeting, small ablation zones and side effects including bowel injury and skin burns. In addition, in renal tumours the overlying ribs and respiratory movements can present a problem [44].

One study applied HIFU to the healthy renal tissue of patients requiring nephrectomy for tumour and found the tissue effects were variable and did not correspond well with the amount of HIFU energy applied [45]. Other studies have also not demonstrated complete tumour ablation [46, 47]. At present therefore, HIFU although very attractive is not recommended as a treatment option.

16. Microwave thermotherapy

Microwave thermotherapy involves the insertion of flexible antennae into tissue and the formation of a rapidly alternating electromagnetic field which in turn causes coagulative necrosis [48]. Experimental studies in rabbits have suggested oncological equivalence with nephrectomy [49].

The disadvantages of the limited zone of ablation and the large antenna size have limited the minimally invasive application of microwave thermotherapy. The technique remains largely experimental although some early clinical experience has been described [50, 51]. The technique has also been described as an adjunct to open partial nephrectomy in order to provide a bloodless plane before resection [52].

17. Interstitial LASER coagulation

Interstitial LASER therapy works by inserting a bare-tip laser fibre directly into tissue. Laser light is converted to heat >55'C and causes tissue necrosis. Nd-YAG and diode lasers have been used. Although the technique has been described experimentally with the laparoscopic approach [53] and in a small number of clinical studies [54] it should still be regarded as experimental.

18. Cyberknife (radiosurgery)

This technique was pioneered in neurosurgery for the treatment of intracranial tumours and uses stereotactic techniques to apply highly focused radiation. The cyberknife is a frameless image-guided radiosurgery device with a linear accelerator on a robotic arm which delivers an adequate conformal dose of radiation by focusing a large number of radiation beams at the target area such that each individual beam does not damage the surrounding normal tissue. Ponsky et al reported initial results in porcine kidneys and demonstrated complete fibrosis of the lesions with preservation of the surrounding normal tissue [55]. A phase 1 study of radiosurgery involving 3 patients showed necrotic tumour in 1 of the 3 patients at subsequent nephrectomy and further trials are awaited [56].

19. Conclusion

In this chapter we have discussed the management of small renal tumours by ablative therapies. These treatments have emerged as an alternative to nephron sparing or radical surgery. The most common ablative techniques are cryotherapy and radiofrequency ablation (RFA). The indications for ablative techniques are the same as for partial nephrectomy and the ideal lesion is a peripheral, enhancing, well circumscribed lesion less than 4cm in diameter (Fig2)

Cryotherapy is most commonly applied laparoscopically and depends upon repeated freeze thaw cycles to achieve tissue destruction. There is good oncological control in the medium term and long term data is continuing to emerge.

Radiofrequency ablation is more commonly applied percutaneously. Several meta-analyses have suggested that short term oncological outcomes are good but that local recurrence, retreatment rates and progression to metastatic disease may be higher than with cryotherapy.

Other ablative techniques include High Intensity Focused Ultrasound (HIFU), Microwave Thermotherapy, Interstitial Laser Coagulation and Radiosurgery (Cyberknife). Although attractive as treatment options these techniques are yet to be established as viable treatments for the small renal mass.

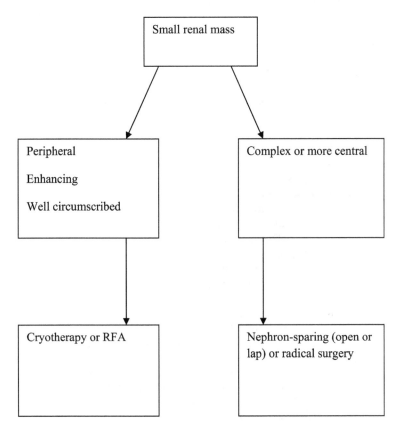

Fig. 2. The Management of Small Renal Tumours by Ablative Therapies

20. References

[1] Ljungberg, B., et al., *EAU guidelines on renal cell carcinoma: the 2010 update.* Eur Urol. 58(3): p. 398-406.

[2] Ferlay, J., D.M. Parkin, and E. Steliarova-Foucher, *Estimates of cancer incidence and mortality in Europe in 2008.* Eur J Cancer. 46(4): p. 765-81.

[3] Jayson, M. and H. Sanders, *Increased incidence of serendipitously discovered renal cell carcinoma.* Urology, 1998. 51(2): p. 203-5.

[4] Chow, W.H., et al., *Rising incidence of renal cell cancer in the United States.* Jama, 1999. 281(17): p. 1628-31.

[5] Crispen, P.L. and R.G. Uzzo, *The natural history of untreated renal masses.* BJU Int, 2007. 99(5 Pt B): p. 1203-7.

[6] Chawla, S.N., et al., *The natural history of observed enhancing renal masses: meta-analysis and review of the world literature.* J Urol, 2006. 175(2): p. 425-31.

[7] Gill, I.S., *Minimally invasive nephron-sparing surgery.* Urol Clin North Am 2003.30:551-579.

[8] Weight, C.J., et al., *The impact of minimally invasive techniques on open partial nephrectomy: a 10-year single institutional experience.* J Urol, 2008. 180(1): p. 84-8.

[9] Rewcastle, J.C., et al., *Considerations during clinical operation of two commercially available cryomachines.* J Surg Oncol 1999.71: p.106-111.

[10] Rehman, J., et al., *Needle- based ablation of renal parenchyma using microwave, cryoablation, impedance- and temperature based monopolar and bipolar radiofrequency, and liquid and gel chemoablation; laboratory studies and review of literature.* J Endourol 2004.18:p.83-104

[11] Ackler, J.P., et al., *Intracellular ice formation is affected by cell interactions.* Cryobiology 1999.38:p.363-371..

[12] Bichof, J.C., et al., *Cryosurgery of Dunning AT-1rat prostate tumour:thermal,biophysical,and viability response at tissue level.* Cryobiology1997.34:p.42-69

[13] Chosy, S.G., et al., *Monitoring kidney cryosurgery: Predictors of tissue necrosis in swine.* J Urol 1998.159:p1370-1374.

[14] Campbell, S.C., et al., *Renal cryosurgery: experimental evaluation of treatment parameters.* 1998. Urology 1998. 52:p29-33.

[15] Daum, P.S.,et al.*Vascular casts demonstrate microcirculatory insufficiency in acute frost bite.*Cryobiology1987.24:p65-73.

[16] Clarke, D.M., et al. *Cryoablation of renal tumours: variables involved in freezing-induced cell death.* Technology in Cancer Research & Treatment.2007.6: P69-79.

[17] Delworth, M.G., et al. *Cryotherapy for renal cell carcinoma and angiomyolipoma.* J Urol 1996.155: p252-254

[18] Janzen, N., et al. *Minimally invasive ablative approaches in the treatment of renal cell carcinoma.* Curr Urol Rep 2002.3:13 p13-320.

[19] Kunkle, D. A, Uzzo, R.G., *Cryoablaion or radiofrequency ablation of the small renal mass.* Cancer 2008.113: p2671-2680.

[20] Beemster, P., et al. *Follow -up of renal masses after cryosurgery using computed tomography; enhancement patterns and cryolesion size.*BJU Int.2008.101:p1237-1242.

[21] Weight, C.J., et al. *Correlation of radiographic imaging and histopathology following cryoablation and radiofrequency ablation for renal tumours.* J Urol.2008.179:p1277-1281.

[22] Berger, A, Kamoi, K, Gill, I.S, Aron M. *Cryoablation of renal tumours the current status.* Curr Opin Urol 2009.19(2):p138-42.

[23] Kunkle, D.A., B.L. Egleston, and R.G. Uzzo, *Excise, ablate or observe: the small renal mass dilemma--a meta-analysis and review.* J Urol, 2008. 179(4): p. 1227-33; discussion 1233-4.

[24] Desai, M.M, Gill, I.S., *Current status of cryoablation and radiofequency ablation in the management of renal tumours.* Curr Opin Urol 2002.12:p387-393

[25] Johnson, D.B., et al. *Defining the complications of cryoablation and radiofrequency ablation of small renal tumours: a multi- institutional study.* J Urol, 2004.172: p874-877.

[26]   Weight, C.J., et al., *The impact of minimally invasive techniques on open partial nephrectomy: a 10-year single institutional experience.* J Urol, 2008. 180(1): p. 84-8.

[27]   Zlotta, A.R., et al., *Radiofrequency interstitial tumor ablation (RITA) is a possible new modality for treatment of renal cancer: ex vivo and in vivo experience.* J Endourol, 1997. 11(4): p. 251-8.

[28]   Goldberg, S.N., G.S. Gazelle, and P.R. Mueller, *Thermal ablation therapy for focal malignancy: a unified approach to underlying principles, techniques, and diagnostic imaging guidance.* AJR Am J Roentgenol, 2000. 174(2): p. 323-31.

[29]   Aron, M. and I.S. Gill, *Minimally invasive nephron-sparing surgery (MINSS) for renal tumours. Part II: probe ablative therapy.* Eur Urol, 2007. 51(2): p. 348-57.

[30]   McDougal, W.S., et al., *Long-term follow up of patients with renal cell carcinoma treated with radio frequency ablation with curative intent.* J Urol, 2005. 174(1): p. 61-3.

[31]   Zagoria, R.J., et al., *Oncologic efficacy of CT-guided percutaneous radiofrequency ablation of renal cell carcinomas.* AJR Am J Roentgenol, 2007. 189(2): p. 429-36.

[32]   Stern, J.M., et al., *Intermediate comparison of partial nephrectomy and radiofrequency ablation for clinical T1a renal tumours.* BJU Int, 2007.100(2): p. 287-90.

[33]   Levinson, A.W., et al., *Long-term oncological and overall outcomes of percutaneous radio frequency ablation in high risk surgical patients with a solitary small renal mass.* J Urol, 2008. 180(2): p. 499-504; discussion 504.

[34]   Weight, C.J., et al., *Correlation of radiographic imaging and histopathology following cryoablation and radio frequency ablation for renal tumors.* J Urol, 2008. 179(4): p. 1277-81; discussion 1281-3.

[35]   Raman, J.D., et al., *Absence of viable renal carcinoma in biopsies performed more than 1 year following radio frequency ablation confirms reliability of axial imaging.* J Urol, 2008. 179(6): p. 2142-5.

[36]   Matin, S.F., et al., *Residual and recurrent disease following renal energy ablative therapy: a multi-institutional study.* J Urol, 2006. 176(5): p. 1973-7.

[37]   Michaels, M.J., et al., *Incomplete renal tumor destruction using radio frequency interstitial ablation.* J Urol, 2002. 168(6): p. 2406-9; discussion 2409-10.

[38]   Kunkle, D.A. and R.G. Uzzo, *Cryoablation or radiofrequency ablation of the small renal mass : a meta-analysis.* Cancer, 2008. 113(10): p. 2671-80.

[39]   Kunkle, D.A., B.L. Egleston, and R.G. Uzzo, *Excise, ablate or observe: the small renal mass dilemma--a meta-analysis and review.* J Urol, 2008. 179(4): p. 1227-33; discussion 1233-4.

[40]   Johnson, D.B., et al., *Defining the complications of cryoablation and radio frequency ablation of small renal tumors: a multi-institutional review.* J Urol, 2004. 172(3): p. 874-7.

[41]   Zagoria, R.J., et al., *Percutaneous CT-guided radiofrequency ablation of renal neoplasms: factors influencing success.* AJR Am J Roentgenol, 2004. 183(1): p. 201-7.

[42]   Chapelon, J.Y., et al., *Effects of high-energy focused ultrasound on kidney tissue in the rat and the dog.* Eur Urol, 1992. 22(2): p. 147-52.

[43]   Vallancien, G., et al., *Focused extracorporeal pyrotherapy: experimental study and feasibility in man.* Semin Urol, 1993. 11(1): p. 7-9.

[44]   Marberger, M., et al., *Extracorporeal ablation of renal tumours with high-intensity focused ultrasound.* BJU Int, 2005. 95 Suppl 2: p. 52-5.

[45]   Hacker, A., et al., *Extracorporeally induced ablation of renal tissue by high-intensity focused ultrasound.* BJU Int, 2006. 97(4): p. 779-85.

[46] Ritchie, R.W., et al., *Extracorporeal high intensity focused ultrasound for renal tumours: a 3-year follow-up.* BJU Int. 106(7): p. 1004-9.

[47] Kohrmann, K.U., et al., *High intensity focused ultrasound as noninvasive therapy for multilocal renal cell carcinoma: case study and review of the literature.* J Urol, 2002. 167(6): p. 2397-403.

[48] Ankem, M.K. and S.Y. Nakada, *Needle-ablative nephron-sparing surgery.* BJU Int, 2005. 95 Suppl 2: p. 46-51.

[49] Kigure, T., et al., *Laparoscopic microwave thermotherapy on small renal tumors: experimental studies using implanted VX-2 tumors in rabbits.* Eur Urol, 1996. 30(3): p. 377-82.

[50] Clark, P.E., et al., *Microwave ablation of renal parenchymal tumors before nephrectomy: phase I study.* AJR Am J Roentgenol, 2007. 188(5): p. 1212-4.

[51] Liang, P., et al., *Ultrasound guided percutaneous microwave ablation for small renal cancer: initial experience.* J Urol,2008. 180(3): p. 844-8; discussion 848.

[52] Naito, S., et al., *Application of microwave tissue coagulator in partial nephrectomy for renal cell carcinoma.* J Urol, 1998. 159(3): p. 960-2.

[53] Lotfi, M.A., P. McCue, and L.G. Gomella, *Laparoscopic interstitial contact laser ablation of renal lesions: an experimental model.* J Endourol, 1994. 8(2): p. 153-6.

[54] Deane, L.A. and R.V. Clayman, *Review of minimally invasive renal therapies: Needle-based and extracorporeal.* Urology, 2006. 68(1 Suppl): p. 26-37.

[55] Ponsky, L.E., et al., *Initial evaluation of Cyberknife technology for extracorporeal renal tissue ablation.* Urology, 2003. 61(3): p. 498-501.

[56] Ponsky, L.E., et al., *Renal radiosurgery: initial clinical experience with histological evaluation.* Surg Innov, 2007. 14(4): p. 265-9.

7

Cancer Treatment with Hyperthermia

Dariush Sardari[1] and Nicolae Verga[2]
[1]College of Engineering, Islamic Azad University
Science and Research Branch, Tehran
[2]Carol Davila University of Medicine and Pharmacy, Bucharest
[1]Iran
[2]Romania

1. Introduction

Broadly speaking, the term hyperthermia refers to either an abnormally high fever or the treatment of a disease by the induction of fever, as by the injection of a foreign protein or the application of heat. Hyperthermia may be defined more precisely as raising the temperature of a part of or the whole body above normal for a defined period of time. The extent of temperature elevation associated with hyperthermia is on the order of a few degrees above normal temperature (41–45°C) (Habash et al. 2006).

Hyperthermia is a type of cancer treatment in which body tissue is exposed to high temperatures, using external and internal heating devices. Hyperthermia is almost always used with other forms of cancer therapy such as radiation and/or chemotherapy. Research has shown that high temperatures can damage and kill cancer cells, usually with minimal injury to normal tissues. It is proposed that by killing cancer cells and damaging proteins and structures within the cells, hyperthermia may shrink tumors making the cells more sensitive to radiation therapy (RT) and/or chemotherapy (ACS 2009).

In some cases if the elevated temperature is utilized as the stand alone technique, tissue temperature above 48 degree would be the objective.

hyperthermia induces almost reversible damage to cells and tissues, but as an adjunct it enhances radiation injury of tumor cells and chemotherapeutic efficacy. Because of the results that high temperature may produce in tissues, one can refer to use of temperatures >50°C as coagulation, 60 to 90°C as thermal ablation, >200°C as charring (Chichel A., et al. 2007). Hyperthermia, as a novel concept for cancer treatment has already entered clinical practice.

2. History

The clinical use of hyperthermia in the system of traditional medicine (Ayurveda) began in India around 3000 years ago. It formed part of a clinical protocol developed called "Panchakarma" that was used in curative and preventive medicine. Hippocrates (540-480 B.C) said that incurable disease is cured by heat, and demonstrated it using the hot sand in the summer. Semantically, hyperthermia comes from the Greek word hyper ("raise") and therme (heat).

Furthermore, Parmenides, Greek philosopher and physician said: "Give me the power to produce fever and I will cure any disease".

Cancer treatment by hyperthermia was first mentioned in ancient Rome by Cornelius Celsus Aulus, Roman encyclopedic doctor (25 BC - 50 AD), who noted that the first stages of cancer are extremely thermosensible.

In the Middle Ages hyperthermia was described by Leonidas - Nicolaus Leonicenus (1428-1524), professor of medicine in Padua. Fever was considered to be an agent of purification and detoxification of the body. After the Renaissance, there were reports of spontaneous tumor regression in patients with smallpox, influenza, tuberculosis and malaria, accompanied by fever.

Enthusiasm for applying heat diminished after 1537, when Ambroise Paré, military surgeon, has demonstrated that medical treatment by cauterization unacceptable consequences. In 1779 Dr Kizowitz described the effect of hyperthermia on malignant tumors caused by malaria.

As in modern ages, the literature on the use of hyperthermia, either as an adjunct to other treatments or as the primary mode of tumor eradication, goes back to the last century. The first paper on hyperthermia was published in 1886 (Bush W., 1886). It was claimed that the sarcoma on the face of a 43-year-old woman was cured when fever was caused by erysipelas. A decade later, (Westermark 1898) used circulating high temperature water for the treatment of an inoperable cancer of uterine cervix with positive results. Hyperthermia was already investigated for the treatment of malignancies more than a hundred years ago. Westermark reported on the use of localized, nonfever-producing heat treatments that resulted in the long-term remission of inoperable cancer of the cervix. Hot baths, electrocautery, and surgical diathermy were employed to locally raise tumor temperature. In the early twentieth century, both applied and basic research on hyperthermia was carried out; however, the heating methods and temperature measuring technologies were not sufficiently advanced at that time and positive clinical application of hyperthermia treatment was not accomplished.

The concept of using heat to treat cancer has been around for a long time, but early attempts to treat cancer with heat had mixed results. Several clinical trials were developed in the 1980s. Given the difficulties with hyperthermia delivery with the available technology and lack of widely applicable quality assurance guidelines enthusiasm for hyperthermia was about to disappear in the late 1980s. Despite little clinical success, research continued in the early 1990s (Hurwitz, 2010).

Worldwide interest in hyperthermia was initiated by the first international congress on hyperthermic oncology in Washington in 1975. Research on hyperthermia rose sharply during 1970's (Kim & Hahn 1979 and references therein). In the 1970's hyperthermia was investigated for the treatment of muscle invasive bladder cancer. More than ten years ago Matzkin performed an in vitro study where solely hyperthermia (43.8C) was used in the treatment of superficial transitional cell carcinoma (TCC) of the bladder . Results of several clinical trials are encouraging [Colombo et al]

In the United States, a hyperthermia group was formed in 1981 and the European Hyperthermia Institute was formed in 1983. In Japan, hyperthermia research started in 1978 and the Japanese Society of Hyperthermia Oncology was established in 1984.

3. Reasons for hyperthermia

The simplest curative application of heat that possess physiological basis (physiological hyperthermia) is treatment of aches, pains, strains, and sprains via   application of temperature below 41°C for approximately an hour and use physiological mechanisms of increasing blood flow and metabolic rates (Roemer RB. 1999).

For cancer treatment purposes, there are reports that malignant cells are more sensitive to heat than are their normal counterparts (Cavalieri, R.et al. and Levine, E.M), although that finding is not universal.

By now, several clinical studies have demonstrated the beneficial effect of regional hyperthermia (ZIB report 2008). Tumor cell environment, such as hypoxia, poor nutrition, and low pH, while detrimental to cell kill by ionizing radiation, is beneficial to heat therapy. Acidic environment of tumor confers resistance to radiation but favors cell kill due to heat. The effect of hyperthermia depends on the temperature and exposure time. For example, it has been demonstrated that with a non-specific HT-applicator already a significant increase in local control (from 24% for RT alone versus 69% for RT plus HT) is achieved for metastatic lymph nodes, without additional toxicity.

Report of long-term follow-up in a randomized trial comparing radiation therapy and radiation therapy plus hyperthermia to metastatic lymph nodes in stage IV head and neck patients (Valdagni R., 1994).

4. Types of cancers

Cancer tumors located in various organs might be treated with different hyperthermia techniques. The chance of successful treatment depends on the stage of cancer development, application of specific technique, and response of patient's physiology to treatment. The cancer types already cured by hyperthermia are:

sarcoma, carcinoma , melanoma, head and neck, Brain

thyroid, lung, esophagus, breast,

kidney, bladder, liver, appendix, stomach,

pancreas, endometrial,

ovarian, prostate, cervix,

peritoneal lining. (mesothelioma).

rectum, appendix

By definition, the term "head and neck cancers" usually excludes tumors that occur in the eyes, in brain and in skin. The most frequently occurring cancers of the head and neck area are located in the oral cavity and the larynx. Worldwide, around 3-5% of patients suffering from cancer have tumors in the head and neck (H&N) region. (Paulides, M., 2007)

5. Physiological and biological phenomena in hyperthermia

First of all, it is noteworthy that there is no individual cellular target of hyperthermia, in contrast to the well known DNA damage after irradiation with x- , gamma or hadron.

In cellular level, reproductive death starts at 40 °C which is progressive with increasing time at the elevated temperature. Cells when heated to a temperature of 45 °C tend to undergo apoptosis or mitotic death process. Heat in the range of 42 °C to 45 °C, can also sensitize cells exposed to ionizing radiation or chemotherapy. The cells' sensitivity to heat shock is a function of their position in the cell cycle but heat-injured cells are capable of repairing sublethal and potentially lethal damage. (Hahn, G., 1974)

Inactivation curves showing duration of hyperthermic shock versus logarithm of surviving fraction have a shape similar to that for X-ray killing, i.e., a shoulder, followed by an approximately linear portion of the survival curve.

The results indicate that the cells in solid tumors that are most difficult to kill with conventional radio-therapy or chemotherapy may be those most readily eliminated by hyperthermia. Data indicate that elevated temperatures (39-43° C) increase the sensitivity of the cells to at least low-dose-rate X-irradiation and probably to some chemotherapeutic agents. One of the important mechanisms of cell death is probably protein denaturation, observed at temperature above 40 °C, leading to changes in enzyme complexes for DNA synthesis and repair as well as alterations in structures like cytoskeleton and membranes. Heating cells at 42 °C for 10 minutes leads inhibition of DNA synthesis by 40 percent while, this figure amounts to 90 percent at 45 °C for 15 minutes. Heat can induce cell death in non-dividing cells by activation of various enzymes. Heat also affects cell membrane, a target not shared with ionizing radiation. Hypoxic cells, which are generally resistant to ionizing radiation, are sensitive to heat.

The cellular and molecular basis for this selective death of cancer cell has been studied. While inhibited RNA synthesis and mitosis arrest are reversible and nonselective results of hyperthermia, an increase in the number of lysosomes and lysosomal enzyme activity are selective effects in malignant cells. These heat-induced lysosomes are more labile in malignant cells and therefore result in increased destructive capacity. Furthermore, the microcirculation in most malignant tumors exhibits a decrease in blood flow or even complete vascular stasis in response to hyperthermia, which is in contrast to an increased flow capacity found in normal tissues. This, in combination with depression or complete inhibition of oxidative metabolism in tumour cells subjected to hyperthermia and unaltered anaerobic glycolysis, leads to accumulation of lactic acid and lower pH in the microenvironment of the malignant cell. (S. González-Moreno, et al, 2010)

Thus hyperthermia in the range of 42 °C-45 °C is good sensitizer of ionizing radiation. It is also shown to have synergistic effects with chemotherapy agents such as Bleomycin, Adriamycin and Platinol derivatives.

Increased perfusion due to warmer environment improves drug delivery to the tumor. It also ensures increased intracellular uptake of the drug as well as repair inhibition of DNA damage due to cytotoxic drugs. Combination of hyperthermia and chemotherapy also has shown decreased drug resistance. Interestingly an enhancement ratio of 23 was shown in cell lines when cell lines were treated with Melphalan and heat at 44 °C. (ACR 2008, ACR 2009).

Most of the biomolecules, especially regulatory proteins involved in cell growth and certain receptor molecules are largely influenced by hyperthermia. New insights from molecular biology have shown that a few minutes after hyperthermia, a special class of proteins are expressed into the cell, the so-called heat shock proteins (HSP). They protect the cell from further heating or subsequent thermal treatments and lead to an increase of cell survival after preheating, an effect called thermotolerance. Additionally, the activity of certain regulatory proteins is influenced by hyperthermia causes alterations in the cell cycle and can even induce apoptosis, the cell death driven by the cell regulatory system itself.

At tissue scale, primary malignant tumors have poor blood circulation, which makes them more vulnerable to changes in temperature (Habash 2006)

Cancer tissues accumulate lactic acid at an extremely increased glucose level, because cancer cells metabolize glucose to great extent into lactic acid, even in the presence of oxygen. This over-acidification makes the cancer cells more sensitive to hyperthermia. On the other hand, the normal cells are stabilized energetically by glucose in the presence of oxygen. Therefore, in a temperature range between 41.9 and 42.5 °C, the cancer cells are destroyed or at least damaged. The normal tissues of the organism, however, are not affected.

HT kills cells itself, implicates radiotherapy by inducing reoxygenation, increases delivery of liposomally encapsulated drugs and macromolecules such as monoclonal antibodies or polymeric peptides, enhances cellular effects of chemotherapeutics and augments immune reactions against the tumor due to thermotolerance mediated by heat shock proteins (HSPs) (Mayerson, 2004).

The generation of free radicals by hyperthermia treatment (HT) in the membrane or cytoplasm of cancer cells, results in peroxidation of intracellular polyunsaturated fatty acids (PUFA), and is considered to be an important source of antitumor activity.

6. Thermal and electrical properties of tissue

	Relative Permitivity	Conductivity [S/m]
Muscle	62.8	0.72
Bone	14.6	0.068
Marrow	6.2	0.024
Skin	63.5	0.53
Blood	72.2	1.25
Tumor	74	0.89
Rest (high water content but includes some fat)	40	0.4

Table 1. Electrical properties of human tissues

	Mass Density [kg/m^3]	Thermal Conductivity [W/(m °C)]	Specific Heat [W/(kg °C)]
Muscle	1047	0.45	3550
Bone	1990	0.29	970
Marrow	1040	0.45	3550
Skin	1125	0.31	3000
Blood	1058	0.49	3550
Tumor	1047	0.55	3560
Rest (high water content but includes some fat)	1020	0.4	3200

Table 2. Thermal properties of human tissues.

7. Definition of radiofrequency, range of frequencies in hyperthermia

Designation	Frequency	Approximate wavelength
Radiofrequency (RF)	100 kHz	1000 m
	1 MHz	100 m
	10 MHz	10 m
	100 MHz	1 m
Microwave	1 GHz	10 cm
X-ray		

Table 3. Concise and approximate definition of frequency ranges in electromagnetic waves.

8. Treatment types: Local, regional, whole body

Depending on the organ bearing the cancerous tissue, stage of cancer development and method of energy delivery to patient's body, three kinds of hyperthermia techniques are recognized. This brings about various equipments and treatment works. These types are:
- Local hyperthermia
- Regional hyperthermia
- Whole-body hyperthermia

9. Local hyperthermia

Primary malignant tumors before the metastases stage are treated with local hyperthermia. Treatment is performed with superficial applicators of different shapes and kinds such as waveguide, spiral and current sheet placed on the surface of superficial tumors with an intervening layer called bolus. Energy sources could be RF, microwave, or ultrasound. When ultrasound is used, the technique is called high intensity focused ultrasound (HIFU). Heat is applied to a small area such as a tumor. The penetration depth depends on the frequency and size of the applicator; the clinical range is typically not more than 3–4 cm and the area is less than 50 cm². In local hyperthermia temperature rises to 42°C for one hour within a cancer tumor, hence the cancer cells will be destroyed.

There are several approaches to local hyperthermia including (ACS, 2009; NCI, 2004):
- External/Superficial: external applicator is used to deliver energy to the tumor below the skin
- Intraluminal or endocavitary: used to treat tumors within or near body cavities (e.g., rectum and esophagus) with placement of radiative probes inside the cavity.
- Interstitial: used to treat tumors deep within the body (e.g., brain tumors) with the use of anesthesia to place probes or needles into the tumor to deliver energy.

Candidates for local hyperthermia include chest wall recurrences, superficial malignant melanoma lesions, and lymph node metastases of head and neck tumors. Therapeutic depth is highly limited in regions with irregular surface, such as the head and neck (Habash et al, 2006)

10. Regional hyperthermia

For large, deeply seated, and inoperable tumors, regional hyperthermia is used. Cervical and bladder cancer are of this type. Another example is treatment of a part of the body, such as a limb, organ, or body cavity.   In regional hyperthermia external applicators using microwave or radiofrequency energy are positioned around the body cavity or organ to be treated. (JJW Lagendijk et al, 1998).

A sub-group of regional hyperthermia is regional perfusion which is used to treat cancers in the arms and legs (e.g., melanoma) or cancers in some organs (e.g., liver and lung). Some of the patient's blood is removed, heated, and then pumped or perfused back into the limb or organ. Anticancer drugs are usually administered during this treatment.

Another kind of regional hyperthermia, hyperthermic intraperitoneal chemotherapy (HIPEC), also referred to as intraperitoneal hyperthermic chemotherapy (IPHC), has been proposed as an alternative for the treatment of cancers within the peritoneal cavity, including primary peritoneal mesothelioma and gastric cancer. The HIPEC is applied during surgery, via an open or closed abdominal approach. The heated chemolytic agent is infused into the peritoneal cavity, raising the temperature of the tissues within the cavity to 41-42ºC. (ACS 2009)

Whole Body Hyperthermia (WBH): WBH, achieved with either radiant heat or extracorporeal technologies, elevates the temperature of the entire body to at least 41 °C. There are various techniques of heating systemically. Immersion in temperature controlled hot water bath and radiant heat with U.V. are the usual techniques for whole body hyperthermia.

In radiant WBH, heat is externally applied to the whole body using hot water blankets, hot wax, inductive coils, or thermal chambers. The patient is sedated throughout the WBH procedure, which lasts less than four hours. The patient reaches target temperature within approximately 1 hour, is maintained at 41.8 °C for one hour, and experiences a one-hour cooling phase. During treatment, the esophageal, rectal, skin and ambient air temperatures are monitored at 10-minute intervals. Small probes may be inserted into the tumor under a local anesthetic to monitor the temperature of the affected tissue and surrounding tissue. Heart rate, respiratory rate, and cardiac rhythm are continuously monitored. Patients are returned to regular situation in patient rooms after hyperthermia and discharged after 20–24 hours of observation (Robins, et al., 1997; Green, 1991).

Extracorporeal WBH is achieved by reinfusion of extracorporeally heated blood. A circuit of blood is created outside the body by accessing an artery, usually the femoral artery, and creating an extracorporeal loop. The circulating blood is passed through a heating device, usually a water bath or hot air, and the heated blood is then reinjected into a major vein. The desired body temperature is adjusted and controlled by changing the volume flow of the warmed reinfused blood (Wiedemann, et al., 1994).

Extracorporeal hyperthermia treatments are conducted under general anesthesia. To counteract the activation of coagulation by the hemodialyzer, high-dose heparin is administered. An extracorporeal WBH treatment session typically lasts four hours. Target temperature is reached in two hours and is maintained for one hour, followed by a cooling period of one hour. Subsequently, the patient is infused with normal saline to maintain systolic blood pressure above 100 mm Hg. The patient is then monitored weekly for complications (Kerner, et al., 2002; Wiedemann, et al., 1994).

11. Treatment planning and simulation

Due to varying tumor location and geometry and different size and shape of patients, individual therapy planning is necessary. The first step of hyperthermia treatment planning is the generation of a patient model by segmentation of images from computerized tomography (CT) or magnetic resonance imaging (MRI) scans. In some cases, online parameter identification based on MRI is performed. A model of the applicator and this segmentation are used to calculate the power absorption (PA, [W/m3]) or specific absorption rate (SAR, [W/kg]) distribution in the patient by electromagnetic models. These EM models for treatment planning are commonly based on the finite-element (FE) method or finite-difference time-domain (FDTD) method. A temperature distribution in the patient can be calculated from the power absorption distribution by applying Pennes' bio-heat equation (PBHE), or more elaborate algorithms including the blood vessel network, i.e. discrete vasculature (DIVA) models, down to vessel sizes in the millimeter range. The main problems with these thermal methods are long time-requirements for the generation of a vessel network and the large, poorly-predictable, variations in thermal properties of tissues. The target in treatment planning is to heat a particular tumor and delivering at least 43°C to 90% of its volume for cumulative in multiple treatments for longer than 10 minutes corresponds to doubling of the probability for complete response and duration of response to hyperthermia and radiotherapy versus radiotherapy alone (Oleson et al. 1993).

The thermal iso-effect dose is an established quantity for assessing the therapeutic benefit of a treatment. As for now CEM 43°C T90 (cumulative equivalent minutes at a standard targeted treatment temperature of 43°C obtained within 90% of the tumour volume) appears to be the most useful dosimetric parameter in clinical research. Treatment planning based on the tumor cell survival has been proposed for thermoseed placement , but up to now rather ad hoc cost functional based on the temperature distribution or on the absorption rate density have been used for regional hyperthermia. (J. van der Zee et al 2007)

In local-regional hyperthermia therapy planning using RF as the heat source the therapeutically optimal antenna parameters for the applicator are determined for each patient. The specific absorption rate values are obtained by solving the Maxwell equations, and the temperature distribution is predicted by variants of the bio-heat transfer equation. Although this can be a demanding task, a planning tool greatly improves the medical treatment quality with a virtual experiment to model, simulate and optimize the therapy with high precision.[J Crezee et al. 2005]

12. Motivations for simulation

-    Provide better heating through treatment preplanning.
-    Optimize setups for treatment cases.
-    Assist new applicator design in the future.

On the other hand, the perfusion depends on the temperature due to autoregulation capabilities of the tissue. Moreover, at least in abdominal hyperthermia, the systemic thermoresponse seems to play a significant role. Different perfusion models have been proposed, covering a broad spectrum of homogenized and discrete vascular models.

A mathematical model of the clinical system (radio frequency applicator with 8 antennas, water bolus, individual patient body) involves Maxwell's equations in inhomogeneous media and a so–called bio–heat transfer PDE describing the temperature distribution in the human body. The electromagnetic field and the thermal phenomena need to be computed at a speed suitable for the clinical environment.

Finaly, in all treatment planning works an upper bound is imposed on the temperature: T <Tlim . Typical values for Tlim are 44 C for muscle, fat, and bone tissues, and 42 C for more sensitive organs such as bladder or intestine. (M. Weiser, 2008).

13. Instrumentation: Applicator, bolus, temperature measurement and monitoring

Hyperthermia can be applied by whole-body, external or interstitial/intracavitary techniques (applicators). External HT applicators use ultrasound (US) or electromagnetic (EM) waves to direct energy to the target region. US provides similar heating options as EM but results in more bone-pain complaints during treatment (Ben-Yosef et al. 1995).

In general, two types of probes are required in hyperthermia. One to deliver energy to the tissue, another to monitor the tissue temperature. The temperature in the tumor is measured by temperature sensors during the treatment. The temperature is then optimized continuously using automatic computer-controlled regulation of the applicator power output. Commercially Available Thermometer probes are :

Thermocouples
Thermistors
Non-perturbing probes
Thermistor sensor with high-resistance plastic leads containing graphite
Optical fibres
Liquid Crystal sensor
Birefringent sensor of LiNbO3
Fluorescent-type sensor made of two phosphorus
Semiconductor crystal, gallium-arsenide (GaAs) as a temperature sensor
Multichannel systems with non-perturbing multisensor probes
Multi-GaAs-sensors as a linear array with up to 8 sensor points in one probe
Multiple fluorescent phosphor sensors
Multiple thermistor sensors with high-resistance leads

Non-invasive thermometry

- Microwave multi-frequency Radiometry
- Computerized tomography (CT) for thermometry in vivo
- Nuclear Magnetic Resonance (NMR)
- Electrical impedance tomography (EIT)

The thermometers based on optical fibers offer the advantage of not possessing metallic components, and therefore they do not disturb the electromagnetic fields

The probe that delivers energy to the patient's body, usually referred to as applicator, ordinarily is in touch with skin. Every applicator includes a bolus which is placed on the patient's skin. For treatment, this bolus is filled with circulating water that can be heated as necessary. The bolus serves to physically couple the electromagnetic waves to the patient's body, and hence reduce the reflection and waste of energy.

Heating could be capacitive or inductive. Heating could be with external antennae or with interstitial and intracavitory probes. Intracellular heating with ferromagnetic material subjected to alternating magnetic field can also generate localized heating. RF at

8-12 MHz is useful for heating of the deep-seated tumor while, microwave heating at 434 MHz to 915 MHz is useful in surface tumors. Heating with ultrasound is also feasible. Mechanical ultrasonic waves delivered at 0.2-5MHz and can effectively heat a small volume at various depth.

In case of shallow tumors, the energy source is microwave 915 MHz generator. Commonly, it has eight channels, with phase and amplitude of each adjustable individually. Using a three-way splitter up to 24 antennas can be powered. The eight signals from the individual channels (each capable of delivering up to 50 watts) can be combined to provide a total output of up to 400 watts.

In order to deliver an optimal therapy, the phased array applicator needs to be controlled in such a way that the tumor is maximally heated without damaging healthy tissue by excessive temperatures. Pain and unpredictable heat deposition at tissue bone or tissue air cavity can be a limiting technological factor. Scanning transducers can overcome this difficulty. Ultrasound heating, unlike imaging has not gained popular use in the clinic.

14. Clinical techniques

Hyperthermia is mostly applied within a department of radiation oncology under the authority of a radiation oncologist and a medical physicist. It is always implemented as part of a multimodal, oncological treatment strategy, i.e., in combination with radiotherapy or chemotherapy. (Habash 2006).

In a hyperthermia clinic, the treatment starts with a comprehensive medical consultation with previous medical-imaging reports such as sonographics, X-rays, CTs, MRIs, nuclear medical images. If further examinations would be prescribed if necessary.

Depending on the indications, the hyperthermia treatment is given once or twice a week. Due to thermotolerance a general phenomenon pertaining to transient resistance to additional heat stress, it is impractical to apply two different HT sessions with an interval shorter than 48–72 hours, until the resistance decays to a negligible level. Total number of sessions depends on the tumor characteristics and varies between 5 and 10 per patient. chemotherapy is administered concurrently; radiation therapy must closely precede or follow the hyperthermia treatment by up to 120 minutes.

First, the patient is placed in a horizontal position. The temperature sensors are affixed to the skin above the tumor or inserted into the tissue through an implantable catheter. The number of temperature sensors used depends on the size of the tumor. The applicator, which is selected on the basis of the size and location of the tumor lesion, is held in the treatment position with the aid of either a support arm or holding straps.

On the day of main treatment, patients come at 8:00 to the hyperthermia-clinic with an empty stomach (on the day prior to the treatment, eating is permitted until 8:00 p.m. and drinking until midnight), a premedication (a sedative injection) is given in the morning before plus the attachment of an indwelling bladder catheter.

During an approximately 60-minute controlled infusion period, still at normal body temperature, the blood glucose level is increased by the three to four-fold of the initial value (by continuing the infusion during the TCHT main treatment, the blood glucose level attains a five to six-fold level of the initial value). Then, the body-warming-up process (hyperthermia) begins at approximately the same time as a moderate anaesthesia (neuroleptic analgesia at maintained spontaneous respiration; intratrachial intubation only if neccessary) which acts over a time frame of approximately 6 hours. By means of infrared-A (short-wave part of the infrared spectrum) the body-core temperature is raised to 42.0°C (107.6 °F) within about 90 to 120 minutes. The chemotherapy is administered during the warming-up phase just before the body reaches 42.0°C

In the following so-called temperature-plateau-phase, a main body temperature of 42.0°C to 42.5°C is constantly maintained over 60 to 90 minutes. The cooling-off phase lasts for approximately another 90 to 120 minutes and uses the same monitoring measures as the warming-up and the plateau phase. An anti-emetic (a means to reduce vomiting) is added to the infusion during the last phase.

During the TCHT main treatment, lasting altogether approx. 8 hours, two doctors and two nurses are constantly at the patient's side(one doctor and a nurse continuously during the night and the next morning) then the patient will be transferred to the adjoining intensive care unit, an intensive care phase follows. The next morning at about midday the patient will be transferred by an accompanying doctor to the convenient private hospital to recover. For about 5 days the patients need infusions and medicines for recovery and initial daily blood sampling.

In a detailed report which you will take along, we recommend the follow-up checks as an outpatient later at the home town.

To make a general sense of external hyperthermia using RF, one could say the heat session is started by applying 80 W of total power with the power and phase control system (Bakker *et al* 2010), using the optimized phase and power settings from HTP.

Power is increased subsequently in steps of 30W, usually around one step per minute, till one of the tolerance limits is reached (40 °C in myelum indicative, 60Wkg–1 in myelum predicted by HTP, 43 °C in other tissues) or the occurrence of a hot spot indicated by the patient at a site without thermometry. Two phases of a treatment are defined for data analysis: (1) 'warm-up phase' and (2) 'plateau-phase', and the transition is assumed to be always after 15 min of heating.

The increased oxygen saturation in the blood results in a stabilization of the cardiac functions, the circulatory system, the respiratory system and the central nervous system. Some cytostatics act better in an acid environment, so that the efficacy of chemotherapy can be increased through overacidification of the tumor. Hyperthermia itself also increases the efficacy of some cytostatics. Some side effects of chemotherapy can be alleviated by relative hyperoxemia. On the basis of this complex interaction, an individually adapted chemotherapy in combination with the hyperthermia is highly effective and, in general, well tolerated.

External local hyperthermia is utilized or heating of small areas (usually up to 50 cm2) to treat tumors in or just below the skin up to 4 cm. This can be used alone or in combination with radiation therapy for the treatment of patients with primary or metastatic cutaneous or subcutaneous superficial tumors (such as superficial recurrent melanoma, chest wall recurrence of breast cancer, and cervical lymph node metastases from head and neck cancer). Heat is usually applied using high-frequency energy waves generated from a source outside the body (such as a microwave or ultrasound source).

Intraluminal or endocavitary methods may be used to treat tumors within or near body cavities. Endocavitary antennas are inserted in natural openings of hollow organs. These include (1) gastrointestinal (esophagus, rectum), (2) gynecological (vagina, cervix, and uterus), (3) genitourinary (prostate, bladder), and (4) pulmonary (trachea, bronchus). Very localized heating is possible with this technique by inserting an endotract electrode into lumens of the human body to deliver energy and heat the area directly.

The transient phase of heat distribution in patient's body takes about 15 minutes, while the duration of a single treatment session is about two hours. For this reason, usually only the steady state of the temperature distribution is optimized, which results in a significantly simpler optimization task.

Hyperthermia is most effective when the area being treated is kept within an exact temperature range for a defined period of time without affecting nearby tissues. This is challenging since not all body tissues respond in the same way to heat. Small thermometers on the ends of probes are placed in the treatment areas to monitor the desired temperature. Magnetic resonance imaging (MRI) is proposed as a replacement of the probes to monitor the temperature (ACS, 2009).

The following measures are taken in order to intensively monitor all the body functions. Two peripheral venous accesses in the form of flexible soft-tip catheters are attached for infusions, intravenous injections and blood sampling. The painless localization of the thermometric probes (rectal, axillary, as well as on the skin of the stomach and the back), of the pulse oxymeter (on the right middle finger) and of the ECG miniature adhesive electrodes complete the intensive medical monitoring. During the whole treatment time, the ECG and oxygen saturation are very closely observed and all the relevant parameters are monitored by means of blood samples every 15 minutes. Continuous blood pressure measurements as well as regular blood-gas analysis are monitored. In this way possible deviations are recognised and corrected early. Serious disturbances can thus be averted to the greatest possible extent.

15. Case studies

In a study involving 109 patients with superficial tumors, patients mostly suffering from breast wall recurrence due to mammary carcinoma, the enhancement effect of hyperthermia in combination with radiation therapy was demonstrated. Previously irradiated patients who underwent a second round of radiation therapy in conjunction with hyperthermia responded significantly better to this therapy. Complete remission was achieved in 68% of those treated with hyperthermia plus radiation while in the control group who did not receive hyperthermia, complete remission was observed in only 24% of the patients. (Jones, E.2005)

The effectiveness of hyperthermia treatment in cases of advanced head and neck tumors has been confirmed (R. Valdagni and M. Amichetti 1994). With radiation therapy alone, complete remission was achieved in 41% of patients, while the combination of radiation therapy and hyperthermia increased the remission rate to 83%. In addition, the 5-year survival rate for these patients was increased from zero to 53% from the addition of hyperthermia to radiation therapy.

There are nearly 24 randomized studies reported to which 18 have reported a positive benefit in combining hyperthermia with radiation. Patients with cervical nodes were randomized to radiation alone to a dose of 64-70 Gy and radiation with hyperthermia. Hyperthermia was delivered twice a week. The initial response was reported to have improved from 41% to 83% with a 5 year overall local control increasing from 245 to 69% and survival from none to 53%9. Addition of hyperthermia to radiation in cancer of cervix was reported to have improved outcome as compared to radiation (N. G. Huilgol)

Bladder cancer at various stages was studied for 358 patients from 1990 to 1996. Patients were divided to two groups. One group underwent radiotherapy (median total dose 65 Gy) alone (n=176) another group radiotherapy plus hyperthermia (n=182). Complete-response rates were 39% after radiotherapy and 55% after radiotherapy plus hyperthermia. The duration of local control was significantly longer with radiotherapy plus hyperthermia than with radiotherapy alone. The 3-year overall survival was 27% in the radiotherapy group and 51% in the radiotherapy plus hyperthermia group (Van der Zee 2000).

For ovarian cancer, in vitro studies have shown that hyperthermia produces a dose-enhancement effect (i.e. a thermal enhancement ratio of approximately 3 for a 60 min heat exposure) besides, it is shown that hyperthermia can overcome acquired drug resistance . (A.M.Westerman 2001)

Around 70% of all initial responders to chemotherapy make no improvement and subsequently require additional therapy. The classic treatment includes aggressive tumor reductive surgery (TRS) followed by platinum based combination chemotherapy, using cisplatin or carboplatin combined with a taxane. As an adjunct to traditional therapy, hyperthermia has been shown to enhance cisplatin cytotoxicity. Mild hyperthermia (39–43°C) has successfully been utilized in combination with chemotherapy to increase cellular sensitivity to anticancer drugs mainly using an intraperitoneal approach. The interaction between heat and chemotherapeutic agents results in increased drug uptake by accelerating the primary step in a drug's efficacy and increasing the intracellular drug concentration. Therefore, the combination of hyperthermia and anti-cancer drugs may reduce the required effective dose of the anti-cancer drug, and it could enhance the response rates in ovarian cancer cells. (Amber P. et al, 2007)

Local recurrence rates of breast cancer after mastectomy alone have been reported as high as 45%. This high rate of failure can be reduced to 2–15% with the addition of postmastectomy radiation therapy (PMRT) and usually chemotherapy as well, with a corresponding improvement in overall survival. With its radiosensitizing properties, hyperthermia presumably lowers the radiation dose needed to achieve durable local control, which in turn has potential implications for decreased long-term toxicities in patients with a prior history of radiotherapy. The addition of concurrent chemotherapy to hyperthermia and radiation therapy, constituting thermochemoradiotherapy (ThChRT)), has been evaluated in phase I/II trials by several researchers and found to be well-tolerated, with moderate success. (Timothy M. Zagar et al 2010)

16. Side effects

The possible side effects of hyperthermia depend of the technique being used and the part of the body being treated. Pain, thermal burns or blisters are the limiting adverse events of the techniques. Fewer side effects are observed with improvement in technology along with better skills and improved technology (ACS, 2009; ECRI, 2007). Post surgical site may be more susceptible to heat due to poorly vascularised state. Skin and subcutaneous tissues are generally susceptible to increased power deposition when heated with microwave and radiofrequency waves. Thermal burns which are superficial and generally heal quickly are seen in 2-15% of the patients (N. G. Huilgol)

In case of thermochemotherapy (TCHT) during the first days after the main treatment, the occurrence of fever up to 39 °C can be observed as an expression of a strong

immunostimulation and is desirable in most cases. At this time, though, exhaustion, weakness,
Nausea, vomiting, headaches, diarrhoea and herpes labialis (blisters on the lips) can also occur.
Cases requiring treatment are, however, observed in less than 3 % of the therapies.
In rare single cases after TCHT treatment, an increased amount of oncolytical products can lead to an overstrain of the excretory mechanism (liver, kidney). As a consequence, temporary jaundice (icterus) as well as an increase of the liver and kidney values may occur. Although the side effects of most of the cytostatics are milder than those of conventional chemotherapy, toxic effects of isolated cytostatics caused by the TCHT are observed in very few cases. Temporary functional disturbances of the peripheral nerves can, though, occur with temporary strength reductions.
During the TCHT main treatment, a moderate anaesthesia is given. The patient is unable to drive for at least three days after the main treatment. In the following days, due to various reasons (e.g. after-effects of the chemotherapy or additional medications), reaction times can be deteriorated and, therefore, driving ability is considerably limited. Most of these side effects are temporary.

17. Engineering aspects of hyperthermia: Modeling, computation of temperature distribution, computer applications

Energy absorption in cancerous tissue provides heat required for temperature increase. Predominantly, electromagnetic waves in various frequency ranges are utilized. Thus, Maxwell's equations must be solved for the specific geometry with estimated electrical properties at the given anatomy. This computation process leads to SAR (Specific Absorption Rate) in Watts per unit mass of tissue. Then heat transfer equation must be solved to reproduce the temperature distribution in cancerous tissue and the adjacent healthy tissue. In contrast to RF ablation and focused ultrasound therapies, electrical and thermal properties of tissue do not change significantly over 37 - 45 temperature range. For this reason, these values are simply taken as constants depending only on tissue type.
Due to irregular geometry, modeling errors for computing the electrical field exists. Thus, even accurate solution of Maxwell's equations will not provide the actual electrical field. As a reliable tool, MRI can be used for monitoring the temperature distribution and identification of the applicator parameters. The 3D voxel data can be obtained approximately every other minute from proton resonance frequency shifts.
When using RF as the energy source, a time-harmonic electrical interference field is generated by a phased array of antennas which can be controlled individually by variations in amplitude and phase of each source.(M. Werser 2008).
A system for local hyperthermia consists of a generator, control computer applicator, and a scheme to measure temperature in the tumor. The therapy system is controlled automatically by the computer, which can be operated either via a touchscreen or by means of a mouse and keyboard.
To produce a visualization of the model from the patient's anatomy, the computer in clinic is equipped with GPU (Graphical Processing Unit). The GPU is the heart of a graphics card. Due to the application in multibillion game market, GPUs have quickly evolved into powerful devices available at a low price. This makes them attractive not only for graphics of video games, but also for scientific computing. GPUs are so fast because they are inherently parallel: while CPUs have 2 to 4 cores, GPUs have up to 128 arithmetic units.

18. Application of nanoparticles in hyperthermia

The difficulty in limiting heating close to the tumor region without damaging the healthy tissue is a technical challenge in hyperthermia. The use of magnetic nanoparticles can overcome the difficulty in spatial adjusting of power absorption by cancerous tissue. Application of magnetic materials in hyperthermia was first proposed in 1957 (Gilchrist R. K., et al. 1957)

Magnetic induction hyperthermia is a technique for destroying cancer cells with the use of a magnetic field. The temperature of the cancer tissue can be raised in the range of 42–46 C, by indirect heating produced by various magnetic materials introduced into the tumor. Depending on increase in temperature, cell damage (necrosis) or even its direct destruction (thermoablation) may be promoted.

A large number of magnetic materials for magnetic induction hyperthermia have been developed. The major part of ferro-, ferri-, as well as superparamagnetic materials are suitable for this specific application. An important requirement of all these materials is biocompatibility. MgO-Fe is common material of choice in recent research.

The heating capacity depends on the material properties, such as magnetocrystalline anisotropy, particles size and microstructure. To enable them to penetrate into smallest part of every tissue or even into cancer cell, magnetic material is made with nanometer size, called magnetic nanoparticle (MNP).

Cancerous cells typically have diameters of 10 to 100 micrometers. This has produced the motivation to use MNP to penetrate into a cell.

The particles used in hyperthermia exhibit ferro- or ferrimagnetic properties. These particles have permanent magnetic orientations or moments and some kinds display magnetism even in the absence of an applied magnetic field (Pankhurst et al.).

Magnetic nanoparticles are designed to selectively be absorbed in tumor. Once in the tumor, they agitate under an alternating magnetic field and generate heat within tumor. Heat generation is due to different magnetic loss processes such as moment relaxation (Ne´ el), mechanical rotation, (Brown) or domain wall displacements), leading to the destruction of the tumor, whereas most of the normal tissue remains relatively unaffected.

Particles with diameters of 10 nanometers or less typically demonstrate superparamagnetic properties. The magnetic moments of superparamagnetic nanoparticles are randomly reoriented by the thermal energy of their environment and do not display magnetism in the absence of a magnetic field. Unlike ferro- and ferrimagnetic materials, they do not aggregate after exposure to an external magnetic field (Berry and Curtis). Aggregation can hinder the body's efforts to remove the nanoparticles. Therefore, superparamagnetic nanoparticles are ideal candidates for hyperthermia cancer treatment.

Nanoparticles can also effectively cross the blood-brain barrier, an essential step in treating brain tumors (Koziara et al.). Finally, nanoparticles can be coupled with viruses (20-450 nm), proteins (5-50 nm), and genes (10-100 nm long) (Pankhurst et al.).

In practice, MNP is introduced into patient's body by injecting a fluid containing magnetic nanoparticles. This technique is called Magnetic fluid hyperthermia (MFH). When placed in an alternating magnetic field with frequencies in tens to hundreds MHz, MNP begin to agitate and produce enough heat inside the tumor. In this technique, only the magnetic nanoparticles absorb the magnetic field. No heat generation in healthy tissue is the advantage of this technique over other hyperthermia techniques such as laser, microwave, and ultrasound.

Magnetic nanoparticles are evenly dispersed in water or a hydrocarbon fluid. Small size of dissolved particles leads to little or no precipitation due to gravitational forces. For medical applications, the biocompatibility of both the fluid and nanoparticles must be considered. The fluid must have a neutral pH and physiological salinity. In addition, the magnetic material should not be toxic. The established biocompatibility of magnetite (Fe3O4) makes it a common choice.

The heating ability of MNPs is expressed by the specific absorption rate (SAR), which is equal to the power loss per material mass. Generally, it is advantageous to achieve the temperature enhancement needed for any application with as low as possible MNPs concentration. For a specific nanoparticle system, SAR is directly related to the applied field amplitude and frequency as well as to geometrical (size, shape) and structural features of the particle. Although various magnetic nanomaterials present high SAR values, the demand for low MNPs concentration and biocompatibility issues restricts significantly materials choice. An alternate route towards larger SAR values is expected to be the enhancement of magnetic moment per particle, e.g. the use of Fe particles coated by a biocompatible shell such as MgO , instead of iron oxides, besides the higher magnetization, it also provides a satisfactory solution to the problem of chemical stability and biocompatibility. Water soluble Fe/MgO nanoparticle is the basis of magnetic hyperthermia. The use of zero-valence iron particles, instead of iron oxides, provides improved magnetization values while the MgO coating serves as a satisfactory solution for the achievement of chemical stability and biocompatibility. The non-toxicity of magnesium-based materials, their corrosion resistance and antimicrobial action are fields of intense research. (A. Chalkidou, et al. 2011) and (O. Bretcanu, et al, 2006)

19. Hyperthermia in combination with other modalities

As an adjunct to traditional cancer therapy, hyperthermia has been shown to enhance cytotoxicity of chemotherapy agents. Since adequate heating of the whole tumor volume is difficult except for superficially located small tumors, and in general the reported response duration is short, the use of hyperthermia alone is not recommended (van der Zee, et al., 2008). Mild hyperthermia (39–43°C) has successfully been utilized in combination with chemotherapy to increase cellular sensitivity to anticancer drugs mainly using an intraperitoneal approach. The interaction between heat and chemotherapeutic agents results in increased drug uptake by accelerating the primary step in a drug's efficacy and increasing the intracellular drug concentration. Therefore, the combination of hyperthermia and anti-cancer drugs may reduce the required effective dose of the anti-cancer drug, and it could enhance the response rates in cancer cells. The results of combined application of chemotherapy and hyperthermia has been satisfactory .

The thermo-chemotherapy (TCHT) is a combined modality treatment with high tolerance for malignant tumors of the mammary gland, of the whole gastric intestinal tract (specially pancreatic cancer), of the lungs, of the urogenital tract (specially ovarian-cancer), of the skin, bones and soft-tissues as well as oral and neck advanced malignant tumors (specially node metastasis). In principle, adenocarcinoma and squamous epithelium carcinoma with metastasis (as well bone metastasis) or without metastasis, osteo sarcoma and soft-tissue sarcoma of nearly all localisations, the malignant melanoma and non-Hodgkin lymphoma and also pleural malignant mesothelioma can be treated. The TCHT main treatment, which lasts several hours, is followed by approximately 24 hours of intensive care treatment in the specially equipped hyperthermia-clinic.

The treatment itself is based on a controlled interaction between whole-body hyperthermia (body warming-up), induced hyperglycaemia (increasing of the blood glucose level), relative hyperoxemia (oxygen enrichment of the blood) and pre-arranged with the patient modified chemotherapy. Thanks to this multistep therapy, one has the chance to positively influence the course of the illness - even when tumors have not previously responded to radiotherapy, to cytostatics or to hormones.

20. A brief overview of important softwares

In order to permit a patient–specific treatment planning, a special software system (HyperPlan) has been developed.

COMSOL is a general purpose software to compute electromagnetic fields interaction with matter.

SEMCAD X takes the segmentation and a CAD implementation of applicators as input and tissue and material properties are assigned to the solid models. With a proper set-up, the electric fields for each antenna are calculated using the electromagnetic solver of SEMCAD X.

The position of tumor in the patient's body along with neighboring organs and tissues can be reconstructed by Ansoft Human-Body Model. The accuracy of this software is at millimeter level. There are more than 300 objects defined in this model including bones, muscles and organs. Frequency-dependent material parameters are included as well.

21. Prospects

-   Heating deep seated tumors effectively still remains an unsolved technical problem.
-   Hyperthermia may find additional indications in gene therapy, stem cell purging, drug targeting with heat sensitive liposomes and potentiation of immunity in HIV.
-   The reliability of the mathematical optimization depends on the accuracy of the models describing the physical situation. In particular the physiological parameters are individually varying to a significant amount, such that a priori models are subject to significant modelling errors.
-   The physical processes of field interference and heat distribution inside the very heterogeneous human body is too complex to be optimized manually. Thus, optimization algorithms are required for therapy planning,

22. Conclusion

Although basically an old and historic approach for treatment of cancer, hyperthermia is not a well-known modality among patients and medical experts. On the other hand, it has proved a very successful therapy method in combination with radiation therapy and / or chemotherapy. The precise mechanism of cancer development and destruction is not known; especially the response of different patients at similar situation is quite unpredictable. At clinical stage, the mathematics behind the treatment planning is difficult to implement for complicated geometry of tumor. The heat transfer and SAR parameters are not identical among patients. Up to the best knowledge of authors of this chapter, these parameters might not be measured with a proper precision, especially at clinical practice.

23. References

AAPM Report No. 27, Hyperthermia Treatment Planning, Report of Task Group No. 2, Hyperthermia Committee , August 1989.

American Cancer Society (ACS). (2009). Hyperthermia. Updated July 17, 2009. Available at URL address:
http://www.cancer.org/docroot/ETO/content/ETO_1_2x_Hyperthermia.asp

American College of Radiology (ACR). (2008). ACR Appropriateness Criteria. Recurrent Rectal Cancer. Available at URL address:
http://www.acr.org/secondarymainmenucategories/quality_safety/app_criteria.aspx

American College of Radiology (ACR). (2009). ACR Practice Guideline for Radiation Oncology. Available at URL address:
http://www.guideline.gov/summary/summary.aspx?ss=15&doc_id=9611&nbr=5 131

Barnes, A. P.; Miller, B. E.; Kucera, G. L. (2007). Cyclooxygenase Inhibition and Hyperthermia for the Potentiation of the Cytotoxic Response in Ovarian Cancer Cells. *Gynecologic Oncology*, Vol. 104, pp. 443–450.

Ben-Yosef, R.; Kapp D. S. (1995). Direct Clinical Comparison of Ultrasound and Radiative Electromagnetic Hyperthermia in the same Tumors. *Int J Hyperthermia*, Vol. 11, pp. 1–10.

Bretcanu, O.; Verne, E.; Coisson, M.; Tiberto, P.; Allia, P. (2006). Magnetic Properties of the Ferrimagnetic Glass-ceramics for Hyperthermia, *Journal of Magnetism and Magnetic Materials* Vol. 305, pp. 529–533.

Bush W. Uber den Finfluss wetchen heftigere Eryspelen zuweilen auf organlsierte Neubildungen dusuben. Verh Natruch Preuss Rhein Westphal. 1886;23:28–30.

Cavalieri, R.; Ciocatto, E. C.; Giovanella, B. C.; Heidelberger, C.; Johnson, R. O.; Margottini, M.; Mondovi, B.; Moricca, G.; & Rossi-Fanelli, A. (1967). Selective Heat Sensitivity of Cancer Cells. *Cancer*, Vol. 20, pp. 1351-1381.

Chichel, A.; Skowronek, J.; Kubaszewska, M.; Kanikowski, M. (2007). Hyperthermia – Description of a Method and a Review of Clinical Applications, *Reports on Practical Oncology and Radiotherapy*; Vol. 12 No.5, pp. 267-275.

Colombo, R.; Brausi, M.; Da Pozzo, L.; Salonia, A.; Montorsi, F.; Scattoni V, et al. (2001). Thermo-chemotherapy and Electromotive   Drug Administration of Mitomycin C in Superficial Bladder Cancer Eradication, A Pilot Study on Marker Lesion. *Eur Urol ;Vol.* 39, pp. 95–100.

Crezee, J.; Kok, H. P.; Wiersma, J.; Van Stam G.; Sijbrands, J.; Bel, A.; & Van Haaren P. M. A. (2005). Improving Loco-regional Hyperthermia Equipment using 3D Power Control: from AMC-4 to AMC-8. *Abstracts of the 22nd Annual Meeting of the ESHO, Graz, Austria (ESHO-05), pages 14–15, June 2005.*

Chalkidou, A.; Simeonidis, K.; Angelakeris, M.; Samaras, T.; Martinez-Boubeta, C.; Balcells, L.; Papazisis, K.; Dendrinou-Samara,C.; Kalogirou, O. (2011). In vitro Application of Fe/Mg on a Noparticles as Magnetically Mediated   Hyperthermia Agents for Cancer Treatment. *Journal of Magnetism and Magnetic Materials*, Vol. 323, pp. 775–780

Dudar T. E.; Jain R. K. (1984). Differential Response of Normal and Tumor Microcirculation to Hyperthermia. Cancer Research, Vol. 44, pp. 605-612.

Gilchrist R. K., et al. "Selective Inductive Heating of Lymph." Annals of Surgery 146 (1957) 596-606.

González-Moreno, S.; González-Bayón, L. A.; Ortega-Pérez, G. (2010). Hyperthermic Intraperitoneal Chemotherapy: Rationale and Technique. *World Journal of Gastrointestinal Oncology*, Vol. 2, No. 2, pp. 68-75.

Green I. ; Hyperthermia in Conjunction with Cancer Chemotherapy. (1991). *Health Technology Assessment, No. 2.* Rockville, MD; U.S. Department of Health and Human Services, Public Health Service, Agency for Health Care Policy and Research. Available at URL address: http://www.ahcpr.gov/clinic/hypther2.htm

Habash, R. W. Y.; Bansal, R.; Krewski, D.; Alhafid, H. T. (2006). Thermal Therapy, Part 2: Hyperthermia Techniques, *Critical Reviews in Biomedical Engineering*, Vol. 34, No.6, pp. 491–542.

Hahn, G. M. (1974). Metabolic Aspects of the Role of Hyperthermia in Mammalian Cell Inactivation and Their Possible Relevance to Cancer Treatment. *Cancer Research*, Vol. 34, pp. 3117-3123.

Huilgol, N. G., Renaissance of Hyperthermia an Addition of a New Therapeutic Option, *Health Administrator* Vol. XVII, Number 1: 158-161,pg.

Hurwitz M. D. (2010). Today's Thermal Therapy: Not Your Father's Hyperthermia: Challenges and Opportunities in Application of Hyperthermia for the 21st Century Cancer Patient. *American Journal of Clinical Oncology*. Vol. 33, No. 1,(Feb. 2010), pp. 96-100.

Jones, E. (2005). A Randomized Trial of Hyperthermia and Radiation for Superficial Tumors. *Journal of Clinical Oncology*., Vol. 23, No. 13, 3079-3085.

Kerner, T.; Deja, M.; Ahlers, O.; Hildebrandt, B.; Dieing, A.; Riess, H. (2002). Monitoring Arterial Blood Pressure during whole Body Hyperthermia. *Acta Anaesthesiol Scand.* Vol. 46, No.5, pp. 561-6.

Koziara, J. M. et al. (2003). In Situ Blood-Brain Barrier Transport of Nanoparticles. *Pharmaceutical Research Vol.* 20, 1772-8.

Lagendijk, J. J. W.; Van Rhoon, G. C.; Hornsleth, S. N.; Wust, P.; De Leeuw, A. C.; Schneider, C. J.; Van Dijk, J. D.; Van Der Zee, J.; Van Heek-Romanowski, R.; Rahman, S. A.; & Gromoll, C. (1998). ESHO Quality Assurance Guidelines for Regional Hyperthermia. *International Journal of Hyperthermia*, Vol. 14, pp. 125–133.

Levine, E.M. & Robbins, E.B. (1969). Differential Temperature Sensitivity of Normal and Cancer Cells in Culture. *Journal of Cellular Physiology*. Vol. 76, pp. 373-380.

Oleson J. R.; Samulski, T.V.; Leopold, K. A. et al. (1993). Sensivity of Hyperthermia Trial Outcomes to Temperature and Time: Implications for Thermal Goals of Treatment. *International Journal of Radiatiation Oncology and Biological Physics* ; 25: 289–97

Pankhurst, Q. A., et al. (2003). Applications of Magnetic Nanoparticles in Biomedicine. *Journal of Physics D: Applied Physics*, Vol. 36, pp. R167-81.

Paulides, M. M.; Wielheesen, D.H.M.; Van der Zee, J.; Van Rhoon, G. C. (2005). Assessment of the Local SAR Distortion by Major Anatomical Structures in a Cylindrical Neck Phantom. *International Journal of Hyperthermia* Vol. 21, pp. 125-140.

Paulides, M. M.; Vossen, S.H.J.A.; Zwamborn, A.P.M.; Van Rhoon, G.C. (2005). Theoretical Investigation into the Feasibility to Deposit RF Energy Centrally in the Head and Neck Region. *International Journal of Radiation Oncology and Biological Physics*, Vol. 63, No. 2, pp. 634-642.

Paulides, M. M. (2007). Development of a Clinical Head and Neck Hyperthermia Applicator, Thesis, Erasmus University Rotterdam.

Robins H. I.; Rushing, D.; Kutz, M.; Tutsch, K. D.; Tiggelaar, C. L.; Paul, D. (1997). Phase I Clinical Trial of Melphalan and 41.8°C Whole-body Hyperthermia in Cancer Patients. *Journal of Clinical Oncology*, Vol. 15, No. 1, pp. 158-64.

Roemer, R. B. (1999). Engineering Aspects of Hyperthermia Therapy. *Annual Review of Biomedical Engineering*, Vol. 1, pp. 347-376.

Satoshi Kokura, Shuji Nakagawa, Taku Hara, Yoshio Boku, Yuji Naito, Norimasa Yoshida, Toshikazu Yoshikawa. (2002). Enhancement of Lipid Peroxidation and of the Antitumor Effect of Hyperthermia upon Combination with Oral Eicosapentaenoic Acid. *Cancer Letters*, Vol. 185, pp. 139-144.

Stauffer, P. R. & Goldberg S. N. (2004). Introduction: Thermal ablation therapy. *International Journal of Hyperthermia*, Vol. 20, No. 7, pp. 671-77.

Valdagni , R.; Amichetti, M. (1994). Report of Long-term Follow-up in a Randomized Trial Comparing Radiation Therapy and Radiation Therapy Plus Hyperthermia to Metastatic Lymph Nodes in Stage IV Head and Neck Patients. *International Journal of Radiatiation Oncology and Biological Physics.* Vol. 28, pp. 163-9.

Van der Zee, J.; de Bruijne, M.; Paulides, M.M.; Franckena, M.; Canters, R.; & Van Rhoon, G. C. (2007). The Use of Hyperthermia Treatment Planning in Clinical Practice, 8th International meeting on progress in radio-oncology ICRO / OGRO, 2007, Salzburg, Austria.

Van der Zee, J.; Gonzlez, D.; Van Rhoon G. C.; Van Dijk,J. D. P.; Van Putten, W. L. J.; Hart A. A. M. (2000). Comparison of Radiotherapy Alone with Radiotherapy Plus Hyperthermia in Locally Advanced Pelvic Tumors: a Prospective, Randomised, Multicentre Trial. *The Lancet*, Vol. 355,

Westermann, A. M. (2001). A Pilot Study of Whole Body Hyperthermia and Carboplatin in Platinum-resistant Ovarian Cancer. *European Journal of Cancer*, Vol. 37, pp. 1111-1117.

Westermark, F. (1898). Uber die Behandlung des ulcerirenden Cervix carcinoma mittels Knonstanter Warme. *Zentralbl Gynkol*, pp. 1335-9.

Weiser, M. (2008). Optimization and Identification in Regional Hyperthermia, ZIB-Report 08-40 (October 2008), Berlin, Germany.

Wiedemann G. J.; d'Oleire, F.; Knop, E.; Eleftheriadis, S.; Bucsky, P.; Feddersen, S.; et al. (1994). Ifosfamide and Carboplatin Combined with 41.8°C Whole-body Hyperthermia in Patients with Refractory Sarcoma and Malignant Teratoma. *Cancer Research*, Vol. 54, No. 20, pp. 5346-50.

Zagar, T. M.; Higgins, K. A.; Miles, E. F.; Vujaskovic, Z.; Dewhirst, M. W.; Clough, R. W.; Prosnitz, L. R.; Jones E. L. (2010). Durable Palliation of Breast Cancer Chest Wall Recurrence with Radiation Therapy, Hyperthermia, and Chemotherapy, *Radiotherapy and Oncology*, Vol. 97, pp. 535-540.

8

Cancer Gene Therapy: The New Targeting Challenge

Walid Touati, Philippe Beaune and Isabelle de Waziers
UMR-S 775 Université Paris Descartes INSERM
France

1. Introduction

Cancer is characterized by genetic alterations due, for instance, to mutations in genomic DNA caused by chemicals (mutagens such as pollutants or nitrosamines, and polycyclic aromatic hydrocarbons), radiations (e.g., prolonged exposure to ultraviolet radiation from the sun, which can lead to melanoma or other skin malignancies), and viral infections (e.g., papilloma virus; human T-cell leukemia viruses 1, 2, 3, and 4; and herpes simplex virus). Mutations in genes involved in cell proliferation, tumor suppressor genes, or proto-oncogenes may lead to uncontrolled cell proliferation into a tumor. Currently, the most widely used treatments for cancer are combinations of surgery, radiotherapy and chemotherapy. However, the effectiveness of these treatments is variable. Consequently, means of potentiating conventional treatments, as well as new strategies, need to be developed.

Gene therapy is generally perceived as a treatment for rare genetic diseases, in which replacing the deficient gene by its normal counterpart has proved successful, most notably in severe combined immunodeficiency (SCID) (Fischer et al., 2010), adrenoleukodystrophy (Cartier et al., 2009), and ß-thalassemia (Cavazzana-Calvo et al., 2010). However, cancer is the main focus of basic and clinical research on gene therapy (http://www.wiley.com//legacy/wileychi/genmed/clinical/). Variable levels of success have been achieved using a broad range of genes encoding tumor suppressor proteins such as p53, antiangiogenic proteins such as anti-vascular endothelial growth factor (VEGF), inflammatory cytokines, and other proteins (Lane et al., 2010), (Candolfi et al., 2010), (Adachi et al., 2010).

One of the main hurdles in gene therapy is selective delivery of recombinant vectors to the target tissue. In cancer gene therapy, administration of the vector within the tumor may be of interest, but some tumors are not readily accessible and vector dissemination to healthy cells cannot be ruled out. Today, accurate tumor targeting is a major goal of cancer gene therapy.

In this chapter, we will focus on the methods developed to improve targeting in cancer gene therapy, most notably gene-directed enzyme prodrug therapy (GDEPT), which is a major focus of research at our laboratory.

2. Gene-directed enzyme prodrug therapy (GDEPT)

Cytotoxic chemotherapy is often associated with severe systemic toxicities. Gene-directed enzyme prodrug therapy (GDEPT) or suicide gene therapy consists in selective delivery to the tumor of a gene encoding a drug-metabolizing enzyme that catalyzes the *in situ* conversion of a non-toxic prodrug to a toxic active drug (Figure 1). GDEPT can be used to increase the levels of an enzyme produced by the tumor or to introduce an enzyme that is not expressed endogenously. The local production of the cytotoxic drug within the tumor is expected to result in greater effectiveness and less toxicity, compared to systemic drug delivery.

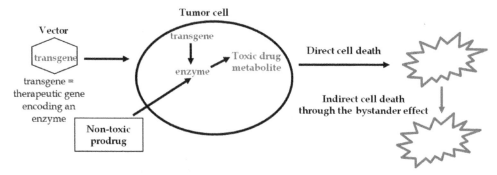

Fig. 1. Principle of gene-directed enzyme prodrug therapy (GDEPT)

Several studies have been performed with different enzyme and prodrug combinations. The most widely studied combinations are herpes simplex thymidine kinase/ganciclovir, cytosine deaminase/5-fluorouracile, and cytochrome P450 (CYP)/ oxazaphosphorines (cyclophosphamide [CPA] and ifosphamide) (Altaner, 2008) (Table 1)

Enzymes	Source	Prodrug	Drug	Indication
Herpes simplex thymidine kinase	Herpes simplex virus	Ganciclovir	Ganciclovir triphosphate (GCV-TP)	Glioma, pancreatic cancer
Cytosine deaminase	*Escherichia coli*	5-Fluorocytosine (5-FC)	5-Fluorouracil (5-FU)	Glioblastoma, Colorectal cancer
Cytochrome P450	Rat/human/dog	Cyclophosphamide (CPA)	4-OH Cyclophospha mide (4-OH CPA)	Head and neck cancer, lung cancer, Burkitt's lymphoma
Nitroreductase	*Escherichia Coli*	CB1954	N-acetoxy derivatives	Cancer cells in general

Table 1. Enzyme/prodrug combinations used in GDEPT

2.1 Cytochrome P450 (CYP)/cyclophosphamide (CPA) combination

The chemotherapeutic prodrug CPA is widely used for the treatment of both solid tumors and hematological malignancies. Enzymatic bioactivation, chiefly via human CYP2B6 (Gervot et al., 1999), produces the metabolite 4'-OH-CPA, which undergoes spontaneous decomposition to acrolein and phosphoramide mustard. Phosphoramide mustard is an electrophilic alkylating agent that causes the formation of intra- and interstrand DNA cross-links, which eventually lead to apoptotic cell death (Schwartz & Waxman, 2001). In patients treated with CPA, this prodrug is activated by CYP2B6 in the liver, and the active metabolites enter the bloodstream, which transports them not only to the tumor but also to healthy tissues where they may cause severe side effects including cardiotoxicity, renal toxicity, bone marrow suppression, and neurotoxicity (Fraiser et al., 1991) (Langford, 1997). To prevent these side effects, CYP2B-based gene-directed enzyme prodrug therapy was developed by D.J. Waxman and colleagues and, more recently, by our group (Waxman et al., 1999), (Jounaidi, 2002), (Jounaidi et al., 2006), (Tychopoulos et al., 2005). CYP2B expressed in tumor cells results in the *in situ* conversion of CPA to cytotoxic metabolites. Moreover, the diffusible 4'-OH-CPA metabolite can enter neighboring cells, where it is converted to phosphoramide mustard, leading to the death of nontransfected tumor cells (Wei et al., 1995), (Tychopoulos et al., 2005). This bystander effect plays a major role in the CYP2B-based GDEPT strategy, and several studies of various suicide gene and prodrug combinations have shown that complete eradication of the tumor is possible even when the suicide gene product is expressed by less than 10% of the cells (Portsmouth et al., 2007)

In our laboratory, we are developing a GDEPT strategy based on human CYP2B6, the human CYP isoform that preferentially metabolizes CPA (Gervot et al., 1999). One of the main difficulties is the relatively low affinity of CYP2B6 for CPA. Modifications aimed at increasing the efficiency of CYP2B6 (V_{max}/K_m) in catalyzing the 4-hydroxylation of CPA have therefore been evaluated. We used site-directed mutagenesis of the active site of CYPB26 to produce a double mutant (I114V/V477W) characterized by a 4-fold increase in CPA-4-hydroxylation efficiency compared to the wild-type CYP2B6 (CYP2B6wt), ascribable chiefly to an increase in enzyme affinity (Nguyen et al., 2008). Recently, we obtained a triple CYP2B6 mutant (CYP2B6TM) that is 8 times more efficient than CYP2B6wt (unpublished results from our laboratory)

Another means of improving the efficiency of CYP2B6-mediated GDEPT is co-expression in the tumor cells of NADPH-cytochrome P450 reductase (RED). RED is a FAD- and FMN-containing enzyme that catalyzes the transfer from NADPH of electrons required for CYP-dependent enzyme reactions. Within tumors, where RED expression is heterogeneous (Fitzsimmons et al., 1996; L. J. Yu et al., 2001), CYP-GDEPT results in high levels of CYP expression, and RED availability can limit the rate of CYP-catalyzed enzyme reactions and, therefore, of prodrug bioactivation. To ensure the production of both CYP2B6 and RED by the same cancer cell, a CYP2B6wt-RED fusion protein having both 4-hydroxylase activity and reductase activity was built. This fusion protein proved more efficient than CYP2B6wt alone for metabolizing CPA in several pulmonary cell lines (Tychopoulos et al., 2005). Recently, we produced a CYP2B6TM-RED fusion protein that is 10 times more efficient than CYP2B6wt-RED in activating CPA (unpublished results from our laboratory).

These studies show that improving the efficiency of CYP2B6 is feasible. This method may allow the use of lower CPA dosages with no loss of cytotoxic effectiveness within the tumor but with less activation by hepatic CYP2B6 and, therefore, a possible decrease in cytotoxic effects on non-tumor tissue. Preliminary results in various human pulmonary and head-and-neck cancer cell lines show that expression of the CYP2B6TM-RED protein sensitized the cancer cells to lower doses of CPA compared to expression of CYP2B6wt-RED (unpublished results from our laboratory).

3. Gene therapy vectors

The most important step in any gene therapy protocol is the development of efficient vectors for delivering the transgene to its target. The ideal vector should be administered by a non-invasive route, penetrate only into the targeted cells in order to limit adverse side effects, and express the transgene in amounts sufficient to produce strong therapeutic effects. A wide range of vectors have been developed including viral vectors, polymers, liposomes, nanoparticles, and bare DNA.

Today, about 70% of clinical gene therapy trials worldwide use viral vectors such as retroviruses, adenoviruses, and adeno-associated viruses (AAV) or lentiviruses (Table 2) to transfer transgenes and 64.5% of these trials are conducted in patients with cancer (http://www.wiley.com//legacy/wileychi/genmed/clinical/).

However, retroviral vectors used to treat SCID have been responsible for leukemia caused by transgene insertion into proto-oncogene regions (Hacein-Bey-Abina et al., 2003). This side effect has severely slowed the development of gene therapy. However, we now have safer vectors such as the lentivirus used for gene therapy of adrenoleukodistrophy (Cartier et al., 2009) and ß-thalassemia (Cavazzana-Calvo et al., 2010). Transgenes from recombinant lentivirus may be integrated mainly within intragenic or intronic regions (S. H. Yang et al., 2008).

Here, we will focus on three viruses that are presently widely used in gene therapy, namely, adenoviruses, AAVs, and lentiviruses.

3.1 Adenoviruses

Adenoviruses cause mild upper airway diseases. They are non-enveloped icosahedral viruses composed of a nucleocapsid and double-stranded linear DNA genome of about 35 kb with inverted terminal repeat (ITR) sequences at each end. There are 51 classified human adenovirus serotypes; serotypes 2 and 5 are those used most widely in *ex vivo* and *in vivo* gene therapy. They are very convenient vectors, because they can accommodate relatively large segments of DNA, up to 8 kb. Moreover, their transduction efficiency is high. To avoid a strong immune response after vector delivery, non-replicative recombinant adenoviruses lacking some of the early genes involved in the immune response are used. Deletion of the E1 sequence renders the virus unable to produce infectious viral particles in infected cells, and the E3 region is not necessary for viral production since it encodes proteins involved in evading host immunity. Thus, deletion of E1 and E3 is used to decrease the host immune response to the viral proteins (Alba et al., 2005).

Adenoviral vectors allow episomal and, therefore, transient transgene expression by infected cells (no integration of the foreign DNA into the genome of the host cell) (Russell, 2009) (Alemany & Curiel, 2001).

To infect cells, adenoviruses use the coxsackie-adenovirus receptor (CAR) and integrins as primary cell surface attachment components (Figure 2). The adenovirus (Ad) fiber knob binds with high-affinity to the CAR receptor and the viral penton base interacts with integrins (Bergelson, 1999). CAR plays a significant role in liver transduction and, consequently, most of the adenoviral particles administered intravenously are sequestered in the liver (Vrancken Peeters et al., 1996). However, the mechanism of adenoviral infection *in vivo* is controversial, especially as the introduction of mutations that abrogate CAR binding does not significantly impact the infectivity of adenoviral vectors.

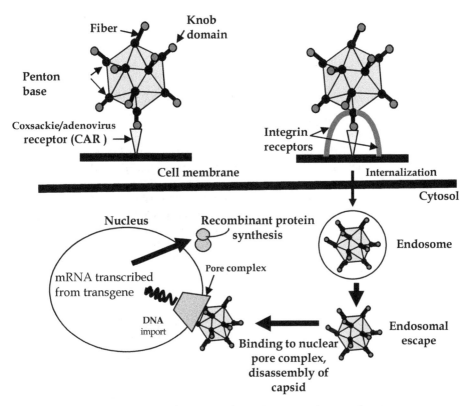

Fig. 2. Schematic representation of adenoviral attachment and internalization

Although immune responses have been limited, they have sometimes restricted the efficiency of adenoviral vectors in clinical trials. Increased immunogenicity has been reported, and many patients have pre-existing immunity to the adenoviral serotypes used in gene therapy. Cell-mediated recognition of the viral capsid components or nucleic acids has received considerable attention and is thought to be chiefly regulated by toll-like receptors (TLRs). Innate immune responses to viruses are initiated by the infected cells, which activate the interferon response to block viral replication, while simultaneously releasing chemokines that attract neutrophils, mononuclear cells, and natural killer cells. In 2010, adenoviruses were still the most widely used vectors for gene therapy. Nevertheless, the use of adenoviral vectors relative to other vectors decreases year on year.

3.2 Adeno-associated viruses (AAV)

Adeno-associated viruses (AAV) are small non-enveloped DNA viruses belonging to the parvovirus family. The single-strand DNA genome of about 4.8 kb comprises two open reading frames (*rep* and *cap*) flanked by inverted terminal repeats (ITRs). Twelve serotypes have been isolated from primate or human tissues (Schmidt et al., 2008). Advantages of AAVs include an apparent lack of pathogenicity, an ability to infect both non-dividing and dividing cells, and stable integration into the host genome at a specific site of the human chromosome 19 when the vector includes the *rep* gene. In the absence of the *rep* gene, chromosomal integration occurs infrequently and at random sites (Huser et al., 2010). The AAV infection cycle is initiated by the binding of the viral capsid to cell surface receptors. One of the main receptors involved is heparan sulfate proteoglycan (HSPG); moreover, several co-receptors contribute to transduction (Asokan et al., 2006). Receptor binding mediates endocytosis, endosomal escape and, finally, transport to the nucleus.

AAV vectors are constructed by replacing the viral DNA with an expression cassette encoding the gene of interest under transcriptional control of a suitable promoter. Vector production is achieved by transfection of a cell line with three plasmids: one contains the expression cassette flanked by the ITRs; another contains *rep cap* helper sequences, and the third is an adenoviral helper plasmid encoding the adenoviral E2a, E4, and VA helper genes (Grimm & Kleinschmidt, 1999).

AAVs have become very popular as gene therapy vectors because of both their ability to mediate stable and efficient gene expression and their good safety profile. The major drawbacks of AAVs are the small amount of DNA that the virus can carry, which results in low capacity; and the difficulty of producing the vector in high titers (Michelfelder & Trepel, 2009). AAVs have been used in at least 80 clinical trials (as of 2011), in strategies based on the delivery of cytotoxic genes, tumor suppressor genes, and other types of genes.

3.3 Lentiviruses

Lentiviruses are retroviruses that include the human immunodeficiency virus 1 (HIV-1). They have a lipid envelope and two identical single-stranded genomic RNA molecules that require a reverse transcriptase for conversion to DNA. The HIV genome is composed of two

	Adenovirus	Adenovirus-associated virus	Retrovirus	Lentivirus
Genome integration	Rarely	No (in absence of *rep* gene) Yes (in presence of *rep* gene)	Yes	Yes
Transgene expression	Transient	Stable	Stable	Stable
Immune response	Marked	According to conditions (animal, transgene, injection conditions,...)	Absent to moderate	Absent to moderate
Target cells	Quiescent or dividing	Quiescent or dividing	Dividing	Quiescent or dividing
Transgene size	up to 8 kb	limited	8-9 kb	8-9 kb
Main use in gene therapy	*in vivo*	*in vivo*	*ex vivo – in vivo*	*ex vivo*
Titer	$>10^{11}$	$>10^{11}$	$>10^8$	$>10^8$
Genotoxicity	No	No	Mutagenesis-related risks	No

Table 2. Characteristics of four viral vectors: adenovirus, adenovirus-associated virus, retrovirus, lentivirus.

regulatory genes, *tat* and *rev*, which are necessary for viral replication; and four accessory genes, *vif, vpr, vpu,* and *nef,* which are not required for *in vitro* replication or growth but are crucial for *in vivo* replication. The tat and rev proteins are involved in regulating HIV gene expression at the transcriptional and post-transcriptional levels, respectively (Pauwels et al., 2009).

Lentiviral particle production involves co-transfection by calcium phosphate precipitation of gag-pol, env, and vector plasmids into HEK 293T cells. Viral particles are then recovered from the cell medium, concentrated, and filtered. Finally, the viral titer is determined (Dull et al., 1998) (Kutner et al., 2009).The transgene present in recombinant lentiviruses is integrated into the host genome via an integrase and is therefore expressed in a stable manner over time. Among retroviruses, lentiviruses efficiently infect both dividing and non-dividing cells (Naldini et al., 1996) without inducing genotoxicity with insertional mutagenesis (Montini et al., 2009), since they are integrated mainly within intragenic or intronic regions. Lentiviruses (e.g., the HIV) use cell receptors such as CD4 and the co-receptors CCR5 or CXCR4 to penetrate the cells. Lentiviral vectors express various types of proteins that are recognized by cell receptors and co-receptors, leading to a very broad tropism.

Since these vectors were first introduced, they have been modified in several ways with the goal of improving their safety profile. Now, these viral vectors are being increasingly used. However, their lack of tissue specificity may limit their use, and several methods have been developed to improve their ability to target the desired site.

4. Current strategies for viral vector targeting

Today, the major goal in cancer gene therapy is to improve tumor targeting, thus preventing transgene expression by normal cells and therefore diminishing the risk of toxic side effects. Initially, the vector was injected directly into the tumor. However, vectors are now available that target the tumor after being administered systemically.

Efforts to improve viral vector targeting can modify the binding of the virus to the cell and entry of the virus into the cell (entry targeting/transductional regulation) or the events that occur once the virus is in the cell (post-entry targeting/transcriptional regulation). Several approaches have been devised such as envelope or capsid modifications, the use of various adapters, placement of transgene expression under specific promoter control, and modifications of the transgene sequence.

4.1 Pseudotyping: Envelope or capsid modification

Viral vectors infect their natural host-cell populations preferentially and with the greatest efficiency. Viral infection occurs when host-cell receptors recognize the viral envelope proteins. Pseudotyping consists in changing the plasmid encoding the expression of envelope proteins. The result is a shift in the range of host cells and, consequently, in the tissue tropism of the viral vector. The vector surface is modified via the incorporation of foreign envelope glycoproteins that have a restricted natural population of host-cell receptors (Frecha et al., 2008). This technique was the first to be used for modifying viral tropism, particularly in retroviruses such as lentiviruses, which have an envelope. Adenoviral vectors have no envelope, and the viral attachment protein must therefore be incorporated into a protein capsid instead of a lipid bilayer.

Lentiviral vector pseudotyping is usually achieved using the vesicular stomatitis virus G (VSV-G) protein, which exhibits a broad tropism for various cell types. Additional advantages of VSV-G-pseudotyped lentivirus are the higher viral titers compared to those obtained with other envelope proteins and the improved vector particle purification due to increased stability of the virus. However, when used in high concentrations, lentiviral vectors bearing VSV-G may exert cytotoxic effects (Chen et al., 1996). Fortunately, this drawback can be overcome either by improving purification of the lentiviral particles using gradient centrifugation to eliminate unincorporated transgene particles (Ricks et al., 2008) or by using other proteins for pseudotyping. VSV-G-pseudotyped particles are convenient to use *ex vivo* to express a transgene in a broad spectrum of cell lines. However, VSV-G-pseudotyped viruses can be inactivated by human serum (DePolo et al., 2000). In clinical trials of cancer gene therapy, the objective is to limit the tropism of the vector to the cancer cells.

Miletic et al., worked on a gene therapy strategy for malignant gliomas, which are the most common primary brain tumors and carry a poor prognosis due to their infiltrative growth (Miletic et al., 2004). Miletic and co-workers compared the expression of various pseudotyped lentiviruses in normal brain cells and malignant glioma cells. VSV-G pseudotyped lentiviruses infected the neurons and astrocytes, whereas the tropism of lymphocytic choriomeningitis virus glycoprotein (LCMV-GP) pseudotypes was virtually confined to the astrocytes. LCMV-G-pseudotyped lentivirus was specifically and efficiently transduced in rat gliomas, whereas VSV-G-pseudotyped lentivirus was considerably less efficient in transducing glioma cells.

Another protein often used to target cancer cells is the modified sindbis virus envelope. Pariente et al., (2007) used it successfully to target prostate cancer cells.

Transduction efficiency is low after tumor cell infection with adenoviruses. One reason is the limited expression of the coxsackievirus-adenovirus receptor (CAR) in tumor cells. To overcome this obstacle, the adenovirus fiber can be modified by removing interactions with both CAR and integrins, the main components involved in adenovirus transduction (Einfeld et al., 2001). This modification diminishes the native tropism and enhances the efficacy of specific targeting ligands in redirecting the adenovirus to the target tissues.

Malignant gliomas are refractory to adenovirus-mediated gene therapy, chiefly because CAR is not expressed by the tumor cells. Zheng et al. identified several receptors that were over-expressed in tumor cells, and they created a series of pseudotyped adenoviral vectors. Some of these vectors enhance gene transfer to tumors and warrant further development for glioma gene therapy. (Zheng et al., 2007)

Yu et al., (L. Yu et al., 2005) reported increased infection of esophageal and oral carcinoma cells with adenoviruses whose Ad5 fiber was substituted with fibers from Ad11 or Ad35, compared to unmodified adenoviruses. Similarly, attaching the Ad3 fiber to the Ad5 backbone was particularly effective for targeting ovarian cancer and squamous cell carcinoma of the head and neck.

The efficacy of pseudotyping may be limited by the lack of tissue specificity and ubiquitous expression of some of the receptors. Furthermore, the viral envelope modifications may diminish viral stability and limit viral production, leading to low titers.

4.2 Use of adapters: Antibody/ligand
Another technique consists in fusing special adapters or proteins to the envelope proteins. These adapters determine the affinity of the vector for the target.

4.2.1 Antibody

A protein can be specifically targeted by the use of specific antibodies, antibody fragments, or single-chain antibodies fused to the viral membrane. There are two main methods for using antibodies to improve targeting by vectors.

- The entire antibody or an antibody fragment directed against both a viral envelope protein and a tumor cell membrane receptor can be used as a bridge to attach the virus to specific cells.
- An antibody fragment (usually the fragment crystallizable region Fc) can be expressed at the viral envelope and the rest of the antibody can be directed against a specific antigen of the target cells.

For prostate cancer gene therapy, Kraaij et al. developed a targeted method based on bi-specific antibodies constructed as conjugates between an anti-adenovirus fiber knob Fab' fragment and an anti-prostate specific membrane antigen (PSMA) (Kraaij et al., 2005). These bi-functional antibodies, used as a bridge between capsid proteins and cell surface receptors, were selective for the prostate cancer cell lines. They may hold promise for gene therapy of prostate cancer.

Another strategy, developed by Zhang et al., consists in binding trastuzumab (or Herceptin®, a monoclonal antibody directed against the human epidermal growth factor receptor (HER-2)) to the lentivirus envelope. Thus, the vector targets cells that overexpress HER-2, such as prostate cancer cells, to which it delivers the transgene. Zhang et al. engineered these lentiviruses to express thymidine kinase and showed that prostate cancer cell lines infected by these lentiviruses became vulnerable to ganciclovir. (Zhang et al., 2009)

Poulin et al. worked on a new adenoviral vector and investigated the usefulness of capsid protein IX (a minor protein of the adenoviral capsid) as a platform for presenting single-chain variable-fragment antibodies and single-domain antibodies for virus targeting. Given the ability of this protein to fuse to large polypeptides, Poulin et al. decided to test large targeting ligands such as antibodies. Presence in the vector of single-chain variable-fragment antibodies was not sufficient to ensure accurate targeting, contrary to the presence of single-domain antibodies (Poulin et al., 2010).

However, this method is still complicated to use, as it requires the production of monoclonal antibodies, which is both time-consuming and costly. In addition, a specific tumor cell antigen must be obtained, which may be difficult. Finally, the titer of vectors that express the antibody in their envelope is sometimes low.

4.2.2 Ligand

The first attempts at inserting a ligand into the viral membrane used various types of ligand such as growth factors, hormones, and peptides, which were inserted at various sites of the viral surface.

Morizono et al., (Morizono et al., 2009) used a strategy based on a lentiviral vector bearing the biotin-adapter-peptide. In earlier studies of adenoviral or AAV vectors, peptides that were biotinylation substrates were inserted and associated with biotinylated sites, bound avidin, neutravidin, or streptavidin. (Parrott et al., 2003; Pereboeva et al., 2007; Stachler et al., 2008)

Similarly, Liu and colleagues (Liu et al., 2011) used a serotype 5 adenoviral vector (Ad5) whose fiber knob was deleted and replaced by a biotin-acceptor peptide. The advantage of this new adenoviral vector is that no CAR-dependent cell uptake and transduction occurs; moreover when the vector is biotinylated, biotinylated antibodies can be used to achieve targeting. AAV vectors can also be biotinylated.

A hybrid approach using an antibody and a protein ligand has been described in two papers by a group working at the University of California, Los Angeles. (Joo & Wang, 2008), (L. Yang et al., 2006). This group of researchers engineered a lentiviral vector whose surface bears two distinct molecules, an antibody conferring target specificity to the engineered vector and a pH-dependent fusogenic protein that allows the engineered vector to penetrate the target cells. Evaluation by image processing showed highly specific incorporation of this lentivirus into the cells.

Hajitou et al. (Hajitou et al., 2006) developed an AAV vector combined with a double cyclic peptide (RGD-4C) of an fd-tet phage. Their aim was to target αV integrins, a cell surface receptor that is overexpressed in tumors and interacts with the RGD peptide. The native tropism of AAV for mammalian cells is eliminated, since there is no AAV capside formation and the ligand peptides allow homing to tissue specific receptors. To obtain chimeric viruses, Hajitou et al. inserted an eukaryotic gene cassette from the AAV into an intergenomic region of the RGD-4C phage. The vector was functional and efficiently targeted human Kaposi sarcoma (KS 1767 cells) grafted in nude mice *in vivo*. Using a ganciclovir cytotoxicity strategy, Hajitou et al. obtained a decrease in tumor volume in mice receiving this vector compared with those given a non-specific vector. Using the same strategy, Bauerschmitz et al. (Bauerschmitz et al., 2002) used an adenovirus modified with a RGD domain to target ovarian cancer cells. As seen with the other approaches involving transductional targeting, limited viral production and stability may occur when the viral envelope is modified.

4.3 Tissue-specific promoter

A promoter is a DNA region that is located upstream of the gene and plays a key role in regulating gene expression. The insertion of a cell-specific regulated promoter upstream from the transgene may limit the expression of the promoter to the targeted cells. Several cancer-specific promoters have been found effective in cancer gene therapy, including prostate stem cell antigen (PSCA) promoter in prostate cancer (Petrigliano et al., 2009), carcinoembryonic antigen (CEA) promoter in gastric cancer (Tanaka et al., 2006), and alpha-fetoprotein (AFP) enhancer and albumin promoter in hepatocellular carcinoma (He et al., 2000).

These promoters are tissue-dependent, however. A universal tumor-specific promoter targeting tumor cells of any origin would be of considerable interest. For instance, given that hypoxia is a common physiological feature of tumor tissue, an optimized hypoxia-responsive promoter (OBHRE) may be effective in increasing the therapeutic window of cytotoxic cancer gene therapy (Binley et al., 2003). In a range of cell types, this promoter expresses high levels of transgene in hypoxic tissue but has minimal activity in normoxia. Moreover, the OBHRE promoter in a recombinant adenovirus allowed high-level expression of the transgene in tumor cells but was not expressed in normal tissues such as the liver, spleen, lung, and kidney. Binley et al. developed a GDEPT strategy using CYP2B6 or thymidine kinase as the transgene in combination with CPA and ganciclovir, respectively. Direct administration of the gene therapy vector containing OBHRE into established tumor models was effective, and this method limited the toxic effects due to hepatic sequestration of the adenovirus.

A characteristic promoter of cancer cells is the prostate stem cell antigen (PSCA) promoter. Petrigliano et al. (Petrigliano et al., 2009) used the PSCA promoter to develop a lentiviral vector targeting prostate cells. PSCA is consistently expressed by high-grade prostate intraepithelial neoplasias and invasive prostate cancers (Watabe et al., 2002). The lentiviral vector carried a cytotoxic thymidine kinase gene and was combined with ganciclovir treatment. Lentiviral gene therapy vector driven by a short PSCA promoter induced prostate-specific cellular toxicity *in vivo* and *in vitro*. This strategy could be used to treat local and advanced metastatic prostate cancer.

However, one of the main problems with the specific promoter strategy is that faithful reconstitution of a complete gene sequence promoter can be difficult. Moreover, transcriptional targeting cannot prevent the sequestration of therapeutic viruses in normal tissues, which may result in toxicity and loss of efficacy.

5. A new strategy for viral vector targeting: micro RNAs (miRNA)

In addition to the above-mentioned methods, microRNAs (miRNAs) may hold potential for improving viral vector targeting, as they are involved in the post-transcriptional regulation of gene expression.

5.1 microRNAs (miRNAs)

The small non-coding RNAs (~20-25 nucleotides) known as miRNAs regulate gene expression at the post-transcriptional level. They are involved in a variety of biological processes including development, differentiation, apoptosis, and cell proliferation. They repress gene expression by binding to their complementary target sites in mRNAs, thereby increasing the degradation or preventing the translation of the transcripts. Thus, cells that express an miRNA complementary to an mRNA do not express the protein coded by this mRNA: miRNAs are endogenous negative gene regulators. (Figure 3).

In 1993, miRNAs were identified for the first time, in the nematode *Caenorhabdtis elegans*, in which they were encoded by the *lin-4* and were complementary to mRNA for the *lin-14* gene (R. C. Lee et al., 1993). The *lin-4* gene product is a small RNA of 22 nucleotides (i.e., na miRNA) that is specific of the 3'UTR of the *lin-14* gene and therefore inhibits the production of the lin-14 protein, thus preventing the transition from larval stage L1 to stage L2. Since the discovery of miRNAs, their mechanisms of action and biogenesis have been studied in detail, and they have been shown to play a major role in physiological processes, development, and disease.

Briefly, miRNA biogenesis involves four stages: transcription of pri-miRNA; cleavage by Drosha to release a precursor pre-miRNA; export of the precursor to the cytoplasm; and cleavage of the pre-miRNA precursor by Dicer. All miRNAs are processed from precursor molecules called pri-miRNAs (Y. Lee et al., 2002), which are transcribed from independent miRNA genes or are portions of introns of protein-coding RNA polymerase II transcripts. Typically, a single pri-miRNA often contains sequences of several different miRNAs.

These pri-miRNAs of about 100 nucleotides are folded into hairpin structures and characterized by imperfectly base-paired stems. These molecules are then processed by a multiprotein complex including the Rnase III type endonuclease Drosha and DiGeorge syndrome critical region gene 8 (DGCR 8). The hairpin structures are recognized in the nucleus by DGCR 8, a double-stranded RNA-binding protein (dsRBP). DGCR8 and the Drosha complex process the pri-miRNAs to pre-miRNA hairpins composed of about 70 nucleotides. Pre-miRNAs are then transported from the nucleus to the cytoplasm by exportin 5. In the cytoplasm, they undergo a final maturation step consisting in cleavage by

Dicer, which is complexed with TAR RNA binding protein (TRBP). This cleavage step releases an miRNA duplex of about 20 nucleotides. Mature miRNAs are integrated into a ribonucleoprotein complex called RNA induced silencing complex (RISC) or miRNA-induced silencing complex (miRISC). The components of miRISC complexes are mature miRNAs, Dicer and TRBP proteins, and proteins of the Argonaute family (AGO).

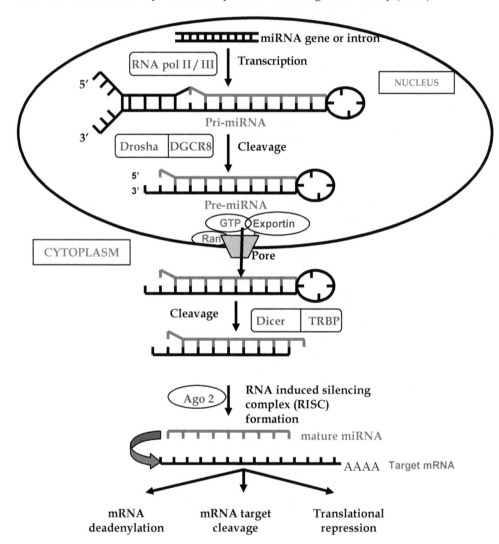

Fig. 3. Principle of miRNA biogenesis

AGO proteins represent the key components of miRISCs; in mammals, four AGO proteins (AGOs 1, 2, 3, and 4) have been identified. They are involved in the miRNA repression function via protein synthesis repression, whereas only AGO2 contributes to the RNA interference (RNAi) function. (Jaskiewicz & Filipowicz, 2008).

Binding of miRNAs to complementary target sites on mRNAs prevents the translation of the transcript or accelerates its decay. The regulation of miRNAs depends on the binding of the first 2 – 8 bases of their mature sequence to the 3'UTR of target genes. To date, 1048 human miRNA precursor sequences have been deposited in the miRBase *(http://www.mirbase.org)* (Kozomara & Griffiths-Jones)

There is now sound evidence that miRNAs are involved in the pathogenesis of conditions such as cancer and inflammatory responses. It has been shown that miRNA expression is deregulated in cancer cells. The differences in miRNA expression between normal and malignant cells may be related to the location of miRNA genes in cancer-associated regions, to epigenetic mechanisms, and to alterations in the miRNA processing machinery (Calin & Croce, 2006). Several studies suggest that miRNAs may contribute to oncogenesis by acting either as tumor suppressors (excessive regulation) or as oncogenes (insufficient regulation).

5.2 Targeting strategy using miRNA

Recently, researchers have started to evaluate endogenous miRNA-mediated regulation as a means of targeting the expression of exogenous genes. Naldini and co-workers demonstrated that endogenous miRNAs could be broadly exploited to regulate transgene expression in various cell lines. This very elegant approach to the control of protein expression relies on the potent regulatory properties of miRNAs. Several studies demonstrated that miRNA expression in cancer cells is deregulated compared to normal cells. The idea is to use this deregulation to modulate the expression of the transgene (B. D. Brown et al., 2007a) (Figure 4). Naldini and colleagues first developed a vector characterized by suppression of transgene expression in hematopoietic cells. The vector contains target sequences for the hematopoietic cell-specific miRNA miR 142-3p; thus, transgene expression is specifically suppressed in all hematopoietic cell lines but is not affected in other cell types. (B. D. Brown et al., 2007a)

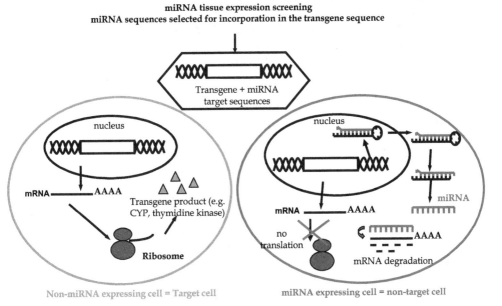

Fig. 4. Principle of miRNA targeting strategy

During the development of this technique, one issue was determination of the amount of endogenous miRNA needed to obtain effective target mRNA suppression. Brown et al., (B. D. Brown et al., 2007b) investigated this issue and concluded that target suppression depended on a threshold miRNA concentration.

Suzuki et al., (Suzuki et al., 2008) worked on a suicide gene therapy strategy based on the herpes simplex virus thymidine kinase (HSVtk) gene and ganciclovir (GCV), with adenoviral vectors. Based on the literature and their experiments, they showed that intratumorally injected adenoviral vectors were disseminated into the systemic circulation and transduced in the liver, resulting in hepatotoxicity. They therefore decided to produce a vector capable of preventing the hepatotoxicity of adenoviruses without altering the antitumor effects of suicide gene therapy. They hypothesized that insertion of sequences complementary to miR122a (which is highly expressed in the liver) into the 3′-UTR of a transgene expression cassette in adenoviral vectors would reduce hepatic transduction without affecting transgene expression in the tumor.

They constructed several vectors; among them, one had four tandem copies of sequences with perfect complementarities to miR122a. The copy number of miRNA target sequences is expected to play an important role in the regulation of transgene expression. An increase in the number of miRNA sequences leads to greater suppression of transgene expression (Doench et al., 2003); thus, four copies are better than two (B. D. Brown et al., 2007b). However, considerable work remains needed to determine the best number of copies and the best spacing elements between tandem copies of miRNA.

Simultaneously, Ylosmaki et al. have developed an adenoviral vector containing sequences complementary to miR 122. They tested the expression of a protein encoded by the vector in Huh7 cells. Huh7 cells resemble normal hepatocytes in that they have a high level of miR 122 expression. As mentioned previously, this strategy prevented transgene expression in the liver, thus avoiding adenovirus-induced hepatotoxicity.

An increasing number of studies combine tissue promoter regulation with miRNA regulation. For instance, Wu C et al. (Wu et al., 2009) developed a baculoviral vector, a strategy that could be extended to other viral vectors. To target glioblastoma cells, they used thymidine kinase/ganciclovir, and a glial fibrillary acidic protein (GFAP) gene promoter. Expression of the herpes simplex virus thymidine kinase gene was controlled by adding the repeated target sequences of three miRNAs that are enriched in astrocytes but downregulated in glioblastoma cells. To determine which miRNA sequences should be used, they reviewed the literature on miRNA expression in gliomas and normal brain tissues.

Downregulated miRNAs are miR 128, 137, 299, 31, 107, 132, 133a, 133b, 154, 323, 330, 127, 134, 181a, and 181b (Ciafre et al., 2005) (Silber et al., 2008); there is only one upregulated miRNA, namely, miR 10b. Wu and colleagues used these results to construct targeting vectors. Suicide gene expression controlled by specific miRNA sequences exerted selective cellular effects *in vitro* and *in vivo*. Glioma cells were specifically targeted, and ganciclovir was toxic in these cells. Wu et al. concluded that incorporating miRNA regulation into a transcriptional targeting vector provided a high level of control over transgene expression. The crucial steps in developing an efficient system include selection of a relevant tissue-specific promoter and determination of relative miRNA expressions in tumor cells and their normal counterparts. The next step is selection of miRNAs that are downregulated in tumor cells and expressed at high levels in normal cells.

This approach has also been studied in another cancer treatment strategy based on oncolytic viruses. Thus, Leja et al., (Leja et al., 2010) worked on an oncolytic adenovirus. Their aim was to abolish the hepatic tropism of the adenovirus, and therefore the occurrence of hepatotoxicity, without altering the antitumoral effects in neuroendocrine cells. They used not only a specific promoter but also miR 122 sequences. Similar to Suzuki et al. (Suzuki et al., 2008) and Ylosmaki et al. (Ylosmaki et al., 2008), Leja et al. found that hepatic tropism and expression were abolished.

Edge et al. (Edge et al., 2008) used another oncolytic virus, the vesicular stomatitis virus (VSV). They incorporated let-7 miRNA complementary sequences within the VSV to eliminate toxicity for normal cells without preventing expression in cancer cells *in vitro* and *in vivo*.

This approach has also been found effective in diseases other than cancer. Thus, an miR 142-3p regulated lentiviral vector has been used in hemophilia B (B. D. Brown et al., 2007a); miR 122 regulated transgene expression improved targeting to the heart (Geisler et al.); and a lentiviral vector containing miR 142 sequences regulated UGT1A1 expression in the liver (Schmitt et al., 2010)).

6. Conclusion

Cancer gene therapy and, in particular, suicide gene therapy holds considerable promise as a substitute for conventional chemotherapy. However, several aspects of gene therapy remain to be improved. In particular, there is a need for developing enzymes such as mutant forms of human enzymes that are more efficient than the wild-type enzyme regarding specificity and kinetics for the prodrugs, as exemplified by our CYP2B6TM-RED and CPA combination.

The viral vectors used to achieve gene transfer may have a broad tropism and may therefore infect healthy tissue. An insufficient ability of vectors to target tumors has contributed to slow the development of cancer gene therapy. Researchers have therefore expended considerable effort to improve viral vector targeting, as discussed in this chapter. Moreover, the accumulation of knowledge about miRNAs has opened up a new field of gene regulation. Using miRNA properties to regulate transgene expression, and therefore targeting, in cancer gene therapy is both extremely elegant and quite simple. Future strategies should combine several targeting methods (Figure 5). Several groups have already constructed vectors characterized by a double targeting system consisting of specific promoters and miRNA. Today, the development of vectors characterized by both transductional and transcriptional targeting is within reach. It is reasonable to hope that safe vectors capable of specifically targeting cancer cells will be available soon and will open up new horizons for cancer gene therapy.

Last, new prodrugs with greater effectiveness are needed. Given that hypoxia is a common environmental feature in solid tumors, prodrugs specifically activated by hypoxia should be designed. For example, our previously described fusion gene expresses both CYP2B6 and RED catalytic activities, and we plan to use CPA treatment in combination with additional prodrugs known to be activated to cytotoxic metabolites under hypoxic conditions, such as AQ4N by CYP 2B6 or mitomycin C and tirapazamine by RED (J. M. Brown & Wang, 1998; Cavazzana-Calvo et al., 2010; Friery et al., 2000; McErlane et al., 2005).

Recent clinical trials confirmed the usefulness of cancer gene therapy and its potential for application in the clinical setting, as a substitute for conventional chemotherapy or, if the result is only a decrease in tumor size, in combination with surgery and radiotherapy. We hope that the expected improvements in cancer gene therapy outlined above will further facilitate the use of this strategy for treating solid tumors.

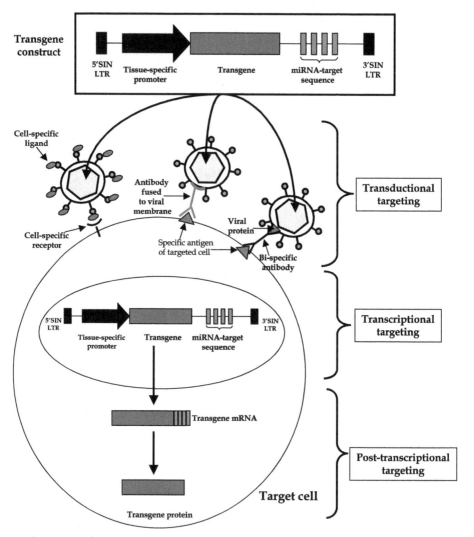

Fig. 5. Summary of various strategies for targeting lentiviral expression to cancer cells

7. References

Adachi, Y., Yoshio-Hoshino, N., Aoki, C., & Nishimoto, N. (2010). VEGF targeting in mesotheliomas using an interleukin-6 signal inhibitor based on adenovirus gene delivery. *Anticancer Res*, 30(6),pp. 1947-1952.

Alba, R., Bosch, A., & Chillon, M. (2005). Gutless adenovirus: last-generation adenovirus for gene therapy. *Gene Ther*, 12 Suppl 1,pp. S18-27.

Alemany, R., & Curiel, D. T. (2001). CAR-binding ablation does not change biodistribution and toxicity of adenoviral vectors. *Gene Ther*, 8(17),pp. 1347-1353.

Altaner, C. (2008). Prodrug cancer gene therapy. *Cancer Lett*, 270(2),pp. 191-201.

Asokan, A., Hamra, J. B., Govindasamy, L., Agbandje-McKenna, M., & Samulski, R. J. (2006). Adeno-associated virus type 2 contains an integrin alpha5beta1 binding domain essential for viral cell entry. *J Virol*, 80(18),pp. 8961-8969.

Bauerschmitz, G. J., Lam, J. T., Kanerva, A., Suzuki, K., Nettelbeck, D. M., Dmitriev, I., Krasnykh, V., Mikheeva, G. V., Barnes, M. N., Alvarez, R. D., Dall, P., Alemany, R., Curiel, D. T., & Hemminki, A. (2002). Treatment of ovarian cancer with a tropism modified oncolytic adenovirus. *Cancer Res*, 62(5),pp. 1266-1270.

Bergelson, J. M. (1999). Receptors mediating adenovirus attachment and internalization. *Biochem Pharmacol*, 57(9),pp. 975-979.

Binley, K., Askham, Z., Martin, L., Spearman, H., Day, D., Kingsman, S., & Naylor, S. (2003). Hypoxia-mediated tumour targeting. *Gene Ther*, 10(7),pp. 540-549.

Brown, B. D., Cantore, A., Annoni, A., Sergi, L. S., Lombardo, A., Della Valle, P., D'Angelo, A., & Naldini, L. (2007a). A microRNA-regulated lentiviral vector mediates stable correction of hemophilia B mice. *Blood*, 110(13),pp. 4144-4152.

Brown, B. D., Gentner, B., Cantore, A., Colleoni, S., Amendola, M., Zingale, A., Baccarini, A., Lazzari, G., Galli, C., & Naldini, L. (2007b). Endogenous microRNA can be broadly exploited to regulate transgene expression according to tissue, lineage and differentiation state. *Nat Biotechnol*, 25(12),pp. 1457-1467.

Brown, J. M., & Wang, L. H. (1998). Tirapazamine: laboratory data relevant to clinical activity. *Anticancer Drug Des*, 13(6),pp. 529-539.

Calin, G. A., & Croce, C. M. (2006). MicroRNA signatures in human cancers. *Nat Rev Cancer*, 6(11),pp. 857-866.

Candolfi, M., Xiong, W., Yagiz, K., Liu, C., Muhammad, A. K., Puntel, M., Foulad, D., Zadmehr, A., Ahlzadeh, G. E., Kroeger, K. M., Tesarfreund, M., Lee, S., Debinski, W., Sareen, D., Svendsen, C. N., Rodriguez, R., Lowenstein, P. R., & Castro, M. G. (2010). Gene therapy-mediated delivery of targeted cytotoxins for glioma therapeutics. *Proc Natl Acad Sci U S A*, 107(46),pp. 20021-20026.

Cartier, N., Hacein-Bey-Abina, S., Bartholomae, C. C., Veres, G., Schmidt, M., Kutschera, I., Vidaud, M., Abel, U., Dal-Cortivo, L., Caccavelli, L., Mahlaoui, N., Kiermer, V., Mittelstaedt, D., Bellesme, C., Lahlou, N., Lefrere, F., Blanche, S., Audit, M., Payen, E., Leboulch, P., l'Homme, B., Bougneres, P., Von Kalle, C., Fischer, A., Cavazzana-Calvo, M., & Aubourg, P. (2009). Hematopoietic stem cell gene therapy with a lentiviral vector in X-linked adrenoleukodystrophy. *Science*, 326(5954),pp. 818-823.

Cavazzana-Calvo, M., Payen, E., Negre, O., Wang, G., Hehir, K., Fusil, F., Down, J., Denaro, M., Brady, T., Westerman, K., Cavallesco, R., Gillet-Legrand, B., Caccavelli, L., Sgarra, R., Maouche-Chretien, L., Bernaudin, F., Girot, R., Dorazio, R., Mulder, G. J., Polack, A., Bank, A., Soulier, J., Larghero, J., Kabbara, N., Dalle, B., Gourmel, B., Socie, G., Chretien, S., Cartier, N., Aubourg, P., Fischer, A., Cornetta, K., Galacteros, F., Beuzard, Y., Gluckman, E., Bushman, F., Hacein-Bey-Abina, S., & Leboulch, P. (2010). Transfusion independence and HMGA2 activation after gene therapy of human beta-thalassaemia. *Nature*, 467(7313),pp. 318-322.

Chen, S. T., Iida, A., Guo, L., Friedmann, T., & Yee, J. K. (1996). Generation of packaging cell lines for pseudotyped retroviral vectors of the G protein of vesicular stomatitis virus by using a modified tetracycline inducible system. *Proc Natl Acad Sci U S A*, 93(19),pp. 10057-10062.

Ciafre, S. A., Galardi, S., Mangiola, A., Ferracin, M., Liu, C. G., Sabatino, G., Negrini, M., Maira, G., Croce, C. M., & Farace, M. G. (2005). Extensive modulation of a set of microRNAs in primary glioblastoma. *Biochem Biophys Res Commun*, 334(4),pp. 1351-1358.

DePolo, N. J., Reed, J. D., Sheridan, P. L., Townsend, K., Sauter, S. L., Jolly, D. J., & Dubensky, T. W., Jr. (2000). VSV-G pseudotyped lentiviral vector particles produced in human cells are inactivated by human serum. *Mol Ther*, 2(3),pp. 218-222.

Doench, J. G., Petersen, C. P., & Sharp, P. A. (2003). siRNAs can function as miRNAs. *Genes Dev*, 17(4),pp. 438-442.

Dull, T., Zufferey, R., Kelly, M., Mandel, R. J., Nguyen, M., Trono, D., & Naldini, L. (1998). A third-generation lentivirus vector with a conditional packaging system. *J Virol*, 72(11),pp. 8463-8471.

Edge, R. E., Falls, T. J., Brown, C. W., Lichty, B. D., Atkins, H., & Bell, J. C. (2008). A let-7 MicroRNA-sensitive vesicular stomatitis virus demonstrates tumor-specific replication. *Mol Ther*, 16(8),pp. 1437-1443.

Einfeld, D. A., Schroeder, R., Roelvink, P. W., Lizonova, A., King, C. R., Kovesdi, I., & Wickham, T. J. (2001). Reducing the native tropism of adenovirus vectors requires removal of both CAR and integrin interactions. *J Virol*, 75(23),pp. 11284-11291.

Fischer, A., Hacein-Bey-Abina, S., & Cavazzana-Calvo, M. (2010). 20 years of gene therapy for SCID. *Nat Immunol*, 11(6),pp. 457-460.

Fitzsimmons, S. A., Workman, P., Grever, M., Paull, K., Camalier, R., & Lewis, A. D. (1996). Reductase enzyme expression across the National Cancer Institute Tumor cell line panel: correlation with sensitivity to mitomycin C and EO9. *J Natl Cancer Inst*, 88(5),pp. 259-269.

Fraiser, L. H., Kanekal, S., & Kehrer, J. P. (1991). Cyclophosphamide toxicity. Characterising and avoiding the problem. *Drugs*, 42(5),pp. 781-795.

Frecha, C., Szecsi, J., Cosset, F. L., & Verhoeyen, E. (2008). Strategies for targeting lentiviral vectors. *Curr Gene Ther*, 8(6),pp. 449-460.

Friery, O. P., Gallagher, R., Murray, M. M., Hughes, C. M., Galligan, E. S., McIntyre, I. A., Patterson, L. H., Hirst, D. G., & McKeown, S. R. (2000). Enhancement of the anti-tumour effect of cyclophosphamide by the bioreductive drugs AQ4N and tirapazamine. *Br J Cancer*, 82(8),pp. 1469-1473.

Geisler, S. B., Green, K. J., Isom, L. L., Meshinchi, S., Martens, J. R., Delmar, M., & Russell, M. W. (2010). Ordered assembly of the adhesive and electrochemical connections within newly formed intercalated disks in primary cultures of adult rat cardiomyocytes. *J Biomed Biotechnol*, 2010,pp. 624719.

Gervot, L., Rochat, B., Gautier, J. C., Bohnenstengel, F., Kroemer, H., de Berardinis, V., Martin, H., Beaune, P., & de Waziers, I. (1999). Human CYP2B6: expression, inducibility and catalytic activities. *Pharmacogenetics*, 9(3),pp. 295-306.

Grimm, D., & Kleinschmidt, J. A. (1999). Progress in adeno-associated virus type 2 vector production: promises and prospects for clinical use. *Hum Gene Ther*, 10(15),pp. 2445-2450.

Hacein-Bey-Abina, S., von Kalle, C., Schmidt, M., Le Deist, F., Wulffraat, N., McIntyre, E., Radford, I., Villeval, J. L., Fraser, C. C., Cavazzana-Calvo, M., & Fischer, A. (2003). A serious adverse event after successful gene therapy for X-linked severe combined immunodeficiency. *N Engl J Med*, 348(3),pp. 255-256.

Hajitou, A., Trepel, M., Lilley, C. E., Soghomonyan, S., Alauddin, M. M., Marini, F. C., 3rd, Restel, B. H., Ozawa, M. G., Moya, C. A., Rangel, R., Sun, Y., Zaoui, K., Schmidt, M., von Kalle, C., Weitzman, M. D., Gelovani, J. G., Pasqualini, R., & Arap, W. (2006). A hybrid vector for ligand-directed tumor targeting and molecular imaging. *Cell*, 125(2),pp. 385-398.

He, P., Tang, Z. Y., Ye, S. L., Liu, B. B., & Liu, Y. K. (2000). The targeted expression of interleukin-2 in human hepatocellular carcinoma cells. *J Exp Clin Cancer Res*, 19(2),pp. 183-187.

Huser, D., Gogol-Doring, A., Lutter, T., Weger, S., Winter, K., Hammer, E. M., Cathomen, T., Reinert, K., & Heilbronn, R. (2010). Integration preferences of wildtype AAV-2 for consensus rep-binding sites at numerous loci in the human genome. *PLoS Pathog*, 6(7),pp. e1000985.

Jaskiewicz, L., & Filipowicz, W. (2008). Role of Dicer in posttranscriptional RNA silencing. *Curr Top Microbiol Immunol*, 320,pp. 77-97.

Joo, K. I., & Wang, P. (2008). Visualization of targeted transduction by engineered lentiviral vectors. *Gene Ther*, 15(20),pp. 1384-1396.

Jounaidi, Y. (2002). Cytochrome P450-based gene therapy for cancer treatment: from concept to the clinic. *Curr Drug Metab*, 3(6),pp. 609-622.

Jounaidi, Y., Chen, C. S., Veal, G. J., & Waxman, D. J. (2006). Enhanced antitumor activity of P450 prodrug-based gene therapy using the low Km cyclophosphamide 4-hydroxylase P450 2B11. *Mol Cancer Ther*, 5(3),pp. 541-555.

Kozomara, A., & Griffiths-Jones, S. (2011). miRBase: integrating microRNA annotation and deep-sequencing data. *Nucleic Acids Res*, 39(Database issue),pp. D152-157.

Kraaij, R., van Rijswijk, A. L., Oomen, M. H., Haisma, H. J., & Bangma, C. H. (2005). Prostate specific membrane antigen (PSMA) is a tissue-specific target for adenoviral transduction of prostate cancer in vitro. *Prostate*, 62(3),pp. 253-259.

Kutner, R. H., Zhang, X. Y., & Reiser, J. (2009). Production, concentration and titration of pseudotyped HIV-1-based lentiviral vectors. *Nat Protoc*, 4(4),pp. 495-505.

Lane, D. P., Cheok, C. F., & Lain, S. (2010). p53-based cancer therapy. *Cold Spring Harb Perspect Biol*, 2(9),pp. a001222.

Langford, C. A. (1997). Complications of cyclophosphamide therapy. *Eur Arch Otorhinolaryngol*, 254(2),pp. 65-72.

Lee, R. C., Feinbaum, R. L., & Ambros, V. (1993). The C. elegans heterochronic gene lin-4 encodes small RNAs with antisense complementarity to lin-14. *Cell*, 75(5),pp. 843-854.

Lee, Y., Jeon, K., Lee, J. T., Kim, S., & Kim, V. N. (2002). MicroRNA maturation: stepwise processing and subcellular localization. *EMBO J*, 21(17),pp. 4663-4670.

Leja, J., Nilsson, B., Yu, D., Gustafson, E., Akerstrom, G., Oberg, K., Giandomenico, V., & Essand, M. (2010). Double-detargeted oncolytic adenovirus shows replication arrest in liver cells and retains neuroendocrine cell killing ability. *PLoS One*, 5(1),pp. e8916.

Liu, H., Wu, L., & Zhou, Z. H. (2011). Model of the trimeric fiber and its interactions with the pentameric penton base of human adenovirus by cryo-electron microscopy. *J Mol Biol*, 406(5),pp. 764-774.

McErlane, V., Yakkundi, A., McCarthy, H. O., Hughes, C. M., Patterson, L. H., Hirst, D. G., Robson, T., & McKeown, S. R. (2005). A cytochrome P450 2B6 meditated gene therapy strategy to enhance the effects of radiation or cyclophosphamide when combined with the bioreductive drug AQ4N. *J Gene Med*, 7(7),pp. 851-859.

Michelfelder, S., & Trepel, M. (2009). Adeno-associated viral vectors and their redirection to cell-type specific receptors. *Adv Genet*, 67,pp. 29-60.

Miletic, H., Fischer, Y. H., Neumann, H., Hans, V., Stenzel, W., Giroglou, T., Hermann, M., Deckert, M., & Von Laer, D. (2004). Selective transduction of malignant glioma by lentiviral vectors pseudotyped with lymphocytic choriomeningitis virus glycoproteins. *Hum Gene Ther*, 15(11),pp. 1091-1100.

Montini, E., Cesana, D., Schmidt, M., Sanvito, F., Bartholomae, C. C., Ranzani, M., Benedicenti, F., Sergi, L. S., Ambrosi, A., Ponzoni, M., Doglioni, C., Di Serio, C., von Kalle, C., & Naldini, L. (2009). The genotoxic potential of retroviral vectors is strongly modulated by vector design and integration site selection in a mouse model of HSC gene therapy. *J Clin Invest*, 119(4),pp. 964-975.

Morizono, K., Xie, Y., Helguera, G., Daniels, T. R., Lane, T. F., Penichet, M. L., & Chen, I. S. (2009). A versatile targeting system with lentiviral vectors bearing the biotin-adaptor peptide. *J Gene Med*, 11(8),pp. 655-663.

Naldini, L., Blomer, U., Gallay, P., Ory, D., Mulligan, R., Gage, F. H., Verma, I. M., & Trono, D. (1996). In vivo gene delivery and stable transduction of nondividing cells by a lentiviral vector. *Science*, 272(5259),pp. 263-267.

Nguyen, T. A., Tychopoulos, M., Bichat, F., Zimmermann, C., Flinois, J. P., Diry, M., Ahlberg, E., Delaforge, M., Corcos, L., Beaune, P., Dansette, P., Andre, F., & de Waziers, I. (2008). Improvement of cyclophosphamide activation by CYP2B6 mutants: from in silico to ex vivo. *Mol Pharmacol*, 73(4),pp. 1122-1133.

Parrott, M. B., Adams, K. E., Mercier, G. T., Mok, H., Campos, S. K., & Barry, M. A. (2003). Metabolically biotinylated adenovirus for cell targeting, ligand screening, and vector purification. *Mol Ther*, 8(4),pp. 688-700.

Pauwels, K., Gijsbers, R., Toelen, J., Schambach, A., Willard-Gallo, K., Verheust, C., Debyser, Z., & Herman, P. (2009). State-of-the-art lentiviral vectors for research use: risk assessment and biosafety recommendations. *Curr Gene Ther*, 9(6),pp. 459-474.

Pereboeva, L., Komarova, S., Roth, J., Ponnazhagan, S., & Curiel, D. T. (2007). Targeting EGFR with metabolically biotinylated fiber-mosaic adenovirus. *Gene Ther*, 14(8),pp. 627-637.

Petrigliano, F. A., Virk, M. S., Liu, N., Sugiyama, O., Yu, D., & Lieberman, J. R. (2009). Targeting of prostate cancer cells by a cytotoxic lentiviral vector containing a prostate stem cell antigen (PSCA) promoter. *Prostate*, 69(13),pp. 1422-1434.

Portsmouth, D., Hlavaty, J., & Renner, M. (2007). Suicide genes for cancer therapy. *Mol Aspects Med*, 28(1),pp. 4-41.

Poulin, K. L., Lanthier, R. M., Smith, A. C., Christou, C., Risco Quiroz, M., Powell, K. L., O'Meara, R. W., Kothary, R., Lorimer, I. A., & Parks, R. J. (2010). Retargeting of adenovirus vectors through genetic fusion of a single-chain or single-domain antibody to capsid protein IX. *J Virol*, 84(19),pp. 10074-10086.

Ricks, D. M., Kutner, R., Zhang, X. Y., Welsh, D. A., & Reiser, J. (2008). Optimized lentiviral transduction of mouse bone marrow-derived mesenchymal stem cells. *Stem Cells Dev*, 17(3),pp. 441-450.

Russell, W. C. (2009). Adenoviruses: update on structure and function. *J Gen Virol*, 90(Pt 1),pp. 1-20.

Schmidt, M., Voutetakis, A., Afione, S., Zheng, C., Mandikian, D., & Chiorini, J. A. (2008). Adeno-associated virus type 12 (AAV12): a novel AAV serotype with sialic acid- and heparan sulfate proteoglycan-independent transduction activity. *J Virol*, 82(3),pp. 1399-1406.

Schmitt, F., Remy, S., Dariel, A., Flageul, M., Pichard, V., Boni, S., Usal, C., Myara, A., Laplanche, S., Anegon, I., Labrune, P., Podevin, G., Ferry, N., & Nguyen, T. H. (2010). Lentiviral vectors that express UGT1A1 in liver and contain miR-142 target sequences normalize hyperbilirubinemia in Gunn rats. *Gastroenterology*, 139(3),pp. 999-1007, 1007 e1001-1002.

Schwartz, P. S., & Waxman, D. J. (2001). Cyclophosphamide induces caspase 9-dependent apoptosis in 9L tumor cells. *Mol Pharmacol*, 60(6),pp. 1268-1279.

Silber, J., Lim, D. A., Petritsch, C., Persson, A. I., Maunakea, A. K., Yu, M., Vandenberg, S. R., Ginzinger, D. G., James, C. D., Costello, J. F., Bergers, G., Weiss, W. A., Alvarez-Buylla, A., & Hodgson, J. G. (2008). miR-124 and miR-137 inhibit proliferation of glioblastoma multiforme cells and induce differentiation of brain tumor stem cells. *BMC Med*, 6,pp. 14.

Stachler, M. D., Chen, I., Ting, A. Y., & Bartlett, J. S. (2008). Site-specific modification of AAV vector particles with biophysical probes and targeting ligands using biotin ligase. *Mol Ther*, 16(8),pp. 1467-1473.

Suzuki, T., Sakurai, F., Nakamura, S., Kouyama, E., Kawabata, K., Kondoh, M., Yagi, K., & Mizuguchi, H. (2008). miR-122a-regulated expression of a suicide gene prevents hepatotoxicity without altering antitumor effects in suicide gene therapy. *Mol Ther*, 16(10),pp. 1719-1726.

Tanaka, T., Huang, J., Hirai, S., Kuroki, M., Watanabe, N., Tomihara, K., Kato, K., & Hamada, H. (2006). Carcinoembryonic antigen-targeted selective gene therapy for gastric cancer through FZ33 fiber-modified adenovirus vectors. *Clin Cancer Res*, 12(12),pp. 3803-3813.

Tychopoulos, M., Corcos, L., Genne, P., Beaune, P., & de Waziers, I. (2005). A virus-directed enzyme prodrug therapy (VDEPT) strategy for lung cancer using a CYP2B6/NADPH-cytochrome P450 reductase fusion protein. *Cancer Gene Ther*, 12(5),pp. 497-508.

Vrancken Peeters, M. J., Perkins, A. L., & Kay, M. A. (1996). Method for multiple portal vein infusions in mice: quantitation of adenovirus-mediated hepatic gene transfer. *Biotechniques*, 20(2),pp. 278-285.

Watabe, T., Lin, M., Ide, H., Donjacour, A. A., Cunha, G. R., Witte, O. N., & Reiter, R. E. (2002). Growth, regeneration, and tumorigenesis of the prostate activates the PSCA promoter. *Proc Natl Acad Sci U S A*, 99(1),pp. 401-406.

Waxman, D. J., Chen, L., Hecht, J. E., & Jounaidi, Y. (1999). Cytochrome P450-based cancer gene therapy: recent advances and future prospects. *Drug Metab Rev*, 31(2),pp. 503-522.

Wei, M. X., Tamiya, T., Rhee, R. J., Breakefield, X. O., & Chiocca, E. A. (1995). Diffusible cytotoxic metabolites contribute to the in vitro bystander effect associated with the cyclophosphamide/cytochrome P450 2B1 cancer gene therapy paradigm. *Clin Cancer Res*, 1(10),pp. 1171-1177.

Wu, Q., Fang, L., Wu, X., Li, B., Luo, R., Yu, Z., Jin, M., Chen, H., & Xiao, S. (2009). A pseudotype baculovirus-mediated vaccine confers protective immunity against lethal challenge with H5N1 avian influenza virus in mice and chickens. *Mol Immunol*, 46(11-12),pp. 2210-2217.

Yang, L., Bailey, L., Baltimore, D., & Wang, P. (2006). Targeting lentiviral vectors to specific cell types in vivo. *Proc Natl Acad Sci U S A*, 103(31),pp. 11479-11484.

Yang, S. H., Cheng, P. H., Sullivan, R. T., Thomas, J. W., & Chan, A. W. (2008). Lentiviral integration preferences in transgenic mice. *Genesis*, 46(12),pp. 711-718.

Ylosmaki, E., Hakkarainen, T., Hemminki, A., Visakorpi, T., Andino, R., & Saksela, K. (2008). Generation of a conditionally replicating adenovirus based on targeted destruction of E1A mRNA by a cell type-specific MicroRNA. *J Virol*, 82(22),pp. 11009-11015.

Yu, L., Takenobu, H., Shimozato, O., Kawamura, K., Nimura, Y., Seki, N., Uzawa, K., Tanzawa, H., Shimada, H., Ochiai, T., & Tagawa, M. (2005). Increased infectivity of adenovirus type 5 bearing type 11 or type 35 fibers to human esophageal and oral carcinoma cells. *Oncol Rep*, 14(4),pp. 831-835.

Yu, L. J., Matias, J., Scudiero, D. A., Hite, K. M., Monks, A., Sausville, E. A., & Waxman, D. J. (2001). P450 enzyme expression patterns in the NCI human tumor cell line panel. *Drug Metab Dispos*, 29(3),pp. 304-312.

Zhang, K. X., Moussavi, M., Kim, C., Chow, E., Chen, I. S., Fazli, L., Jia, W., & Rennie, P. S. (2009). Lentiviruses with trastuzumab bound to their envelopes can target and kill prostate cancer cells. *Cancer Gene Ther*, 16(11),pp. 820-831.

Zheng, S., Ulasov, I. V., Han, Y., Tyler, M. A., Zhu, Z. B., & Lesniak, M. S. (2007). Fiber-knob modifications enhance adenoviral tropism and gene transfer in malignant glioma. *J Gene Med*, 9(3),pp. 151-160.

9

Photodynamic Therapy in Combination with Antiangiogenic Approaches Improve Tumor Inhibition

Ramaswamy Bhuvaneswari[1], Malini Olivo[1,2,3,4],
Gan Yik Yuen[5] and Soo Khee Chee[1]
[1]*National Cancer Centre Singapore, 11 Hospital Drive,*
[2]*School of Physics, National University of Ireland Galway, University Road, Galway,*
[3]*Department of Pharmacy, National University of Singapore,*
[4]*Singapore Bioimaging Consortium, Biomedical Sciences Institutes,*
[5]*Natural Sciences and Science Education, National Institute of Education,*
Nanyang Technological University,
[1,3,4,5]*Singapore*
[2]*Ireland*

1. Introduction

Photodynamic therapy is a non-surgical and minimally invasive procedure that is rapidly developing as a cancer treatment modality. It involves the administration of a photosensitizer that selectively accumulates in the tumor tissue, which is subsequently activated with light of specific wavelength that interacts with molecular oxygen to form toxic, short-lived species known as singlet oxygen, which causes tumor cell death (Macdonald & Dougherty, 2001). The evident advantage of PDT over other conventional cancer treatments such as chemotherapy and radiotherapy is its selective targeting and reduced toxicity (Dolmans et al., 2003). The treatment is relatively non-invasive as it usually only requires targeted illumination of the tumor site. PDT can also be repeated without detrimental consequences to the patients. Currently, PDT is being successfully used for the treatment of early lung cancers (Moghissi et al., 2007; Usuda et al., 2006) and in dermatology for the treatment of non-melanoma skin cancers and precancerous diseases (Klein et al., 2008). PDT has also been successfully employed to treat early carcinomas of the oral cavity and larynx to preserve normal tissue and improve cure rates (Biel, 2007). In the past 20 years, PDT has been successfully used for the treatment of dermatological diseases, ophthalmic diseases, head and neck cancers, brain tumors, pulmonary and pleural mesothelial cancer, cardiovascular disease, gastroenterological cancer, urological disease and gynaecological cancer (Z. Huang, 2005).

However, PDT is an oxygen consuming modality, and an inherent consequence of PDT is local hypoxia. This condition arises either due to direct oxygen consumption during treatment or indirectly due to the destruction of tumor vasculature. As a result, cells under hypoxic stress may switch to an adaptive response by inducing hypoxia inducible factor like

HIF-1α thus triggering angiogenesis. Angiogenesis is the formation of new blood vessels from pre-existing vessels. It is a vital process in the progression of cancer from small, localized neoplasms to larger, growing, and potentially metastatic tumors (Folkman, 2002). Therefore, the process of tumor angiogenesis is triggered by the tumor's release of pro-angiogenic signals such as vascular endothelial growth factor (VEGF), which bind to receptors on nearby vessel endothelial cells. VEGF is a potent regulator of tumor angiogenesis that plays a critical role by increasing blood vessel permeability, endothelial cell growth, proliferation, migration and differentiation (Ferrara, 2004). It is upregulated in response to hypoxic conditions in tumor via the transcription of hypoxia-inducible factor (HIF-1) (Pugh & Ratcliffe, 2003). Cellular and circulating levels of VEGF have been elevated in haematological malignancies and are adversely associated with prognosis (Giles, 2001).

Reports on tumors treated with PDT showed an upregulation of various angiogenic factors like VEGF, HIF-1α, cyclooxygenase-2 (COX-2), basic fibroblast growth factor (bFGF) and matrix metalloproteinases (MMPs) (Solban et al., 2006; Yee et al., 2005). Studies have shown the upregulation of HIF-1α, VEGF, COX-2 and bFGF after hypericin-mediated PDT treated tumors, suggesting that PDT-induced damage to tumor microvasculature and the resultant hypoxia upregulated the expression of certain proangiogenic factors (Zhou et al., 2005). They also reported that the inclusion of various angiogenic inhibitors along with PDT treatment enhanced the PDT effectiveness. Currently, anti-angiogenesis agents are being developed to target different growth factors and molecular pathways that play a major role in tumor angiogenesis.

This chapter evaluates expression of VEGF after PDT and also the efficacy of PDT by combining monoclonal antibodies (angiogenesis inhibitors) against VEGF and epidermal growth factor receptor (EGFR) to improve the overall bladder tumor responsiveness. The following approaches were adapted in this study: (i) evaluating the expression of VEGF after PDT, (ii) targeting the VEGF pathway using monoclonal antibody, Avastin, to inhibit tumor angiogenesis and also to study the effect of Avastin on other angiogenic growth factors; (ii) targeting the EGFR pathway, using the monoclonal antibody Erbitux to inhibit tumor angiogenesis and to assess its effect on the EGFR pathway and finally (iii) combining both Avastin and Erbitux with PDT to assess the importance of blocking the two major angiogenic pathways, VEGF and EGFR, to improve treatment outcome.

PDT followed by Avastin inhibited VEGF expression and other important growth factors to improve tumor response in bladder carcinoma xenografts. In a similar way, PDT and Erbitux suppressed growth factors related to the EGFR pathway to produce better treatment outcome. It was noticed that PDT induced tumor destruction can be maintained and significantly enhanced by the administration of Erbitux. VEGF and EGFR pathways play a major role in angiogenesis of bladder tumors. Combining angiogenic inhibitors with PDT protocol to block VEGF and EGFR pathways has proven to be effective in controlling tumor regrowth. Therefore, antiangiogenesis agents may augment the activity of PDT by inhibiting its counterproductive upregulation of VEGF and EGFR. The success achieved by combining angiogenic inhibitors with PDT can provide information for potential target mechanisms, which can be translated into clinical studies with better response rate, less local and systemic toxicity and improved overall survival in patients.

2. Photodynamic therapy induced VEGF

Vascular endothelial growth factor is one of the most important regulators of angiogenesis that acts as a switch to trigger tumor recurrence by promoting proliferation, migration and tube formation of endothelial cells. Moreover, VEGF binds to the tyrosine kinase receptors, VEGFR-1 and VEGFR-2 thus initiating a downstream signaling cascade that promotes angiogenesis (Kowanetz & Ferrara, 2006). In vitro studies have clearly demonstrated that VEGF is a potent mediator of angiogenesis as it helps in the proliferation and migration of the endothelial cells to form tube like capillaries (Bernatchez et al., 1999). Studies have reported that hypoxia plays a major role in the expression of VEGF in tumor tissue (Robbins et al., 1997). It has also been reported that PDT produced significant increases in VEGF within treated lesion (Ferrario & Gomer, 2006). The expression of VEGF in areas surrounding tumor necrosis has also suggested that hypoxia within tumors played a major role in angiogenesis (Senger et al., 1986; Shweiki et al., 1992).

Photodynamic therapy can produce a significant effect on the expression profile of VEGF in serum and tumors. Experiments were conducted in a xenograft model to evaluate VEGF expression at 24 h, 48 h and 72 h after treatment to understand the initiation of regrowth post hypericin PDT (Bhuvaneswari, Gan et al., 2007). Controls in the experiments were animals with untreated tumors. As human nasopharyngeal carcinoma cells was used as xenografts in a mouse model, both human and mouse VEGF were estimated in serum and tumor tissue. The decrease in mouse VEGF in serum immediately post treatment was not significant, but it reached control levels within 72 h. Greater amount of mouse VEGF compared to human VEGF in serum could indicate the involvement of host environment in modulating the PDT response of the tumor (Figure 1). At 24 h post PDT, both the mouse and human VEGF levels in tumor tissue decreased compared to the control group but elevated by 72 h (Figure 2). The decrease of VEGF observed at 24 h post PDT could be explained through the postulation that the residual tumor cells from the initial PDT treatment could be reoxygenated after 24 h following PDT (Uehara et al., 2001) or may be due to reversal of temporary vascular occlusion (Tsutsui et al., 2002). Downregulation of VEGF immediately after PDT and its subsequent upregulation at 72 h could indicate that regrowth in tumors after PDT begins as early as 72 h. It can be argued that both tumor angiogenesis and recurrence may therefore be mediated by PDT via the enhancement of VEGF expression within the treated tumor mass (Tsutsui et al., 2002).

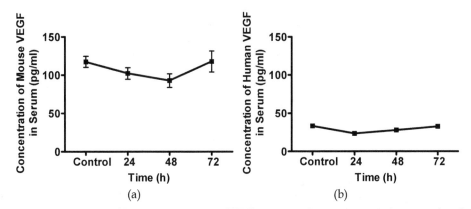

Fig. 1. Concentration of (a) mouse VEGF and (b) human VEGF in serum in the control and at 24 h, 48 h and 72 h post PDT. Error bars represent the standard error of the mean concentration of mouse VEGF in serum at 24 h, 48 h and 72 h, n = 8. The mouse VEGF in serum decreased at 24 h and 48 h post treatment compared to the control group. However at 72 h post PDT the mouse VEGF levels increased and were comparable to the control group.

Mouse VEGF levels were found to be significantly lower than human VEGF in the tumor tissue and this could be attributed to the number of host cells versus the number of tumor cells present within the treated region. Similar observations were reported by Gomer et al. (Gomer et al., 2006). Detection of VEGF has long been known as a potential serum diagnostic marker for malignant diseases. Increased serum VEGF concentrations have been measured in various types of cancer, including brain, lung, renal and ovarian cancer (Kondo et al., 1994). High serum VEGF has been strongly associated with poor clinical outcome in lymphoma patients (Salven et al., 2000). Overexpression of VEGF is known to be common in NPC, which is related to hypoxia up-regulated expression involving a HIF-dependent pathway, and is associated with poor prognosis. Targeting the hypoxia pathway may be useful in the treatment of NPC (Hui et al., 2002). Patients with nasopharyngeal carcinoma having high VEGF levels in serum have been associated with a worse progression-free survival. A recent study has also shown increased microvessel density in oral cancer tissues in VEGF-positive tumors and indicated that upregulation of VEGF was correlated with tumor angiogenesis and disease progression (Shang et al., 2007).

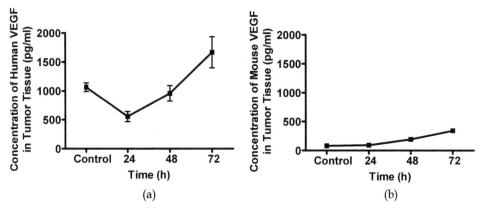

Fig. 2. Concentration of (a) mouse VEGF and (b) human VEGF in tumor tissue in control and at 24 h, 48 h and 72 h points post PDT. Error bars represent the standard error of the mean concentration of human VEGF in tumor tissue at 24 h, 48 h and 72 h, n = 8. Mouse and human VEGF were significantly higher in the tumor tissue (320-1700 pg/ml) compared to serum (33-110 pg/ml). Mouse VEGF in tumor tissue increased at 48 h and 72 h post PDT. The increase in VEGF levels from 24 h to 72 h was found to be statistically significant (p<0.05) (Figure 2b). Controls were animals with untreated tumors.

Immunofluorescence results also confirmed the increased expression of VEGF post PDT in the tumor tissue (Figure 3). Several groups have reported the upregulation of VEGF following PDT (Bhuvaneswari, Gan et al., 2007; Ferrario et al., 2006; Uehara et al., 2001; Yee et al., 2005). Ferrario et al. revealed that PDT-mediated hypoxia and oxidative stress could be involved in photofrin-mediated PDT induced expression of HIF-1α and also increased protein levels of the HIF-1 target gene VEGF, in treated mouse mammary carcinoma xenografts (Ferrario et al., 2000). In a similar study, the same group also reported significant overexpression of HIF-1α and VEGF after photofrin-mediated PDT in a xenograft model of Kaposi's sarcoma (Ferrario et al., 2006). Increased expression of VEGF was noticed from 0 h to 6 h in tumors treated with haematoporphyrin mediated PDT compared to control tumor

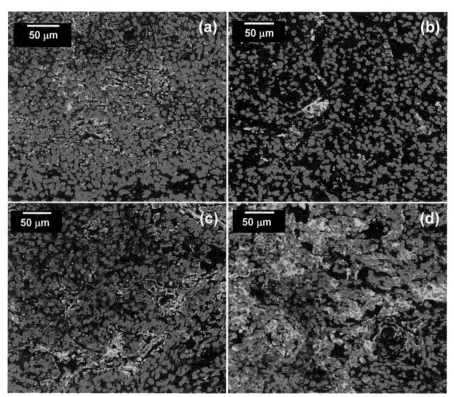

Fig. 3. Immunofluorescence was performed to confirm the expression of VEGF in tumor tissue at different time points post PDT. In the confocal images, the green FITC fluorescence staining indicated the expression of VEGF. (a) control, (b) 24 h post PDT, (c) 48 h post PDT and (d) 72 h post PDT. Magnification: 200X, scale bar = 50 mm. Around 13% and 15% (IF score 2) of scattered staining in certain regions of the cytoplasm was observed in the control (Figure 3a) and at 48 h post PDT (Figure 3c). Minimum VEGF expression of 5% (IF score 1) was observed at 24 h post PDT (Figure 3b). Maximum VEGF staining of 26% (IF score 3) was noticed at 72 h time point (Figure 3d).

in a mouse squamous cell carcinoma model (Uehara et al., 2001). Similar observations were noted by Jiang et al. whereby VEGF levels significantly increased after photofrin-PDT in intracranial glioblastoma xenografts (Jiang et al., 2008). In earlier studies, the same research group had reported increased VEGF levels in normal rat brain that induced the formation of aberrant new vessels following treatment with high dose PDT. In another study it was demonstrated that low dose PDT increases endothelial cell proliferation and VEGF expression in nude mice brain (Zhang et al., 2005). In addition, the upregulation of VEGF in photofrin mediated PDT was also observed in the brain tissue adjacent to tumor in a dose dependent manner (Jiang et al., 2004). Solban et al. investigated the effect of subcurative PDT using photosensitizer benzoporphyrin derivative (BPD) in an *in vivo* orthotopic model of human prostate cancer that demonstrated increased VEGF secretion 24 h following PDT and suggested vascular damage and/or a direct effect of BPD to be responsible for this increase (Solban et al., 2006). Kosharskyy et al. observed increases in not only VEGF secretion but also incidences of lymph node metastases after subcurative PDT in an orthotopic model of prostate cancer (LNCaP), that created conditions favorable for enhanced tumor growth and metastasis (Kosharskyy et al., 2006). The same group also investigated the use of an optical molecular imaging strategy to monitor VEGF expression *in vivo* and effectively labeled and imaged bound VEGF released from the extracellular matrix in response to photodynamic therapy (Chang et al., 2008). Increased secretion of HIF-1α and its target gene VEGF has been observed in hypericin-mediated PDT in both nasopharyngeal and bladder carcinoma (Bhuvaneswari, Gan et al., 2007; Bhuvaneswari, Yuen et al., 2007). Moreover, cellular mediated long drug light interval (DLI) hypericin-PDT induced greater expression of pro-angiogenic growth factors compared to vascular mediated short drug light interval PDT in bladder carcinoma (Bhuvaneswari et al., 2008). Zhou et al. (Zhou et al., 2005) demonstrated that the expression of HIF-1α and VEGF increased in PDT-treated tumor samples collected 24 h post-PDT in a mouse model of human nasopharyngeal carcinoma. Mono-L-aspartyl chlorin e6 (NPe6) PDT of cytokine-overexpressing Lewis lung carcinoma (LLC/IL-2) tumors revealed that the expression of GADD-5alpha and VEGF are induced after PDT and in particular the expression levels were much higher as compared with those in LLC tumors, 12 h after PDT (Ohtani et al., 2008). However, the application of ALA-PDT resulted in a lowered rate of metastatic spreading and decreased VEGF level in blood serum of 3LL-bearing mice that has been attributed to vascularization disturbances in tumor tissue (Lisnjak et al., 2005). Hypocrellin mediated PDT in human brain tumor cells induced expression of proangiogenic VEGF and of antiangiogenic SFH-1, angiostatin, p43, allograft inflammatory factor-1 and connective tissue growth factor suggesting favorable and deleterious effects of hypocrellin-PDT on tumor outgrowth (Deininger et al., 2002). Based on the above studies, it can be inferred that PDT using photosensitizers i.e., photofrins, hypericin, hypocrellins and chlorin e6 increases VEGF concentrations within the tumor tissue and acts as a key regulator of angiogenesis and tumor recurrence post treatment.

3. PDT in combination with Avastin

Combination of anti-angiogenic agents with the PDT regime has been shown to be effective in inhibiting tumor regrowth and improving tumor response (Bhuvaneswari et al., 2009). Studies have reported that transplantable BA mouse mammary carcinoma treated with PDT and non-specific antiangiogenic peptides, IM862, a dipeptide and EMAP-II, a single chain polypeptide, increased tumor regression by inducing apoptosis and inhibiting VEGF production. However, the anti-angiogenic agents by themselves did not produce the desired outcome (Ferrario et al., 2000). Use of novel antiangiogenic monoclonal antibodies, MF1 and DC101 along with PDT against vascular endothelial growth factor receptors VEGFR-1 and VEGFR-2, respectively, reduced the tumor volume significantly and prolonged the survival time of glioma-implanted animals (Jiang et al., 2008). PDT followed by administration of an antiangiogenic agent, TNP-470, abolished the increase in VEGF levels caused by subcurative PDT and reduced local tumor growth in an orthotopic model of prostate cancer (LNCaP) (Kosharskyy et al., 2006). Synthetic RTK inhibitors SU5416 and SU6668 when combined with hypericin PDT significantly extended survival of tumor-bearing host mice (Zhou et al., 2005). Combining PDT with humanized monoclonal antibody Avastin (bevacizumab) resulted in significant increase in long-term responsiveness of treated Kaposi's sarcoma tumors when compared to monotherapies (Ferrario et al., 2006). Chang et al. (Chang et al., 2008) used an *in vivo* optical imaging technique that produces wavelength-resolved fluorescence hyperspectral images to study changes in tumoral VEGF concentration following PDT and Avastin treatment. The *in vivo* antigen blocking experiment showed that Avastin pretreatment before imaging blocked the tumoral VEGF, and also that VEGF-specific contrast agent labeling decreased in tandem with the pretreated Avastin dose, demonstrating that VEGF-specific contrast agent specifically binds to the VEGF protein.

Since VEGF and its receptors represent central molecular targets for antiangiogenic intervention, addition of Avastin (bevacizumab) along with PDT can increase the treatment efficacy. Avastin is a recombinant, partially humanized, monoclonal IgG1 antibody that binds to and inhibits the biological activity of human VEGF thus preventing interaction with its receptors. Avastin along with chemotherapy has been approved in the United States of America (USA) for the treatment of colorectal cancer and NSCLC and in other countries for the treatment of breast cancer, prostate cancer and renal cell carcinoma (Shih & Lindley, 2006).

In this study, the potential of combining anti-angiogenic agent Avastin that is specific to VEGF, with photodynamic therapy to enhance treatment efficacy by improving the tumor responsiveness was investigated. As Balb/c nude mice are immunocompromised, human bladder carcinoma cells were injected to establish subcutaneous tumor grafts. Subcutaneous models were used for our experiments because of the simple inoculation procedure, reproducibility of tumor growth and easy accessibility of the tumor for measurement and treatment. MGH bladder tumors form vascularized solid tumors.

The tumor regression experiments conducted in the xenograft model clearly indicated that combining Avastin with PDT can impede the angiogenesis process and improve the response of treated tumors. This has been demonstrated by the significant decrease in the tumor volume of the combination therapy group of PDT + Avastin compared to the control and high dose PDT groups (Figure 4). This demonstrates that by targeting the VEGF pathway, post-PDT angiogenesis can be reduced. It should be noted that Avastin is a monoclonal antibody that targets human VEGF and not mouse VEGF. The tumor volume of high dose PDT treated group was significantly greater than the low dose PDT group and this could be due to the difference in fluence rates administered. High fluence rate can deplete tumor oxygen to a greater extent, thereby reducing the primary cytotoxic processes of PDT and affecting tumor control. On the other hand, low fluence rate treatments can be more effective in decreasing vascular lesions even if the same overall fluence is maintained. Other studies have concluded that lower fluence rate treatments can preserve the status of oxygen for a more effective PDT (Chen et al., 2002; Sitnik et al., 1998; Tromberg et al., 1990) and it is well recognized that light fluence rates play a major role in the tumor oxygenation status during PDT exposure. But we should also understand that oxygen-conserving low fluence rate PDT cannot always be effective if it is unable to produce the desired tumor damage and it is essential to estimate the lower limits of fluence rate that would be required for effective treatment thus potentially allowing the tailoring of treatment to specific situations (Henderson et al., 2006; H. W. Wang et al., 2004). The group of animals that were administered only Avastin showed greater tumor response compared to the high dose PDT and control groups, this could be due to the fact that Avastin by itself can target and bind to human VEGF. Though not statistically significant, better tumor response was observed in the combination therapy group compared to Avastin only and low dose PDT groups, however a greater sample size would be required to establish these findings. Complete cure was not achieved in these groups by end of 30-day post treatment, as Avastin does not target mouse VEGF produced by the host environment. Tumors were excised to analyze the expression of VEGF and other angiogenic proteins at the end of the 30-day tumor growth experiments. This time point was chosen to study the long-term effect of Avastin on the expression profile of angiogenic proteins.

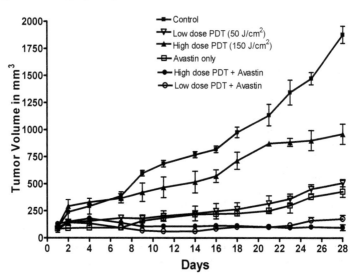

Fig. 4. Tumor volume charted against days, to assess the tumor response in various treatment groups. The combination therapy group of PDT and Avastin exhibited greater tumor response in comparison with other groups. Each group represents the mean (bars, SE) of 10 animals.

Next, circulating human VEGF concentrations in mice was investigated to analyze tumor-derived VEGF. A low but detectable amount of human VEGF was observed in most tumors (Figure 5). It has been shown that high fluence rates during PDT can influence the inflammatory responses associated with PDT (Henderson et al., 2004). In the same way, the results also suggest that high dose PDT could have triggered inflammatory responses within the treated tumors that may enhance VEGF secretion. Though it was expected that Avastin would specifically bind to the circulating human VEGF, measurable amount of VEGF was documented in the animals that received Avastin alone. One of the reasons for detecting circulating VEGF in all the treatment groups could be the extended period of VEGF transcriptional activation, (Liang et al., 2006) and it is likely that low level of VEGF can be generated, continuously or in pulses, during the angiogenesis process that could vary significantly from tumor to tumor. Also, the data did not seem to exhibit any correlation between VEGF secretion and tumor volume. The smaller tumors in the Avastin only group expressed relatively greater amount of VEGF compared to the tumors in the control and high dose PDT treated groups, this observation can be attributed to multiple factors such as tumor vascularization, tumor invasiveness, tumor infiltrating macrophages and the production of cytokine IL-1α that has been shown to influence the secretion of VEGF (Borg et al., 2005).

Immunohistochemistry was performed to detect VEGF and this method has been used in earlier studies for quantifying VEGF (Harper et al., 1996; Saito et al., 1999). As VEGF is a secreted protein, it was observed mainly in the cytoplasm and the extracellular matrix (Figure 6). These data demonstrate that tumors under oxidative stress express greater amounts of VEGF. Also, significantly lower occurrence of VEGF was observed in the combination therapy of PDT and Avastin. These results are consistent with an earlier report by Solban et al. (Solban et al., 2006) on subcurative PDT performed on an orthotopic model of prostate cancer that showed increased VEGF secretion and also demonstrated that VEGF induction can be abolished by administering p38 MAPK inhibitor along with PDT.

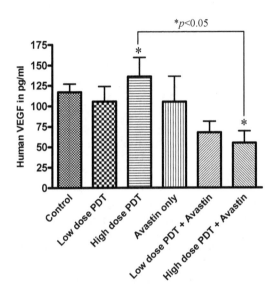

Fig. 5. Relative concentration of human VEGF measured in pg/ml in serum for various treatment groups. Greater expression of VEGF was observed in the high dose PDT group compared to the combination therapy group of high dose PDT + Avastin. Each group represents the mean (bars, SE) of 10 animals.

The effect of different treatment regimes on the expression profiles of angiogenic proteins was also investigated. The study established differential expression of proteins in the angiogenesis pathway as different PDT combinations were administered (Figure 7). The protein angiogenin initiates cell migration, proliferation and induces neovascularization *in vivo* (Hartmann et al., 1999). In our experiments it was upregulated in high-dose PDT treated tumors compared to all other groups and this may be due to hypoxia induced production of angiogenin. Similarly studies have established positive correlation between hypoxia and angiogenin expression in human malignant melanoma, (Hartmann et al., 1999) and human primary breast carcinoma (Campo et al., 2005). A study on gastric carcinoma cancer has shown angiogenin expression in cancer tissues to be positively correlated with VEGF (Chen et al., 2002) and our results show that blocking the VEGF pathway using PDT with Avastin does downregulate the expression of angiogenin. Both bFGF and VEGF seem to differentially activate the Raf pathway in the angiogenesis process (Alavi et al., 2003) and as bFGF has shown to promote angiogenesis indirectly by the upregulation of VEGF in endothelial cells, (Pepper et al., 1992) the reduced expression of bFGF in the combination

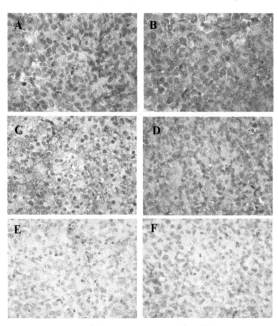

Fig. 6. VEGF expression was assessed in tumors treated with various treatment regimens using immunohistochemistry A - Control (untreated tumor), B - Low dose PDT, C - High dose PDT, D - Avastin only, E -Low dose PDT + Avastin and F - High dose PDT + Avastin. VEGF, a secreted protein was observed in the cytoplasm and extracellular matrix. 30% Immunostaining for VEGF was observed in high dose PDT treated tumors. Control, low dose PDT and Avastin only groups exhibited <5% of staining. Minimal staining of less that 2% was observed in the combination therapy groups of PDT and Avastin. All sections are shown at a magnification of × 630.

therapy groups could mean that inhibiting VEGF may possibly attenuate bFGF expression as well. Amplication of bFGF by a HIF-1α-dependent pathway, (Calvani et al., 2006) may be one of the reasons for the upregulation of bFGF in PDT treated tumors. Similary EGF, a key EGFR ligand that promotes angiogenesis (Ciardiello, 2005) and was upregulated in high dose PDT treated tumors, is known to be HIF-1α regulated (Vaupel, 2004). We observed downregulation of EGF in the combination therapy groups suggesting that VEGF and EGFR pathways are closely related, sharing common downstream signaling pathways. (Tabernero, 2007) PlGF-1 is expressed in placental tissues, colon and mammary carcinomas and it belongs to the VEGF family (Cao et al., 1996). No PlGF expression was noted in the low dose PDT treated group as the oxidative stress in these tumors was expected to be minimal due to low fluence rate administered during PDT. However, the Avastin only and combination therapy treated tumors expressed minimal PlGF, which may suggest that Avastin, which binds to VEGF, has negligible effect on PlGF. Furthermore as PlGF binds only to VEGF receptors, it has been documented that PlGF can be downregulated by blocking the VEGFR-1/FLT1 receptor pathway (Ahmed et al., 2000). As both EGF and PlGF was not observed in the control tumors and induced only post PDT treatment, we conjecture that these proteins may not play a major role in angiogenesis of MGH bladder tumors, based on our experimental data that show increased tumor volume in control groups. After PDT treatment, the tumors are in hypoxic condition which is one of the factors causing cytokine expression (Gomer et al., 2006). The role of IL-6 in angiogenesis is mediated through the induction of VEGF (T. Cohen et al., 1996). The increased expression of interleukins in the control and PDT treated groups may have resulted due to greater tumor volume and PDT induced inflammation, respectively. Compared to high dose PDT group, the tumors in combination therapy group produced lower levels of cytokines and this we theorize to be the role of Avastin in reducing angiogenesis by binding to VEGF, thus reducing the expression of post PDT inflammatory proteins. Expression of IL-6 was elevated in most of the treatment groups compared to IL-8 suggesting its importance in PDT-induced inflammation.

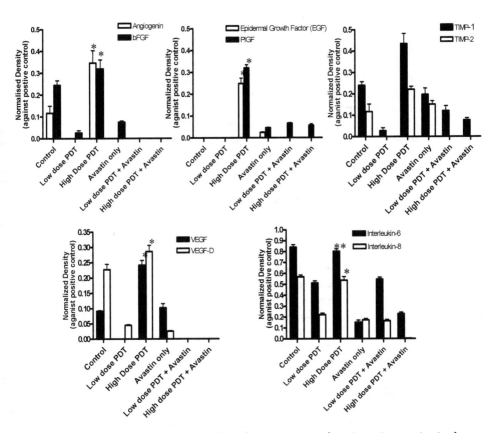

Fig. 7. Antibody arrays were used to analyze the expression of angiogenic proteins in the treated tumors. Density of proteins was plotted and normalized against the positive control Actin, (a) Angiogenin and bFGF, (b) EGF and PIGF, (c) TIMP-1 and TIMP-2, (d) VEGF and VEGF-D and (e) IL-6 and IL-8. Each group represents the mean (bars, SE) of 5 tumors (i.e. one membrane was used per tumor). Statistical analysis was performed using one-way ANOVA with Bonferroni's multiple comparison tests. $* = p<0.001$, $** = p<0.01$ when high dose PDT group was compared with the combination therapy groups of low dose PDT + Avastin and high dose PDT + Avastin.

On the other hand, TIMPs are natural inhibitors of MMPs. A stimulatory role of TIMP-1 in angiogenesis has been proposed in an earlier study (Wurtz et al., 2005) which reports that by inhibiting MMPs, TIMP-1 may prevent angiostatin and endostatin production, thus playing a positive role in tumor angiogenesis. In contradiction to an earlier report (Ferrario et al., 2004) that PDT suppresses TIMP-1 expression in mouse mammary carcinoma, we noticed upregulation of TIMP-1 in the high dose PDT treated tumors. Nevertheless, this dissimilarity can be attributed to the different tumor systems and the PDT protocol administered. VEGF which is also known as VEGF-A is involved in angiogenesis and lymphangiogenesis and VEGF-D, a secreted protein stimulates lymphangiogenesis and metastasis in tumors (Hoeben et al., 2004). Reports have shown that subcurative PDT in an orthotopic model of prostate cancer increases VEGF secretion and also cause lymph node metastasis. It was also demonstrated that the administration of anti-angiogenic agent TNP-40 abolished this increase and reduced tumor growth (Kosharskyy et al., 2006). In our study VEGF was not detected in low dose PDT group and that could be due to lower oxidative insult to the tumor tissue compared to the high dose PDT group. Furthermore, downregulation of VEGF levels was observed in the PDT + Avastin treated tumor as the combination treatment effectively suppressed the VEGF signalling cascade. However, we noticed minimal expression of VEGF using IHC and ELISA and this we attribute to the different tumor microenvironment as tumors were collected from different animals though they were treated with the same treatment protocol. In conclusion, the results demonstrate that by targeting the VEGF pathway, post-PDT angiogenesis can be inhibited. Furthermore, suppressing the VEGF pathway can also downregulate other angiogenic mediators.

4. PDT in combination with Erbitux

Erbitux was approved by the US Food and Drug Administration (FDA) for use in combination with irinotecan for the treatment of metastatic colorectal cancer and it is also being used for the treatment of metastatic squamous cell carcinoma of the head and neck (SCCHN) (Wong, 2005). Results of a large phase II study on irinotecan-refractory, colorectal cancer patients have shown a significant response of 22.9% when Erbitiux was combined with chemotherapy agent, irinotecan (Cunningham et al., 2004). In another study, the response rate was significantly improved when Erbitux was combined with cisplatin in the first-line treatment of recurrent or metastatic SCCHN (Burtness, 2005). A randomized trial that compared radiotherapy plus Erbitux with radiotherapy alone in patients with stage III or IV non-metastatic SCCHN, demonstrated significantly longer locoregional control with radiotherapy plus Erbitux than with radiotherapy alone; moreover, progression-free survival were significantly longer and the overall response rate was significantly better with the combination therapy (Griffin et al., 2009). Erbitux given concurrently with radiotherapy yields a significant clinical benefit over radiotherapy alone without any increase in radiotherapy-associated toxicity, this was demonstrated in the results of a recent phase III randomized study (Bernier & Schneider, 2007).

In the *in vivo* tumor regression study, we demonstrate that the combination therapy of Erbitux with PDT can improve the tumor response by attenuating the angiogenic process (Figure 8). A similar study conducted on a mouse model of human ovarian cancer in which C225 (Erbitux) was combined with PDT regimen produced synergistic reductions in mean tumor burden and significantly greater median survival (del Carmen et al., 2005). In this study, PDT treated tumors did not exhibit significant tumor regression compared to combination therapy groups and this could be attributed to the high fluence rate that was administered during PDT. High fluence rate can deplete tumor oxygen to a large extent, thereby stimulating the production of stress induced survival molecules that reduce the effectiveness of PDT and affect tumor control (Henderson et al., 2004). More importantly, the use of high light dose for this experiment was to test our hypothesis that combining PDT with Erbitux can improve tumor control and also to evaluate the effectiveness of Erbitux in reducing EGFR concentrations. The investigations have indicated that Erbitux alone as monotherapy was not effective in controlling tumor growth. One of the possible reasons for this observation could be the fact that tumors overexpressing EGFR might not be sensitive to Erbitux. Although we would assume that tumors overexpressing EGFR would respond well to anti-EGFR therapy, studies have demonstrated that the level of EGFR expression does not have any impact on tumor response rates as a significant number of EGFR-positive tumors could be resistant to Erbitux (Ellis & Hoff, 2004; Vallbohmer et al., 2005). The group that received the combination therapy of PDT and Erbitux exhibited accelerated growth a week after PDT which could be due an increase in the expression of angiogenic growth factors either due to hypoxia induced by oxygen depletion during PDT light irradiation or incomplete treatment. Our earlier results have shown increased expression of angiogenic growth factor VEGF at 72 h post PDT (Vallbohmer et al., 2005). In this study, the regular administration of Erbitux after PDT treatment could have blocked the EGFR pathway and reduced angiogenesis. Therefore, our data supports the hypothesis that combination therapy of PDT and Erbitux would be more effective in preventing angiogenesis compared to monotherapy alone.

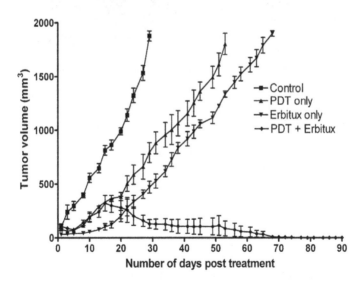

Fig. 8. Mean tumor volume charted against number of days post treatment, to assess the tumor response in various treatment groups. The combination therapy group of PDT and Erbitux exhibited greatest tumor response in comparison with all other groups. Each group represents the mean response (bars, SE) of 10 animals.

To further substantiate our results we performed western blotting and immunohistochemistry to determine the EGFR levels in all the treatment groups. EGFR immunoreactivity was localized mainly in the cell membranes and to a lower extent in the cytoplasm as well (Figure 9). It has been well established that the core of solid tumors is hypoxic, and that hypoxic tumor environment is sufficient to trigger EGFR expression in tumors (Franovic et al., 2007). Previous studies have reported the downregulation of EGFR after PDT (Ahmad et al., 2001; Tsai et al., 2009); in marked contrast our results demonstrated an increase in EGFR expression post hypericin-mediated PDT. This observation could be attributed to numerous reasons such as the light/drug dosage, the complexity of tumor microenvironment and the properties of the photosensitizer (Henderson et al., 2004). Combined antitumor activity of Erbitux with standard chemotherapy and radiotherapy is well documented in the treatment of different types of tumors and is reported to be more efficacious than individual monotherapies (E. E. Vokes & Chu, 2006). In this study, combination modality of PDT and Erbitux was effective in reducing the expression of EGFR and that could have lead to the regression of tumors in this group.

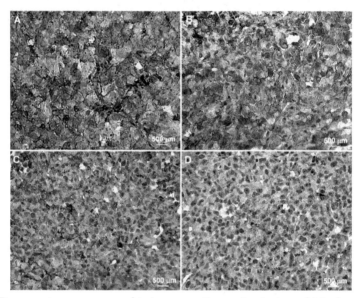

Fig. 9. EGFR expression was assessed in tumor sections using immunohistochemistry. The brown colored membrane staining indicates EGFR positive immunoreactivity. (A: Control, B: PDT, C: Erbitux and D: PDT +Erbitux). PDT and Erbitux (D) resulted in significant reduction of EGFR expression of 4-6% (EGFR score 1) compared to monotherapy (B: PDT and C: Erbitux) and control groups (A). Maximum EGFR tumor cell membrane staining of 21-24% (EGFR score 3) noticed in the untreated tumors. The monotherapy groups of PDT only and Erbitux only, exhibited 15-17% (EGFR score 2) and 11-13% (EGFR score 2) staining respectively. Magnification: 630X.

In the current study, we have also shown that PDT plus Erbitux increased apoptosis in the treated tumors compared to PDT only and inhibitor only monotherapies (Figure 10). Erbitux has been known to increase apoptosis in various tumor models by different mechanisms, including upregulation of pro-apoptotic Bax protein (Mahtani & Macdonald, 2008), decrease in the expression of anti-apoptotic molecule Bcl-2 (S. M. Huang et al., 1999) and the activation of pro-apoptotic caspases (Iwase et al., 2008). Hypericin-PDT is also known to induce apoptosis in a dose-dependent manner with higher doses leading to necrosis. Based on the lack of tumor inhibition in the monotherapy groups, it can be noted that tumors treated with PDT alone and Erbitux alone induced limited apoptosis in bladder carcinoma tumors. Therefore in this investigation, we observe that the combination therapy has significantly increased tumor cell apoptosis and inhibited tumor progression. Preclinically, many studies have shown that treatment with Erbitux in combination with radiotherapy or chemotherapy enhances apoptotic cell death than individual therapies. In a similar manner, PDT induced apoptosis, could have been enhanced by the combination of Erbitux to the treatment regime.

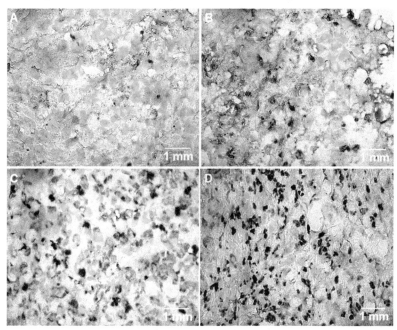

Fig. 10. The tunnel assay was performed on the tumors that were harvested from the animals at the end of the treatment. Few isolated positive nuclei were noticed in (A) untreated tumors, (Apoptotic index (AI) – 6%). Both (B) PDT only (AI - 14%) and (C) Erbitux only (AI - 16%) treated tumors showed increased apoptosis compared to control. High levels of apoptotic nuclei were clearly exhibited by tumors treated with the (D) PDT plus Erbitux combination therapy (AI - 32%, p <0.001). Magnification: 630X.

By using EGF phosphorylation antibody array membranes, we examined the relative level of phosphorylation of specific sites for human EGFR receptors. Interestingly, we noted the phosphorylation of Threonine 686 site of ErbB2 in all the groups. Studies have suggested that the dysregulation of cellular protein kinase C (Ouyang et al., 1996) and protein kinase A (Monje et al., 2008) activity could phosphorylate ErbB2 on Thr-686 for the activation and proliferation of tumor cells (Figure 11). However, our findings suggest that ErB2 on Thr-686 may not be essential for regulation of tumor proliferation, as tumor control was observed in the PDT + Erbitux treated group. Phosphorylation of EGFR tyrosine 845, only noticed in control tumors, is implicated in the stabilization of the activation loop, providing a binding surface for substrate proteins and is capable of regulating receptor function and tumor progression (Cooper & Howell, 1993). c-Src is known to be involved in the phosphorylation of EGFR at Tyr845 (Biscardi et al., 1999). The major autophosphorylation sites of ErbB2 are Tyr1248 and Tyr1221/1222 that lead to Ras-Raf-MAP kinase signal transduction pathway (Kwon et al., 1997). In control tumors, ErbB2 was phosphorylated at tyrosine 1221/1222 and is associated with high tumor grade and with shorter disease-free survival and overall survival (Frogne et al., 2009). Similarly, ErbB4 is able to induce phosphorylation of phosphatidylinositol 3-kinase regulatory subunit which is a pro-survival protein that prevents apoptosis (B. D. Cohen et al., 1996; Gallo et al., 2006). Our data suggests that dephosphorylation of ErbB4 tyrosine 1284 is critical for tumor regression in the dual treatment group.

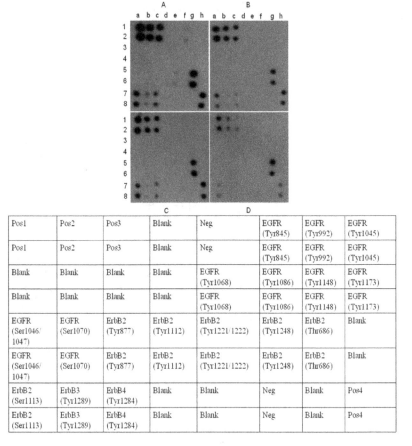

Pos1	Pos2	Pos3	Blank	Neg	EGFR (Tyr845)	EGFR (Tyr992)	EGFR (Tyr1045)
Pos1	Pos2	Pos3	Blank	Neg	EGFR (Tyr845)	EGFR (Tyr992)	EGFR (Tyr1045)
Blank	Blank	Blank	Blank	EGFR (Tyr1068)	EGFR (Tyr1086)	EGFR (Tyr1148)	EGFR (Tyr1173)
Blank	Blank	Blank	Blank	EGFR (Tyr1068)	EGFR (Tyr1086)	EGFR (Tyr1148)	EGFR (Tyr1173)
EGFR (Ser1046/1047)	EGFR (Ser1070)	ErbB2 (Tyr877)	ErbB2 (Tyr1112)	ErbB2 (Tyr1221/1222)	ErbB2 (Tyr1248)	ErbB2 (Thr686)	Blank
EGFR (Ser1046/1047)	EGFR (Ser1070)	ErbB2 (Tyr877)	ErbB2 (Tyr1112)	ErbB2 (Tyr1221/1222)	ErbB2 (Tyr1248)	ErbB2 (Thr686)	Blank
ErbB2 (Ser1113)	ErbB3 (Tyr1289)	ErbB4 (Tyr1284)	Blank	Blank	Neg	Blank	Pos4
ErbB2 (Ser1113)	ErbB3 (Tyr1289)	ErbB4 (Tyr1284)	Blank	Blank	Neg	Blank	Pos4

Fig. 11. Phosphorylation statuses of EGFR sites were determined using antibody arrays. Increased phosphorylation of ErbB2(Thr686), ErbB2(Ser1113) and limited phosphorylation of EGFR(Thy845), ErbB2(Tyr1221/1222), ErbB3(Tyr1289) and ErbB4(Tyr1284) sites was seen in the control group. In the monotherapy groups, ErbB2(Thr686), (Ser113) and ErbB4(Tyr1284) sites were phosphorylated. Inhibition of most of the EGFR phosphorylation sites was observed in combination therapy groups except for ErbB2(Thr686) and (ser1113).

EGFR-mediated Ras-Raf-MEK-ERK and PI3K-PTEN-AKT pathways play an important role in transmission of signals from membrane receptors to downstream targets that regulate apoptosis, cell growth and angiogenesis. Components of these pathways include genes such as Ras, B-Raf, PI3K, PTEN and Akt that can be mutated or aberrantly expressed in human cancer. Though we did not investigate these genes, it should be noted that they could cause resistance to anti-EGFR therapy. Numerous studies have reported Kras mutations as a predictor of resistance to Erbitux therapy and are associated with poor prognosis in colorectal cancer (Lievre et al., 2006) and non-small cell lung carcinoma (Riely et al., 2009). In a similar way, Braf mutation is also known to cause resistance to anti-EGFR therapy in colorectal cancers (Li et al., 2006) and primary lung adenocarcinomas (Schmid et al., 2009). Mutation of PTEN tumor suppressor gene in human cancer cells leads to activated EGFR downstream signaling including PI3-kinase/AKT and have been linked to resistance to anti-EGFR targeted therapies (M. Y. Wang et al., 2006). However, in this study we investigated the role of EGFR target genes cyclin D1 and c-myc that are involved in cell proliferation. Our RT-PCR results showed downregulation of cyclin D1 and c-myc in the tumors treated with the combination therapy (Figure 12). Amplification of cyclin D1, a key cell cycle regulatory protein, appears to be an important event in bladder cancer and is often associated with cell proliferation and poor prognosis in human tumors (Le Marchand et al., 2003). In our study, downregulation of EGFR also resulted in reduction of cyclin D1. This observation could be due to the administration of Erbitux, that is known to cause cell cycle arrest in the G(1)/G(0)-phase, also increases the expression of cyclin-dependent kinase inhibitors (Huether et al., 2005). c-myc, another EGFR target gene that can obstruct the induction of apoptosis in tumor cells and lead to uncontrolled cell growth was reduced in the PDT + Erbitux treated tumors. Over-expression and amplification of c-myc can play an important role in metastatic progression that indicates poor prognosis in different cancers (Peng et al., 1997). These results suggest that EGFR target genes could play a role in tumor inhibition in bladder cancer by arresting cell cycle growth and inducing apoptosis.

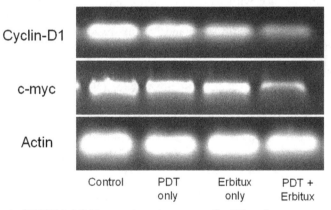

Fig. 12. The effect of EGFR inhibition on target genes cyclin-D1 and c-myc was evaluated at the RNA level. Cyclin D1 is an important regulator of G1 to S-phase transition and overexpression of cyclin D1 has been linked to the development and progression of cancer. c-Myc is activated in a variety of tumor cells and plays an important role in cellular proliferation, differentiation, apoptosis and cell cycle progression. Downregulation of cyclin-D1 and c-myc was observed in the tumors treated with PDT and Erbitux ($p < 0.05$) when compared with the other groups.

5. PDT in combination with Avastin and Erbitux

In this study, the potential of combining anti-angiogenic agent Avastin that is specific to VEGF and Erbitux that targets EGFR along with PDT to improve bladder tumor response was investigated. To achieve this, the inhibitory effect of the anti-angiogenic compounds was tested using angiogenic assays. Cell migration is a highly integrated multistep process that is essential for invasion and metastasis of tumors. Directed cell migration is normally initiated in response to extracellular cues such as chemoattractants, growth factors and the extracellular matrix (Ridley et al., 2003). In this study, stimulation with VEGF, a proangiogenic protein, increased the migration of tumor cells. On the other hand, antiangiogenic agents, Avastin and Erbitux reduced the migratory potential of the tumor cells. Avastin is known to significantly reduce proliferation and migration capacity, and increase apoptotic rates in endothelial cells (Carneiro et al., 2009). A similar study has reported 40-60% inhibition of cell migration of SCC cells when incubated with Erbitux in a dose dependent manner (S. M. Huang et al., 2002). One of the most important and crucial events in cancer metastasis is the invasion of basement membrane. The invasion assay results in this study have clearly demonstrated the stimulatory effect of VEGF on endothelial cell migration (Figure 13). VEGF plays an important role in tumor invasion and metastasis through its specific action on endothelial cells in tumor tissue (Khosravi Shahi & Fernandez Pineda, 2008). In vitro studies have clearly demonstrated that VEGF is a potent mediator of angiogenesis as it helps in the proliferation and migration of the endothelial cells to form tube-like capillaries (Bernatchez et al., 1999). Tumor cells exposed to hypoxia induced by PDT triggers the expression of VEGF mRNA that in turn releases the VEGF protein (Dvorak et al., 1995; Shweiki et al., 1992).

Endothelial barrier disruption by VEGF-mediated Src activity has been shown to potentiate tumor cell extravazation and metastasis (Weis et al., 2004). Another study has reported that interference with VEGF function could be sufficient to abrogate tumor invasion (Skobe et al., 1997). Reduced invasion of endothelial cells through the basement membrane was observed in the Avastin and Erbitux treated cells, suggesting their role in preventing the disruption of the basement membrane. Another important step in angiogenesis is the formation of a functional vascular system for tumor growth and metastasis. Endothelial cell tube formation is a consequence of various biological activities, including cell migration, vacuolization, cell-cell junction formation and cell elongation. It is well established that VEGF plays an important role in the process of angiogenesis by facilitating endothelial cell migration and tube formation similar to the observations in this study (Ferrara, 2004). Another report has also identified Hedgehog signaling as an important component of the molecular pathway leading to vascular tube formation (S. A. Vokes et al., 2004). Avastin and Erbitux were used successfully to reduce and inhibit tube formation, thus signifying their role in blocking major angiogenic processes. Similarly, another study demonstrated that bevacizumab could significantly impair tube formation capabilities in tumor derived endothelial cells and also noted a continuing effect after 14 days of treatment even after omitting the antibody (Grau et al., 2011). Treatment with Cetuximab has also shown to reduce cell-to-cell interaction of human umbilical vascular endothelial cells (HUVEC), resulting in disruption of tube formation (S. M. Huang et al., 2002). Further substantiating these in vitro findings, Avastin and Erbitux also inhibited angiogenesis in a mouse plug matrigel assay, as evaluated by haemoglobin content levels.

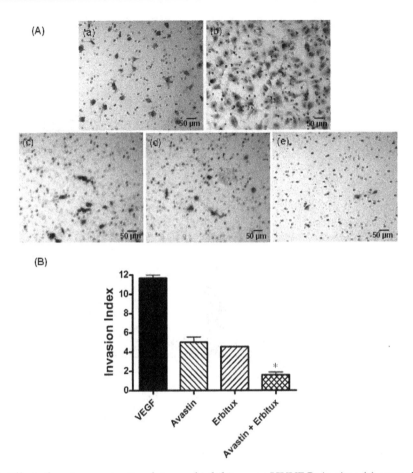

Fig. 13. Effect of angiogenesis stimulator and inhibitors on HUVECs *in vitro*. (a) control, (b) VEGF, (c) Avastin (d) Erbitux and is (e) Avastin + Erbitux. (A) High invasion of endothelial cells through basement membrane were noticed in VEGF treated wells Avastin and Erbitux inhibited the migration of endothelial cells. The figures are representative of the results from three separate experiments. (B) The invasion index was calculated based on the number of cells in the test samples compared to the control samples. Calculations for each group were performed in triplicate. Invasion index for VEGF was high and was lowest for the combination of angiogenesis inhibitors (*=p<0.001). Error bars represent the standard error of the mean invasion index in comparison to control in all the groups, n = 6.

Avastin and Erbitux monotherapies and also Avastin + Erbitux remarkably suppressed the sprouting of endothelial cells and induction of new blood formation in the matrigel plugs (Figure 14). It has been demonstrated that the effects of blocking angiogenesis can be observed on tumor transplanted onto animals (O'Reilly et al., 1994). The antiangiogenic activities of Avastin and Erbitux may be explained by their inhibitory action on the proliferation, migration and differentiation of the tumor cells, by inhibiting VEGF and EGFR respectively.

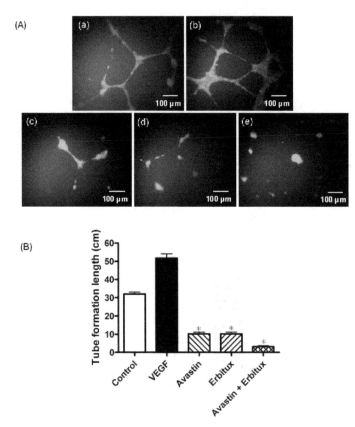

Fig. 14. (A) Endothelial cell tube formation was assessed using VEGF, Avastin and Erbitux. (a) control, (b) VEGF, (c) Avastin (d) Erbitux and (e) Avastin + Erbitux. VEGF induced tube formation and Avastin and Erbitux decreased growth inhibited tube formation of endothelial cells. Combining Avastin and Erbitux, almost completely abrogated tube formation (B) The total tube length of each treatment group was quantified by the software, Datinf Measure (Tubingen, GmbH, Germany). The figures are representative of the results from three separate experiments. Error bars represent the standard error of the mean invasion index in comparison to control in all the groups, n = 8.

The tumor regression data demonstrated that combining Avastin + Erbitux with PDT can impede the angiogenic process and improve the response of treated tumors (Figure 15). The tumor volume of the PDT treated group was significantly greater than the Avastin treated and Erbitux treated groups as high fluence administered during treatment can deplete tumor oxygen to a large extent, releasing stress induced survival molecules that reduce the effectiveness of PDT and affect tumor control (Gomer et al., 2006). Although tumor regression was also observed in Avastin + Erbitux only treated group, complete cure was not observed. Thus targeting EGFR and VEGF without PDT treatment might not be sufficient to cause regression of most bulky tumors. One of the possible explanations for this observation may be related to pericytes that respond to angiogenic stimuli and promote endothelial stability through matrix deposition, and have macrophage-like function (Lu et al., 2007). Also, the tumors overexpressing EGFR might not be sensitive to Erbitux. Although it is normally assumed that tumors overexpressing EGFR would respond well to anti-EGFR therapy, studies have demonstrated that the level of EGFR expression does not have enough impact on tumor response rates as a significant number of EGFR-positive tumors could be resistant to Erbitux (Ellis et al., 2004; Vallbohmer et al., 2005). Complete cure was noted in tumors treated with PDT and continued Avastin + Erbitux therapy. Thus the data from the present study supported the hypothesis that Avastin and Erbitux are capable of binding and neutralizing secreted VEGF and EGFR respectively, thus causing regression of tumor vessels, and preventing tumor recurrence.

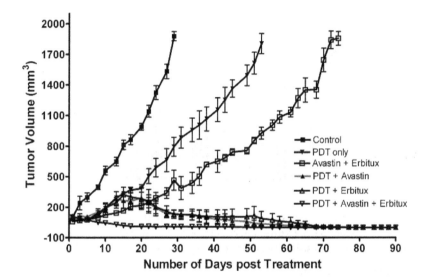

Fig. 15. Tumor volumes were charted against days to assess the tumor response in various treatment groups. The combination therapy groups of PDT + Avastin, PDT + Erbitux and PDT + Avastin + Erbitux exhibited greater tumor response in comparison with other groups. Each group represents the mean (error bars, SE) of 10 animals.

VEGF and EGFR expression was suppressed in the tumors treated with PDT and inhibitors (Figure 16). The data in this study demonstrate that tumors treated with PDT expressed greater amounts of VEGF, which is consistent with an earlier report by Solban et al. (Tortora et al., 2008) on subcurative PDT performed on an orthotopic model of prostate cancer that showed increased VEGF secretion. Also, significantly lower occurrence of VEGF was observed in the combination therapy of PDT and Avastin. On the other hand, previous studies have reported the downregulation of EGFR after PDT (Ciardiello et al., 2006), in marked contrast the results of this study demonstrated an increase in EGFR expression post hypericin-mediated PDT. This observation could be attributed to numerous reasons such as the light/drug dosage, the complexity of tumor microenvironment and the properties of the photosensitizer (Henderson et al., 2004). Combined antitumor activity of Avastin and Erbitux with standard chemotherapy and radiotherapy is well documented in the treatment of different types of tumors and is reported to be more efficacious than individual monotherapies (Press & Lenz, 2007).

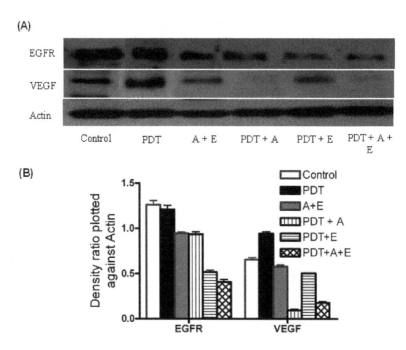

Fig. 16. (A) Expression of EGFR and VEGF was detected in the treatment groups using western immunoblot analysis. Expression of actin was used to monitor protein loading. (B) Ratio of EGFR and VEGF density was plotted against actin.

In this study, combination modality of PDT + Avastin + Erbitux was effective in reducing the expression of VEGF and EGFR which could have led to the greater tumor regression in this group. Combination of Avastin and Erbitux with PDT also improved treatment efficacy by suppressing angiogenic proteins. Though immediate tumor inhibition was noticed in the groups treated with both the inhibitors and PDT, the overall outcome post 90-day treatment for both single agent and double-agent inhibition remained the same. Although tumor regression was also observed in Avastin + Erbitux only treated groups, complete cure was not observed. Thus targeting EGFR and VEGF without PDT treatment might not be sufficient to cause regression of most bulky tumors. One of the possible explanations for this observation may be related to pericytes that respond to angiogenic stimuli and promote endothelial stability through matrix deposition, and have macrophage-like function. Also, the tumors overexpressing EGFR might not be sensitive to Erbitux. Although it is normally assumed that tumors overexpressing EGFR would respond well to anti-EGFR therapy, studies have demonstrated that the level of EGFR expression does not have enough impact on tumor response rates as a significant number of EGFR-positive tumors could be resistant to Erbitux. Complete cure was noted in tumors treated with PDT and continued Avastin + Erbitux therapy.

6. Conclusion

In conclusion, it has been demonstrated that VEGF is upregulated due to hypoxic conditions induced by hypericin-mediated PDT. Also, VEGF acts as a potent angiogenesis-stimulating factor that has potential as a tumor biomarker to determine the outcome of photodynamic therapy. Combination treatment of PDT with Avastin that binds to VEGF and blocks receptor binding improved the tumor response of bladder carcinoma xenografts and suppressed the VEGF pathway by causing the downregulation of important angiogenic mediators. In the similar way, the regular administration of Erbitux, an EGFR inhibitor after PDT treatment can block the EGFR pathway and reduce angiogenesis. Therefore, the combination therapy of PDT and Erbitux was more effective in preventing angiogenesis compared to monotherapy alone. In another study the combination of both Avastin and Erbitux with PDT was capable of binding and neutralizing secreted VEGF and EGFR respectively, thus causing regression of tumor vessels, normalizing surviving mature vasculature and preventing tumor recurrence.

To summarize, combining angiogenesis inhibitors with PDT increased therapeutic efficacy and this method is a promising approach to cancer therapy. The challenge is to choose the appropriate anti-angiogenic agent in combination with optimal light dosimetry PDT for potential clinical application. The success seen with the combination of inhibitors with conventional treatments can provide information for potential target mechanisms, which may translate into better response rate with less local and systemic toxicity and improved overall survival rates.

7. Acknowledgements

The authors would like to thank the National Medical Research Council for funding this research work and the National Cancer Centre Singapore where all the experiments were performed.

8. References

Ahmad, N., Kalka, K., & Mukhtar, H. (2001). In vitro and in vivo inhibition of epidermal growth factor receptor-tyrosine kinase pathway by photodynamic therapy. *Oncogene, 20*(18), 2314-2317.

Ahmed, A., Dunk, C., Ahmad, S., & Khaliq, A. (2000). Regulation of placental vascular endothelial growth factor (VEGF) and placenta growth factor (PlGF) and soluble Flt-1 by oxygen--a review. *Placenta, 21 Suppl A,* S16-24.

Alavi, A., Hood, J. D., Frausto, R., Stupack, D. G., & Cheresh, D. A. (2003). Role of Raf in vascular protection from distinct apoptotic stimuli. *Science, 301*(5629), 94-96.

Bernatchez, P. N., Soker, S., & Sirois, M. G. (1999). Vascular endothelial growth factor effect on endothelial cell proliferation, migration, and platelet-activating factor synthesis is Flk-1-dependent. *J Biol Chem, 274*(43), 31047-31054.

Bernier, J., & Schneider, D. (2007). Cetuximab combined with radiotherapy: an alternative to chemoradiotherapy for patients with locally advanced squamous cell carcinomas of the head and neck? *Eur J Cancer, 43*(1), 35-45.

Bhuvaneswari, R., Gan, Y. Y., Lucky, S. S., Chin, W. W., Ali, S. M., Soo, K. C., et al. (2008). Molecular profiling of angiogenesis in hypericin mediated photodynamic therapy. *Mol. Cancer, 7*, 56.

Bhuvaneswari, R., Gan, Y. Y., Soo, K. C., & Olivo, M. (2009). The effect of photodynamic therapy on tumor angiogenesis. *Cell Mol Life Sci, 66*(14), 2275-2283.

Bhuvaneswari, R., Gan, Y. Y., Yee, K. K., Soo, K. C., & Olivo, M. (2007). Effect of hypericin-mediated photodynamic therapy on the expression of vascular endothelial growth factor in human nasopharyngeal carcinoma. *Int. J. Mol. Med., 20*(4), 421-428.

Bhuvaneswari, R., Yuen, G. Y., Chee, S. K., & Olivo, M. (2007). Hypericin-mediated photodynamic therapy in combination with Avastin (bevacizumab) improves tumor response by downregulating angiogenic proteins. *Photochem. Photobiol. Sci., 6*(12), 1275-1283.

Biel, M. A. (2007). Photodynamic therapy treatment of early oral and laryngeal cancers. *Photochem. Photobiol., 83*(5), 1063-1068.

Biscardi, J. S., Maa, M. C., Tice, D. A., Cox, M. E., Leu, T. H., & Parsons, S. J. (1999). c-Src-mediated phosphorylation of the epidermal growth factor receptor on Tyr845 and Tyr1101 is associated with modulation of receptor function. *J Biol Chem, 274*(12), 8335-8343.

Borg, S. A., Kerry, K. E., Royds, J. A., Battersby, R. D., & Jones, T. H. (2005). Correlation of VEGF production with IL1 alpha and IL6 secretion by human pituitary adenoma cells. *Eur J Endocrinol, 152*(2), 293-300.

Burtness, B. (2005). The role of cetuximab in the treatment of squamous cell cancer of the head and neck. *Expert Opin Biol Ther, 5*(8), 1085-1093.

Calvani, M., Rapisarda, A., Uranchimeg, B., Shoemaker, R. H., & Melillo, G. (2006). Hypoxic induction of an HIF-1alpha-dependent bFGF autocrine loop drives angiogenesis in human endothelial cells. *Blood, 107*(7), 2705-2712.

Campo, L., Turley, H., Han, C., Pezzella, F., Gatter, K. C., Harris, A. L., et al. (2005). Angiogenin is up-regulated in the nucleus and cytoplasm in human primary breast carcinoma and is associated with markers of hypoxia but not survival. *J Pathol, 205*(5), 585-591.

Cao, Y., Linden, P., Shima, D., Browne, F., & Folkman, J. (1996). In vivo angiogenic activity and hypoxia induction of heterodimers of placenta growth factor/vascular endothelial growth factor. *J Clin Invest, 98*(11), 2507-2511.

Carneiro, A., Falcao, M., Azevedo, I., Falcao Reis, F., & Soares, R. (2009). Multiple effects of bevacizumab in angiogenesis: implications for its use in age-related macular degeneration. *Acta Ophthalmol, 87*(5), 517-523.

Chang, S. K., Rizvi, I., Solban, N., & Hasan, T. (2008). In vivo optical molecular imaging of vascular endothelial growth factor for monitoring cancer treatment. *Clin. Cancer Res., 14*(13), 4146-4153.

Chen, Q., Huang, Z., Chen, H., Shapiro, H., Beckers, J., & Hetzel, F. W. (2002). Improvement of tumor response by manipulation of tumor oxygenation during photodynamic therapy. *Photochem Photobiol, 76*(2), 197-203.

Ciardiello, F. (2005). Epidermal growth factor receptor inhibitors in cancer treatment. *Future Oncol, 1*(2), 221-234.

Ciardiello, F., Troiani, T., Bianco, R., Orditura, M., Morgillo, F., Martinelli, E., et al. (2006). Interaction between the epidermal growth factor receptor (EGFR) and the vascular endothelial growth factor (VEGF) pathways: a rational approach for multi-target anticancer therapy. *Ann Oncol, 17 Suppl 7,* vii109-114.

Cohen, B. D., Green, J. M., Foy, L., & Fell, H. P. (1996). HER4-mediated biological and biochemical properties in NIH 3T3 cells. Evidence for HER1-HER4 heterodimers. *J Biol Chem, 271*(9), 4813-4818.

Cohen, T., Nahari, D., Cerem, L. W., Neufeld, G., & Levi, B. Z. (1996). Interleukin 6 induces the expression of vascular endothelial growth factor. *J Biol Chem, 271*(2), 736-741.

Cooper, J. A., & Howell, B. (1993). The when and how of Src regulation. *Cell, 73*(6), 1051-1054.

Cunningham, D., Humblet, Y., Siena, S., Khayat, D., Bleiberg, H., Santoro, A., et al. (2004). Cetuximab monotherapy and cetuximab plus irinotecan in irinotecan-refractory metastatic colorectal cancer. *N Engl J Med, 351*(4), 337-345.

Deininger, M. H., Weinschenk, T., Morgalla, M. H., Meyermann, R., & Schluesener, H. J. (2002). Release of regulators of angiogenesis following Hypocrellin-A and -B photodynamic therapy of human brain tumor cells. *Biochem. Biophys. Res. Commun., 298*(4), 520-530. del Carmen, M. G., Rizvi, I., Chang, Y., Moor, A. C., Oliva, E., Sherwood, M., et al. (2005). Synergism of epidermal growth factor receptor-targeted immunotherapy with photodynamic treatment of ovarian cancer in vivo. *J Natl Cancer Inst, 97*(20), 1516-1524.

Dolmans, D. E., Fukumura, D., & Jain, R. K. (2003). Photodynamic therapy for cancer. *Nat. Rev. Cancer, 3*(5), 380-387.

Dvorak, H. F., Brown, L. F., Detmar, M., & Dvorak, A. M. (1995). Vascular permeability factor/vascular endothelial growth factor, microvascular hyperpermeability, and angiogenesis. *Am J Pathol, 146*(5), 1029-1039.

Ellis, L. M., & Hoff, P. M. (2004). Targeting the epidermal growth factor receptor: an important incremental step in the battle against colorectal cancer. *J Clin Oncol, 22*(7), 1177-1179.

Ferrara, N. (2004). Vascular endothelial growth factor as a target for anticancer therapy. *Oncologist, 9 Suppl 1,* 2-10.

Ferrario, A., Chantrain, C. F., von Tiehl, K., Buckley, S., Rucker, N., Shalinsky, D. R., et al. (2004). The matrix metalloproteinase inhibitor prinomastat enhances photodynamic therapy responsiveness in a mouse tumor model. *Cancer Res, 64*(7), 2328-2332.

Ferrario, A., & Gomer, C. J. (2006). Avastin enhances photodynamic therapy treatment of Kaposi's sarcoma in a mouse tumor model. *J. Environ. Pathol. Toxicol. Oncol., 25*(1-2), 251-259.

Ferrario, A., von Tiehl, K. F., Rucker, N., Schwarz, M. A., Gill, P. S., & Gomer, C. J. (2000). Antiangiogenic treatment enhances photodynamic therapy responsiveness in a mouse mammary carcinoma. *Cancer Res., 60*(15), 4066-4069.

Folkman, J. (2002). Role of angiogenesis in tumor growth and metastasis. *Semin. Oncol., 29*(6 Suppl 16), 15-18.

Franovic, A., Gunaratnam, L., Smith, K., Robert, I., Patten, D., & Lee, S. (2007). Translational up-regulation of the EGFR by tumor hypoxia provides a nonmutational explanation for its overexpression in human cancer. *Proc Natl Acad Sci U S A, 104*(32), 13092-13097.

Frogne, T., Laenkholm, A. V., Lyng, M. B., Henriksen, K. L., & Lykkesfeldt, A. E. (2009). Determination of HER2 phosphorylation at tyrosine 1221/1222 improves prediction of poor survival for breast cancer patients with hormone receptor-positive tumors. *Breast Cancer Res, 11*(1), R11.

Gallo, R. M., Bryant, I., Fry, R., Williams, E. E., & Riese, D. J., 2nd. (2006). Phosphorylation of ErbB4 on Tyr1056 is critical for inhibition of colony formation by prostate tumor cell lines. *Biochem Biophys Res Commun, 349*(1), 372-382.

Giles, F. J. (2001). The vascular endothelial growth factor (VEGF) signaling pathway: a therapeutic target in patients with hematologic malignancies. *Oncologist, 6 Suppl 5*, 32-39.

Gomer, C. J., Ferrario, A., Luna, M., Rucker, N., & Wong, S. (2006). Photodynamic therapy: combined modality approaches targeting the tumor microenvironment. *Lasers Surg Med, 38*(5), 516-521.

Grau, S., Thorsteinsdottir, J., von Baumgarten, L., Winkler, F., Tonn, J. C., & Schichor, C. (2011). Bevacizumab can induce reactivity to VEGF-C and -D in human brain and tumour derived endothelial cells. *J Neurooncol*.

Griffin, S., Walker, S., Sculpher, M., White, S., Erhorn, S., Brent, S., et al. (2009). Cetuximab plus radiotherapy for the treatment of locally advanced squamous cell carcinoma of the head and neck. *Health Technol Assess, 13 Suppl 1*, 49-54.

Harper, M. E., Glynne-Jones, E., Goddard, L., Thurston, V. J., & Griffiths, K. (1996). Vascular endothelial growth factor (VEGF) expression in prostatic tumours and its relationship to neuroendocrine cells. *Br J Cancer, 74*(6), 910-916.

Hartmann, A., Kunz, M., Kostlin, S., Gillitzer, R., Toksoy, A., Brocker, E. B., et al. (1999). Hypoxia-induced up-regulation of angiogenin in human malignant melanoma. *Cancer Res, 59*(7), 1578-1583.

Henderson, B. W., Busch, T. M., & Snyder, J. W. (2006). Fluence rate as a modulator of PDT mechanisms. *Lasers Surg Med, 38*(5), 489-493.

Henderson, B. W., Gollnick, S. O., Snyder, J. W., Busch, T. M., Kousis, P. C., Cheney, R. T., et al. (2004). Choice of oxygen-conserving treatment regimen determines the inflammatory response and outcome of photodynamic therapy of tumors. *Cancer Res, 64*(6), 2120-2126.

Hoeben, A., Landuyt, B., Highley, M. S., Wildiers, H., Van Oosterom, A. T., & De Bruijn, E. A. (2004). Vascular endothelial growth factor and angiogenesis. *Pharmacol Rev, 56*(4), 549-580.

Huang, S. M., Bock, J. M., & Harari, P. M. (1999). Epidermal growth factor receptor blockade with C225 modulates proliferation, apoptosis, and radiosensitivity in squamous cell carcinomas of the head and neck. *Cancer Res, 59*(8), 1935-1940.

Huang, S. M., Li, J., & Harari, P. M. (2002). Molecular inhibition of angiogenesis and metastatic potential in human squamous cell carcinomas after epidermal growth factor receptor blockade. *Mol Cancer Ther, 1*(7), 507-514.

Huang, Z. (2005). A review of progress in clinical photodynamic therapy. *Technol Cancer Res Treat, 4*(3), 283-293.

Huether, A., Hopfner, M., Baradari, V., Schuppan, D., & Scherubl, H. (2005). EGFR blockade by cetuximab alone or as combination therapy for growth control of hepatocellular cancer. *Biochem Pharmacol, 70*(11), 1568-1578.

Hui, E. P., Chan, A. T., Pezzella, F., Turley, H., To, K. F., Poon, T. C., et al. (2002). Coexpression of hypoxia-inducible factors 1alpha and 2alpha, carbonic anhydrase

IX, and vascular endothelial growth factor in nasopharyngeal carcinoma and relationship to survival. *Clin Cancer Res, 8*(8), 2595-2604.

Iwase, M., Takaoka, S., Uchida, M., Yoshiba, S., Kondo, G., Watanabe, H., et al. (2008). Epidermal growth factor receptor inhibitors enhance susceptibility to Fas-mediated apoptosis in oral squamous cell carcinoma cells. *Oral Oncol, 44*(4), 361-368.

Jiang, F., Zhang, X., Kalkanis, S. N., Zhang, Z., Yang, H., Katakowski, M., et al. (2008). Combination therapy with antiangiogenic treatment and photodynamic therapy for the nude mouse bearing U87 glioblastoma. *Photochem. Photobiol., 84*(1), 128-137.

Jiang, F., Zhang, Z. G., Katakowski, M., Robin, A. M., Faber, M., Zhang, F., et al. (2004). Angiogenesis induced by photodynamic therapy in normal rat brains. *Photochem. Photobiol., 79*(6), 494-498.

Khosravi Shahi, P., & Fernandez Pineda, I. (2008). Tumoral angiogenesis: review of the literature. *Cancer Invest, 26*(1), 104-108.

Klein, A., Babilas, P., Karrer, S., Landthaler, M., & Szeimies, R. M. (2008). Photodynamic Therapy in Dermatology - an Update 2008. *J. Dtsch. Dermatol. Ges.*

Kondo, S., Asano, M., Matsuo, K., Ohmori, I., & Suzuki, H. (1994). Vascular endothelial growth factor/vascular permeability factor is detectable in the sera of tumor-bearing mice and cancer patients. *Biochim Biophys Acta, 1221*(2), 211-214.

Kosharskyy, B., Solban, N., Chang, S. K., Rizvi, I., Chang, Y., & Hasan, T. (2006). A mechanism-based combination therapy reduces local tumor growth and metastasis in an orthotopic model of prostate cancer. *Cancer Res., 66*(22), 10953-10958.

Kowanetz, M., & Ferrara, N. (2006). Vascular endothelial growth factor signaling pathways: therapeutic perspective. *Clin Cancer Res, 12*(17), 5018-5022.

Kwon, Y. K., Bhattacharyya, A., Alberta, J. A., Giannobile, W. V., Cheon, K., Stiles, C. D., et al. (1997). Activation of ErbB2 during wallerian degeneration of sciatic nerve. *J Neurosci, 17*(21), 8293-8299.

Le Marchand, L., Seifried, A., Lum-Jones, A., Donlon, T., & Wilkens, L. R. (2003). Association of the cyclin D1 A870G polymorphism with advanced colorectal cancer. *JAMA, 290*(21), 2843-2848.

Li, W. Q., Kawakami, K., Ruszkiewicz, A., Bennett, G., Moore, J., & Iacopetta, B. (2006). BRAF mutations are associated with distinctive clinical, pathological and molecular features of colorectal cancer independently of microsatellite instability status. *Mol Cancer, 5*, 2.

Liang, W. C., Wu, X., Peale, F. V., Lee, C. V., Meng, Y. G., Gutierrez, J., et al. (2006). Cross-species vascular endothelial growth factor (VEGF)-blocking antibodies completely inhibit the growth of human tumor xenografts and measure the contribution of stromal VEGF. *J Biol Chem, 281*(2), 951-961.

Lievre, A., Bachet, J. B., Le Corre, D., Boige, V., Landi, B., Emile, J. F., et al. (2006). KRAS mutation status is predictive of response to cetuximab therapy in colorectal cancer. *Cancer Res, 66*(8), 3992-3995.

Lisnjak, I. O., Kutsenok, V. V., Polyschuk, L. Z., Gorobets, O. B., & Gamaleia, N. F. (2005). Effect of photodynamic therapy on tumor angiogenesis and metastasis in mice bearing Lewis lung carcinoma. *Exp. Oncol., 27*(4), 333-335.

Lu, C., Kamat, A. A., Lin, Y. G., Merritt, W. M., Landen, C. N., Kim, T. J., et al. (2007). Dual targeting of endothelial cells and pericytes in antivascular therapy for ovarian carcinoma. *Clin Cancer Res, 13*(14), 4209-4217.

Macdonald, I. J., & Dougherty, T. J. (2001). Basic principles of photodynamic therapy. *J Porphyr Phthalocyanines, 5*, 105-129.

Mahtani, R. L., & Macdonald, J. S. (2008). Synergy between cetuximab and chemotherapy in tumors of the gastrointestinal tract. *Oncologist, 13*(1), 39-50.

Moghissi, K., Dixon, K., Thorpe, J. A., Stringer, M., & Oxtoby, C. (2007). Photodynamic therapy (PDT) in early central lung cancer: a treatment option for patients ineligible for surgical resection. *Thorax, 62*(5), 391-395.

Monje, P. V., Athauda, G., & Wood, P. M. (2008). Protein kinase A-mediated gating of neuregulin-dependent ErbB2-ErbB3 activation underlies the synergistic action of cAMP on Schwann cell proliferation. *J Biol Chem, 283*(49), 34087-34100.

O'Reilly, M. S., Holmgren, L., Shing, Y., Chen, C., Rosenthal, R. A., Moses, M., et al. (1994). Angiostatin: a novel angiogenesis inhibitor that mediates the suppression of metastases by a Lewis lung carcinoma. *Cell, 79*(2), 315-328.

Ohtani, K., Usuda, J., Ichinose, S., Ishizumi, T., Hirata, T., Inoue, T., et al. (2008). High expression of GADD-45alpha and VEGF induced tumor recurrence via upregulation of IL-2 after photodynamic therapy using NPe6. *Int. J. Oncol., 32*(2), 397-403.

Ouyang, X., Gulliford, T., Zhang, H., Huang, G. C., & Epstein, R. (1996). Human cancer cells exhibit protein kinase C-dependent c-erbB-2 transmodulation that correlates with phosphatase sensitivity and kinase activity. *J Biol Chem, 271*(36), 21786-21792.

Peng, H., Diss, T., Isaacson, P. G., & Pan, L. (1997). c-myc gene abnormalities in mucosa-associated lymphoid tissue (MALT) lymphomas. *J Pathol, 181*(4), 381-386.

Pepper, M. S., Ferrara, N., Orci, L., & Montesano, R. (1992). Potent synergism between vascular endothelial growth factor and basic fibroblast growth factor in the induction of angiogenesis in vitro. *Biochem Biophys Res Commun, 189*(2), 824-831.

Press, M. F., & Lenz, H. J. (2007). EGFR, HER2 and VEGF pathways: validated targets for cancer treatment. *Drugs, 67*(14), 2045-2075.

Pugh, C. W., & Ratcliffe, P. J. (2003). Regulation of angiogenesis by hypoxia: role of the HIF system. *Nat Med, 9*(6), 677-684.

Ridley, A. J., Schwartz, M. A., Burridge, K., Firtel, R. A., Ginsberg, M. H., Borisy, G., et al. (2003). Cell migration: integrating signals from front to back. *Science, 302*(5651), 1704-1709.

Riely, G. J., Marks, J., & Pao, W. (2009). KRAS mutations in non-small cell lung cancer. *Proc Am Thorac Soc, 6*(2), 201-205.

Robbins, S. G., Conaway, J. R., Ford, B. L., Roberto, K. A., & Penn, J. S. (1997). Detection of vascular endothelial growth factor (VEGF) protein in vascular and non-vascular cells of the normal and oxygen-injured rat retina. *Growth Factors, 14*(4), 229-241.

Saito, H., Tsujitani, S., Kondo, A., Ikeguchi, M., Maeta, M., & Kaibara, N. (1999). Expression of vascular endothelial growth factor correlates with hematogenous recurrence in gastric carcinoma. *Surgery, 125*(2), 195-201.

Salven, P., Orpana, A., Teerenhovi, L., & Joensuu, H. (2000). Simultaneous elevation in the serum concentrations of the angiogenic growth factors VEGF and bFGF is an independent predictor of poor prognosis in non-Hodgkin lymphoma: a single-institution study of 200 patients. *Blood, 96*(12), 3712-3718.

Schmid, K., Oehl, N., Wrba, F., Pirker, R., Pirker, C., & Filipits, M. (2009). EGFR/KRAS/BRAF mutations in primary lung adenocarcinomas and corresponding locoregional lymph node metastases. *Clin Cancer Res, 15*(14), 4554-4560.

Senger, D. R., Perruzzi, C. A., Feder, J., & Dvorak, H. F. (1986). A highly conserved vascular permeability factor secreted by a variety of human and rodent tumor cell lines. *Cancer Res, 46*(11), 5629-5632.

Shang, Z. J., Li, J. R., & Li, Z. B. (2007). Upregulation of serum and tissue vascular endothelial growth factor correlates with angiogenesis and prognosis of oral squamous cell carcinoma. *J Oral Maxillofac Surg, 65*(1), 17-21.

Shih, T., & Lindley, C. (2006). Bevacizumab: an angiogenesis inhibitor for the treatment of solid malignancies. *Clin Ther, 28*(11), 1779-1802.

Shweiki, D., Itin, A., Soffer, D., & Keshet, E. (1992). Vascular endothelial growth factor induced by hypoxia may mediate hypoxia-initiated angiogenesis. *Nature, 359*(6398), 843-845.

Sitnik, T. M., Hampton, J. A., & Henderson, B. W. (1998). Reduction of tumour oxygenation during and after photodynamic therapy in vivo: effects of fluence rate. *Br J Cancer, 77*(9), 1386-1394.

Skobe, M., Rockwell, P., Goldstein, N., Vosseler, S., & Fusenig, N. E. (1997). Halting angiogenesis suppresses carcinoma cell invasion. *Nat Med, 3*(11), 1222-1227.

Solban, N., Selbo, P. K., Sinha, A. K., Chang, S. K., & Hasan, T. (2006). Mechanistic investigation and implications of photodynamic therapy induction of vascular endothelial growth factor in prostate cancer. *Cancer Res., 66*(11), 5633-5640.

Tabernero, J. (2007). The role of VEGF and EGFR inhibition: implications for combining anti-VEGF and anti-EGFR agents. *Mol Cancer Res, 5*(3), 203-220.

Tortora, G., Ciardiello, F., & Gasparini, G. (2008). Combined targeting of EGFR-dependent and VEGF-dependent pathways: rationale, preclinical studies and clinical applications. *Nat Clin Pract Oncol, 5*(9), 521-530.

Tromberg, B. J., Orenstein, A., Kimel, S., Barker, S. J., Hyatt, J., Nelson, J. S., et al. (1990). In vivo tumor oxygen tension measurements for the evaluation of the efficiency of photodynamic therapy. *Photochem Photobiol, 52*(2), 375-385.

Tsai, T., Ji, H. T., Chiang, P. C., Chou, R. H., Chang, W. S., & Chen, C. T. (2009). ALA-PDT results in phenotypic changes and decreased cellular invasion in surviving cancer cells. *Lasers Surg Med, 41*(4), 305-315.

Tsutsui, H., MacRobert, A. J., Curnow, A., Rogowska, A., Buonaccorsi, G., Kato, H., et al. (2002). Optimisation of illumination for photodynamic therapy with mTHPC on normal colon and a transplantable tumour in rats. *Lasers Med Sci, 17*(2), 101-109.

Uehara, M., Inokuchi, T., Sano, K., & ZuoLin, W. (2001). Expression of vascular endothelial growth factor in mouse tumours subjected to photodynamic therapy. *Eur. J. Cancer, 37*(16), 2111-2115.

Usuda, J., Kato, H., Okunaka, T., Furukawa, K., Tsutsui, H., Yamada, K., et al. (2006). Photodynamic therapy (PDT) for lung cancers. *J. Thorac. Oncol., 1*(5), 489-493.

Vallbohmer, D., Zhang, W., Gordon, M., Yang, D. Y., Yun, J., Press, O. A., et al. (2005). Molecular determinants of cetuximab efficacy. *J Clin Oncol, 23*(15), 3536-3544.

Vaupel, P. (2004). The role of hypoxia-induced factors in tumor progression. *Oncologist, 9 Suppl 5*, 10-17.

Vokes, E. E., & Chu, E. (2006). Anti-EGFR therapies: clinical experience in colorectal, lung, and head and neck cancers. *Oncology (Williston Park), 20*(5 Suppl 2), 15-25.

Vokes, S. A., Yatskievych, T. A., Heimark, R. L., McMahon, J., McMahon, A. P., Antin, P. B., et al. (2004). Hedgehog signaling is essential for endothelial tube formation during vasculogenesis. *Development, 131*(17), 4371-4380.

Wang, H. W., Putt, M. E., Emanuele, M. J., Shin, D. B., Glatstein, E., Yodh, A. G., et al. (2004). Treatment-induced changes in tumor oxygenation predict photodynamic therapy outcome. *Cancer Res, 64*(20), 7553-7561.

Wang, M. Y., Lu, K. V., Zhu, S., Dia, E. Q., Vivanco, I., Shackleford, G. M., et al. (2006). Mammalian target of rapamycin inhibition promotes response to epidermal growth factor receptor kinase inhibitors in PTEN-deficient and PTEN-intact glioblastoma cells. *Cancer Res, 66*(16), 7864-7869.

Weis, S., Cui, J., Barnes, L., & Cheresh, D. (2004). Endothelial barrier disruption by VEGF-mediated Src activity potentiates tumor cell extravasation and metastasis. *J Cell Biol, 167*(2), 223-229.

Wong, S. F. (2005). Cetuximab: an epidermal growth factor receptor monoclonal antibody for the treatment of colorectal cancer. *Clin Ther, 27*(6), 684-694.

Wurtz, S. O., Schrohl, A. S., Sorensen, N. M., Lademann, U., Christensen, I. J., Mouridsen, H., et al. (2005). Tissue inhibitor of metalloproteinases-1 in breast cancer. *Endocr Relat Cancer, 12*(2), 215-227.

Yee, K. K., Soo, K. C., & Olivo, M. (2005). Anti-angiogenic effects of Hypericin-photodynamic therapy in combination with Celebrex in the treatment of human nasopharyngeal carcinoma. *Int. J. Mol. Med., 16*(6), 993-1002.

Zhang, X., Jiang, F., Zhang, Z. G., Kalkanis, S. N., Hong, X., deCarvalho, A. C., et al. (2005). Low-dose photodynamic therapy increases endothelial cell proliferation and VEGF expression in nude mice brain. *Lasers Med. Sci., 20*(2), 74-79.

Zhou, Q., Olivo, M., Lye, K. Y., Moore, S., Sharma, A., & Chowbay, B. (2005). Enhancing the therapeutic responsiveness of photodynamic therapy with the antiangiogenic agents SU5416 and SU6668 in murine nasopharyngeal carcinoma models. *Cancer Chemother. Pharmacol., 56*(6), 569-577.

10

Epigenetic Therapies for Cancer

Pasano Bojang, Jr. and Kenneth S. Ramos
*Department of Biochemistry and Molecular Biology,
University of Louisville, Louisville, KY,
USA*

1. Introduction

At the cellular level, cancers originate from the monoclonal expansion of a mutant cell leading to accumulation of aberrant cells that continue to lose differentiated features and acquire different biological properties in their progression toward disseminated or metastatic disease. The onset and progression of cancer involves genomic derangements that can be manifested in two ways: 1) Genetic and gross structural defects (e.g. single nucleotide polymorphism (SNP), classic deletion, insertion mutation, chromosomal deletion/inversion/translocation, allelic loss/gain, gene amplification/ deletion), and 2) Aberrant epigenetic covalent modifications (e.g. DNA methylation, histone acetylation, methylation, phosphorylation, citrullination, sumolyation, and ADP ribosylation).

Genomic instability can be triggered by chemical carcinogens, radiation, stress, oncogenic DNA viruses and the aging process. In almost all cancers, genomic instability in the form of genetic alterations or epigenetic modifications affects four classes of genes: oncogenes, tumor suppressor genes, apoptotic genes and/or DNA repair genes. Oncogenes encode proteins that function as positive proliferative signals for tumors. Tumor suppressor genes negatively regulate cell proliferation and are inactivated in many tumors. Apoptotic genes encode proteins that instruct the cell to commit suicide, while DNA repair genes encode proteins that maintain the fidelity of DNA sequences during transcription and replication. The uncontrolled expression of oncogenes or the silencing of tumor suppressor genes can lead to immortalization of cells. For example, in neuroblastoma, the overexpresssion of N-myc oncogene correlates with aggressive tumor behavior (Seeger et al., 1985). The ras oncogene is activated in more than half of the tumors studied in humans (Barbacid et al., 1987), and both relapse and decreased survival in breast cancer patients have been associated with overexpression of Her-2 oncogene (Slamon et al., 1987). The tumor suppressor and cell cycle regulator gene, p53, is mutated or deleted in more than 50% of human tumors (Hollstein M et al., 1991). p53 gene is described as the guardian of the genome because it can activate DNA repair genes when DNA is damaged, or induce apoptosis when DNA damage is sensed to be irreparable.

Despite the presence of defective genes in tumors, tumors actually arise through many different combinations of genetic alterations. The phenotypic diversity observed between normal and cancer cells cannot be explained simply by structural and genetic alterations. Epigenetic mechanisms have been shown to activate or inactivate genes. Conrad Waddington first coined the term epigenetic to mean changes above and beyond (epi) the primary DNA sequence (Waddington, 1939). The term epigenetic refers to heritable genetic variations that give rise to distinct patterns of terminal differentiation phenotypes (Waddington, 1952; Ruden et al., 2005; Goldberg et al., 2007). These heritable variations are independent of the DNA sequence, can be reversible, and often are self-perpetuating (Bonasia et al 2010). Epigenetic modifications can include DNA methylation, histone acetylation, histone methylation, histone phosphorylation, citrullination, sumoylation, and ADP ribosylation. A classic example of epigenetic control is seen as cells undergo differentiation during development (Figure 1). While every cell in the human body has identical DNA sequence (except for T and B cells), epigenetic patterns lead the same cells to differentiate into a wide array of cell types and the formation of different tissues or organs (Figure 1). Also, animals cloned from the same donor DNA are not identical and develop diseases with different penetrance from the donor parent (Esteller, 2008; Rideout 3rd et al., 2001). The methylation patterns (Fraga et al., 2005b; Kaminsky et al., 2009), and histone modification profiles (Kaminsky et al., 2009), are different in monozygote twins, indicating that while epigenetic patterns are stable and heritable, they are also dynamic in the sense that genes can be silenced or activated due to changes in cellular environment (Figure 1). In normal cells, epigenetic patterns are in dynamic equilibrium (Szyf, 2007). Many diseases, of which cancer is no exception, arise when different types of epigenetic patterns are introduced at the wrong time, and/or the wrong place. For example, the hypermethylation of tumor suppressor genes, $t16^{INK4a}$, $p14^{ARF}$ and $MGMT$, has been reported as an early event

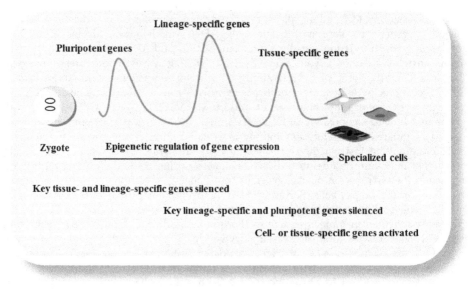

Fig. 1. Epigenetic changes leading to activation or silencing of genes during development. Depicted in the figure is the time dependent activation or inactivation of key genes during development (i.e. from zygote to specialized cells). While every cell has exactly the same DNA composition, the interplay between epigenetic modifications such as DNA methylation or histone modifications (e.g. histone methylation, acetylation, phosphorylation, ubiquitination and sumoylation) can lead to the expression or silencing of pluriponent genes, lineage specific genes or tissue specific genes during development leading to the formation of specialized cells or organs. Peaks depict activation and troughs denote silencing.

in tumorigenesis (Esteller et a., 2007). Because such epigenetic changes are reversible, the epigenome of cancer cells represents an ideal target for cancer treatments. Tumor suppressor genes turned off can be switch back on, and oncogenes turned on can be switched off to restore the epigenetic balance of cancer cells. How epigenetic modifications occur, and how epigenetic profiles define the genomic landscape of cancerous cells and their response to treatment will be the focus of this chapter.

2. Fundamentals of epigenetics

Epigenetic modifications can broadly be classified into three categories: DNA methylation, histone modification and nucleosome positioning. Epigenetic phenotypes result from the interplay between these three categories. Within the microenvironment of the cell, epigenetic patterns are established by transiently activated, and/or stably expressed factors that respond to environmental stimuli, developmental cues, or internal events. Of particular importance within the context of cancer, is the impact of exogenous substances on epigenetic modifications of gene regulation. Since the treatment of many cancers involves exposure to toxic substances, it is important to understand how some of these substances regulate epigenetic modifications. Hence the trajectory of cancer treatment is leaning toward a treatment regimen that includes epigenetic drugs capable of modifying the neoplastic phenotypes to induce shifts in phenotypic expression rather than cytotoxic alterations.

2.1 DNA methylation

DNA methylation was the first identified epigenetic regulation of gene expression in mammals (Holliday and Pugh, 1975; Riggs, 1975). It occurs by enzymatic transfer of a methyl group to carbon 5 of the pyrimidine base, cytosine, in the 5'-3' cytosine guanine (CpG) dinucleotide sequence. Mainly, S-adenosylmethionine (SAM) acts as methyl donor in this reaction. DNA methylation can be classified into four categories based on the region of the genome where methylation occurs. The first identified DNA methylation occurs exclusively in CpG dinucleotides. CpG dinucleotides normally cluster in regions of DNA called CpG islands. They are regions of DNA approximately 200-500 bases long with a G + C content greater than 50% and CpG to GC ratio of at least 0.6 (Bird, 1986; Gardiner-Garden and Frommer, 1987). CpG dinucleotides constitute 1% of the genome and are normally found in the promoter region of genes (Figures 2a and 2b). For example, the promoters of 50-70% of known human genes contain CpG dinucleotides (Bird et al., 1987; Larson et al., 1982; Wang and Lung, 2004). The second kind of DNA methylation is called gene body methylation (Hellman and Chess, 2007). This type of methylation occurs in the open reading frame of genes (Figure 2b) and functions to prevent spurious transcriptional initiation (Hellman and Chess, 2007), or alternative splicing of mainly ubiquitously expressed genes (Zilberman et al., 2007). Recently it has been suggested that gene body methylation also occurs at non CpG dinucleotides (i.e. CHG or CHH sites where H =A, C or T) (Lister et al., 2009; Laurent et al., 2010). A third kind of DNA methylation occurs at CpG island shores (Irizarry et al., 2009; Doi et al., 2009). The term CpG island shores refers to regions of the genome with lower density of CpG dinucleotides that lay approximately 2000 bases away from the CpG islands (Figure 2d). The CpG island shores determines the methylation pattern of tissues (Irizarry et al., 2009; Doi et al., 2009), and the reprogramming of stem cells (Doi et al., 2009; Ji et al., 2010). A fourth kind of DNA methylation occurs at repetitive sequences (e.g. transposable elements and microsatellite regions) (Figure 2e and 2f). The transposable sequences constitute about 47% of the entire genome (Babushok and Kazazian, 2007). Examples of transposable elements are the DNA transposons (e.g. Mer1/2) and retrotransposons (e.g. non-terminal repeat retrotransposon, such as Lines and Sines and long terminal repeat retrotransposon, such as HERVs and IAPs). When activated, these repetitive sequences can move from one region of the genome to another through a so called "cut and paste" or "copy and paste" mechanisms, respectively. Microsatellites are tandem repeats of DNA embedded in various regions of the genome, and their methylation can result in either gene silencing or chromosome instability if it occurs in centromeric regions of the chromosome.

All four types of DNA methylation are catalyzed by a class of enzymes called DNA methyltransferases (DNMT). In mammals, there are five DNMT isoforms: DNMT1, DNMT2, DNMT3a, DNMT3b and DNMT3L (Siedlecki and Zielenkiewicz, 2006). The catalytic domain is conserved between the DNMTs (except DNMT3L), while the regulatory domain responsible for a protein-protein interaction is variable. DNMT1 is a maintenance methyltransferase that ensures the pattern of DNA methylation is transferred from daughter to parent. DNMT1 and proliferating cell nuclear antigen (PCNA) colocalize to DNA replication foci in early S phase (Chuang et al., 1997). Loss of DNMT1 causes cell cycle arrest and apoptosis (Chen et al., 2007). DNMT2 has little DNA methylation activity and DNMT2 knockout mice display no aberrant DNA methylation patterns (Okano et al., 1998). Studies by Goll et al. (2006) have shown that the main function of DNMT2 is to methylate tRNA outside the nucleus. DNMT3a and DNMT3b are *de novo* methyltransferases responsible for establishing methylation patterns during early development. These *de novo* DNMTs are highly expressed in embryonic stem cells and their expression is downregulated after differentiation (Esteller et al., 2007). DNMT3L lacks the catalytic domain and is involved in establishing maternal genomic imprinting by acting as a stimulatory factor for DNMT3a and DNMT3b (Bourc'his et al., 2001). DNMT3L has been shown to interact and colocalize with both DNMT3a and DNMT3b in the nucleus (Chen et al 2005; Holt-Schietinger et al., 2010).

In general, DNA methylations (except gene body methylation) inhibit gene expression. DNA methylation at CpG islands, CpG island shores and repetitive sequence alters the conformation of the DNA in such a way that it prevents recruitment of transcription factors and positive regulators. In addition, methylated DNA promotes the recruitment of Methyl-CpG binding (MBD) proteins (Lopez-Serra and Esteller, 2008). Five classes of MBDs have been identified: MeCP2, MBD1, MBD2, MBD3, and MBD4. MBDs recruit histone deacetylases (HDACs) and histone methyltransferase (HMTs). HMTs methylate histone, with methylated histones being recognized and bound by heterochromatin complexes, such as heterochromatin protein 1 (HP1). These conditions combine to create a chromatin structure (heterochromatin) that favors transcriptional repression. Conversely, unmethylated DNA favors the formation of active chromatin (euchromatin). The formation of active chromatin results in recruitment of histone acetyltansferases and methyltrasferases which create domains characterized by high levels of acetylation and trimethylation at H3K4, H3K36 and H3K79 leading to unwinding of chromatin and binding of transcriptional factors that lead to gene expression.

Compared to normal cells, cancer cells are characterized by global hypomethylation (overall 20-60 less CpG methylation) (Goel et al., 1985). Hypomethylation in cancer cells results in the induction of oncogenic genes, loss of imprinting, activation of transposable elements and microsatellite instability (Dunn, 2003; Esteller, 2008) (Figure 2). Hypomethylation at specific promoters can lead to aberrant expression of oncogenes and loss of imprinting (Figure 2a).

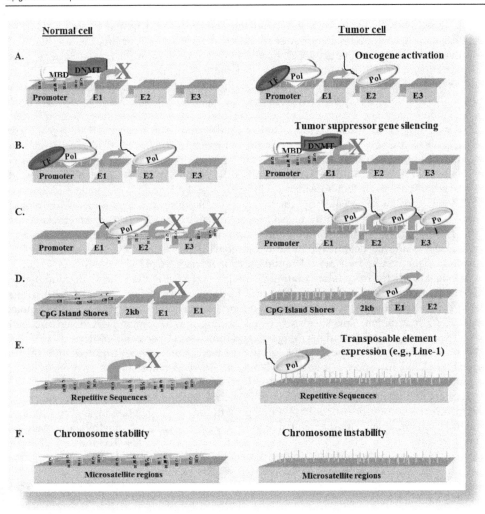

Fig. 2. Methylation patterns in normal versus cancer cells. A. Hypomethylation of oncogene leads to their activation in cancer cells. B. Hypermethylation at the promoter region of a tumor suppressor gene leads to their silencing in cancer cells. C. Gene body hypomethylation leads to spurious transcription initiation in ubiquitously expressed genes. D. Hypomethylation at CpG island shores leads to ubiquitous expression of key regulatory genes. E & F. Hypomethylation at repetitive or microsatellite sequences leads to expression of transoposable elements and chromosomal instability, respectively.

Oncogenes such as S100P, SNCG, melanoma-associated gene (MAGE) and dipeptidyl peptidase 6 (DPP6) are hypomethylated in pancreatic cancer, breast cancer and melanomas, respectively (Wilson et al., 2007; Irizarry et al., 2009). This hypomethylation converts the expression of these genes into aberrantly expressed genes leading to increase growth and metastatic advantage. Loss of imprinting due to hypomethylation has been reported for insulin-like growth factor 2 (IGF2) gene in breast, liver, lung and colon cancers (Ito et al.,

2008). Repetitive sequences are hypomethylated and reactivated in many cancers (Goel et al., 1985; Gaudet et al., 2003; Futscher et al., 2004), as documented for lung, breast, bladder, and liver cancers (Wilson et al., 2007). Lastly, hypomethylation of microsatellite regions at the pericentromeric region leads to genomic instability (Kuismanen et al., 1999).

While the genomes of cancer cells are globally hypomethylated, some aberrant DNA methylation occurs at specific regions of the genome (Figure 2b). These aberrant methylations affect the expression of genes involved in cell cycle control (e.g. p53, Rb, p16^{INK4a}, p15^{INK4b}), apoptosis (TMSI, DAPKI, WIF-1 and SERP1) and DNA repair (e.g. BRAC1, WRN, MGMT, hMLH1). For example, hypermethylation of the CpG dinucleotide in the promoter region of the tumor suppressor gene p16 occurs in 20% of human cancers (Merlo et al., 1995). In addition, the guardian of the genome, p53, is epigenetically silenced in a large proportion of human cancers (Hollstein et al 1991; Jirtle, 1999, Jirtle and Skinner 2007; Jones and Baylin, 2004). Hypermethylation of the promoter region of MASPIN gene was reported as an early event in breast cancer (Futcher et al., 2004). Hypermethylation at CpG regions is also prone to spontaneous point mutations. Methylated cytosines can undergo spontaneous deamination and a subsequent conversion to uracil leading to C-T transition. This results in a rate of mutation at methylated CpG regions that is 42 times higher than predicted for random mutation (Cooper and Youssoufian, 1998). Point mutation (C-T) is frequently seen in p53 and Rb genes leading to loss of function of these proteins (Cooper and Youssoufian, 1988; Magewu and Jone, 1994; Tornaletti and Pfeifer, 1995; Manici et al., 1997). In addition, CpG sites are favored binding sites for carcinogens which also lead to increase rates of CpG mutations (Magewu and Jone, 1994; Yoon et al., 2001).

The question of why some regions of the genome are hypermethylated and others hypomethylated in cancer is poorly understood. However, most of the hypomethylated regions in tumors lie outside the so called CpG islands. In normal cells, these non CpG regions are methylated. Also the patterns of hypermethylation are tumor-specific leading to the idea that selection pressures in favor of growth for clonal cells might lead to different patterns of methylation. Another explanation for the site-specific hypermethylation could be due to recruitment of DNMTs by accessory proteins in cancer cells. The identity of these accessory proteins may be unique to the cancer cell phenotype, and also exhibit specificity for different cancer subtypes. Finally, epigenetic profiles in cancer may involve dysregulation of DNMT expression. This suggestion is consistent with the finding that DNMT1 and DNMT3b are overexpressed in many tumors (Miremadi et al., 2007). In addition, many tumors are characterized by downregulation of miRNAs due to methylation at their promoters (Saito et al., 2006; Melo et al., 2009). Conversely, miRNAs have also been shown to target DNMTs. In fact, miR-29 has been shown to target and downregulate both DNMT3a and DNMT3b, and indirectly DNMT3L (Garzon et al., 2009). Compared to normal cells, it is possible that regulation of DNMTs by miRNAs is dysregulated in cancer cells resulting in unique patterns of DNMT expression.

2.2 Nucleasome positioning

Total eukaryotic DNA is 2m long and must fit into the nucleus which has an approximate size of 2μm³. This is accomplished by an elaborate interaction between DNA, four core histone proteins (i.e. H2A, H2B, H3 and H4) and one linker histone. The core histone proteins are arranged into two sets of H3/H4 and H2A/H2B heterodimers. This arrangement forms into an octomer shaped structure, called the nucleosome, around which ~146bp of DNA is wrapped (Kornberg 1974). The interaction between the nucleosome and

DNA is facilitated by the positively charged amino acids of the histone proteins and the negatively charged phosphate backbone of the DNA. Nucleosomes are separated from each other by 20-100 bp linker regions. The linker region is bound by another histone protein called histone 1 (H1). H1 and its variants function to promote the coiling of nucleosomes into fiber like structures in cells (Bedner et al., 1998). Linker histones are distinguished from other histones because of special modifications at key amino acids, or in their tail regions or domain structures (Li et al., 2007). Nucleosomes, DNA and linker histones are packaged to form chromatin. The conformation of chromatin is determined by the positioning of the nucleosome and its level of modification. For example, loss of nucleosomes at the transcription start site is directly correlated to gene expression (Figure 3), and occlusion of the nucleosome at transcription start sites is correlated with transcriptional repression (Schomes et al., 2008; Cairns et al., 2009). At this level, nucleosomes act as barriers to transcription because they block access to binding sites for transcription factors and regulators (Figure 3), or block elongation by sterically hindering the movement of RNA polymerase II. The precise position of the nucleosome is influenced by linker histones (Zilberman et al., 2007), and chromatin remodeling complexes (Clapier et al., 2009). Incorporation of different histone variants can influence transcription and the methylation landscape in eukaryotic cells (Chodavarapu et al., 2010). For example, incorporation of histone linker H2A.Z protects genes against DNA methylation (Zilberman et al., 2008), thereby playing a role in epigenetic activation of transcription.

The chromatin remodeling complexes are classified into four families: mating type switch/sucrose non-fermenting (SWI/SNF) family, chromodomain helicase DNA-binding (CHD) family, Imitation SWItch (ISWI) family and Inositol/choline responsive element dependent gene activation mutant-80 (INO80) family. These four families are distinguished by unique features within their catalytic subunits that allow them to read specific histone post-translational modifications that stabilize their interaction with chromatin. They also differ in the composition of the other subunits (Ho and Crabtree, 2010). Chromatin remodeling complexes function by moving, ejecting, destabilizing or restructuring the nucleosome in an ATP dependent manner. The remodeling machinery is also influenced by both DNA methylation (Harikrisnan et al., 2005), and histone modifications (Wysoca et al., 2006).

Mammalian SWI/SNF enzymes are multisubunit complexes of 1-2MDa and consist of 9-12 subunits, one of which is an ATPase (De la Serna et al., 2006). The ATPase subunit is identified as either Brahma (BRM) or brama/swi2-related gene-1(BRGI) which have been recognized as human homologs. The BRGI subunit is 75% identical between SWI/SNF family members. Functionally, SWI/SNFs are master regulators of gene expression. For example, SWI/SNFs are involved in regulating the expression of FOS, CRYAB, MIM-1, p21 and CSF-1. These complexes are also involved in alternative splicing (Reisman et al., 2009).

The CHD family of chromatin remodeling complexes is distinguished by having two chromodomains that have affinity for methylated histones (Marfella et al., 2007). There are nine CHD proteins that can be divided into three subfamilies based on the presence of other conserved domains and interacting factors: I. (CHD1 and 2), II. (CHD3 and 4), III. (CHD 5-9). Some CHD family members are involved in the sliding and ejection of the nucleosome thereby promoting transcriptional activation. Others like Mi-2/NuRD have HDAC activity and can also act as methyl binding protein (Clapier et al., 2009). These family members at this role act as transcriptional repressors.

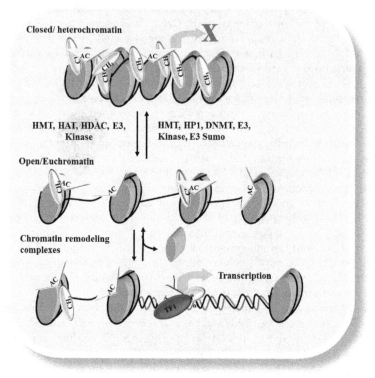

Fig. 3. Chromatin exists in a transcriptionally repressed (heterochromatin) or transcriptionally active (Euchromatin) states. Epigenetic modifications such as DNA methylation, histone methylation, phosphorylation, sumoylation and ubiquination favor the formation of heterochromatin and lead to transcriptional repression. Conversely, histone acetylation, methylation, phosphorylation and ubiquitination favor the formation of euchromatin and transcriptional activation. Note that epigenetic modifications, such as histone methylation, phosphorylation and ubiquitination, favor both the formation of euchromatin and heterochromatin. This depends on the composition of trans-acting factors, cross talk between histone marks, microdomain created by the histone marks and the chromatin remodeling complexes. Additional details can be found in the text. HMT: Histone methyltranferase, HAT: Histone acetyltransferase; DNMT: DNA methyltransferase; E3: E3 ubiquitin ligase: E3 Sumo: E3 sumo ligase; HP1: heterochromatin protein 1; TF: transcription factor; Pol: Polymerase; Ac: Acetylation mark; CH_3: Methylation mark.

Imitation SWItch (ISWI) complexes were initially identified and purified from Drosophila embryo extracts as NUcleosome Remodeling Factor (NURF), ATP dependent Chromatin assembly and remodeling Factor (ACF), and CHRomatin Accessibility Complex (CHRAC) complexes. Currently ISWI complexes have been found in a variety of organisms from yeast to humans (Tsukiyama and Wu, 1995; Tsukiyama et al., 1995; Ito et al., 1997; Varga-Weisz et al., 1997). The ISWI family members such as ACT and CHRAC are involved in promoting chromatin assembly, thus acting as transcriptional repressors. However, the NURF complex has been shown to activate RNA polymerase II, thus acting as a transcriptional activator.

INO80 was identified as a gene encoding an ATPase that is incorporated into a large multisubunit complex (Ebbert et al., 1999). Biochemical characterization of the yeast INO80 complex has revealed the presence of chromatin remodeling activity and 3'-5' helicase activity (Shen et al., 2000). Yeast cells that lack either INO80 or one of its core subunits (Arp5 andArp8) exhibit hypersensitivity to DNA damaging agents, suggesting that the INO80 complex is involved in DNA repair (Morrison et al., 2004; van Attikum et al., 2004). In accord with these findings, the INO80 complex is recruited to sites of double strand DNA breaks through interaction with phosphorylated H2A. From these findings and others, members of the INO80 family are believed to be involved in DNA repair, chromosomal segregation, DNA replication, telomere regulation and transcriptional activation (Ho et al., 2010). However, SWRI functions to restructure the nucleosome by removing the H2A-H2B dimers and replacing them with H2A.Z-H2B dimers (Clapier et al., 2009).

All four families of chromatin remodeling complexes are believed to be involved in tumorigenesis. For example, the BRGI subunit of the SWI/SNF families has been characterized as a tumor suppressor, and is silenced in about 20% of non-small lung cancer (Medina et al., 2008). BRGI subunit also functions to destabilize p53 hence acting as a tumor suppressor (Naidu et al., 2009). SWI/SNF complexes have been shown to interact with oncogenes, such as Rb, Myc, p53, breast cancer 1(BRCA1) and myeloid/lymphoid or mixed–lineage leukemia (MLL) (Roberts et al., 2004). Point mutations in the SNF subunit of the SWI/SNF complex have been implicated in renal tumors, choroid plexus carcinomas, meduloblastoma and neurorectodermal tumors (Robert et al., 2004). In colon cancer, promoter hypermethylation of the *MLH1* gene results in occlusion of the transcription start site by nucleosomes (Lin et al., 2007). The CHD5 complexes are targets of CpG hypermethylation (Mulero-Navarro and Esteller, 2008) resulting in downregulation of these complexes. In addition, crosstalk between chromatin remodeling complexes and histone modifications is vital to transcription regulation and tumorigenesis. For example, members of the CHD family are components of the NRD deacetylating and the SAGA acetyltransferase complexes (Tong et al., 1998). In accord with these findings, The H3K4 methyltransferase MLL has been shown to interact with SNF5/BRG1-associated factors (BAF) 47 (Rozenblatt-Rosen et al., 1998), and H3K4 methylation has been shown to recruit and mediate association of ISWI with chromatin to initiate transcription (Santos-Rosa et al., 2003). Acetylation of H3K56 leads to recruitment of SWI/SNF complexes (Xu et al., 2005). Linker histones have also been shown to play a role in tumorigenesis, with increased expression of linker histone macroH2A in senescent lung cells (Sporn et al., 2009), indicating that lung tumors with high expression of macroH2A have a better prognosis.

2.3 Histone modifications

As noted, chromatin is made of DNA and its associated proteins which are in turn classified into histone and non-histone proteins. Non-histone proteins transiently interact with the DNA to regulate function after which they dropout or are removed. For example, non-histone proteins transiently interact with DNA during transcription, replication, and DNA repair mechanisms. Such proteins include polymerases, co-activators, co-repressors, chromatin remodeling complexes, structural proteins and histone like proteins (e.g. CENPS). On the other hand, histone proteins stably interact with DNA except during transcription, replication or DNA repair during which they are temporally displaced from the DNA as nucleosomes. Each histone can be divided into three segments: a basic N-terminal histone tail, a globular histone fold and a C-terminal tail. The conformation of chromatin is dependent on posttranslational modifications at the tails of all histones which normally protrude from the nucleosome. Posttranslational modifications function by contouring the secondary structures of chromatin so as to allow or disallow accessibility to transcription and regulation sites. Posttranslational modification on histone can be classified as transient or stable. Transient posttranslational modifications include: phosphorylation, sumoylation and ubiquitination, and represent modifications that correlate with transient changes in gene regulation. Acetylation and methylation are fairly stable modifications that reflect the conformation of chromatin (e.g. closed/heterochromatin and open/euchromatin).

2.3.1 Histone acetylation

All histones are subjected to acetylation, and the process is catalyzed by histone acetyltransferase (HAT) complexes (Allfrey et al., 1964). Histone acetylation involves the transfer of acetyl groups from acetyl Coenzyme A to the imino group of lysine. HATs do not acetylate lysine moieties on histone randomly, a potential recognition motif (GKxxP) was revealed by crystal structure analysis (Rojas et al., 1999; Bannister et al., 2000). However, this motif is not a predictor of non-histone protein acetylation as a proteomic survey has identified different sets of preferentially acetylated amino acid stretches (Kim et al., 2006). Functionally, histone acetylation induces the so called open/euchromatin conformation via steric hinderance, changes in the positive charges of histones (Hong et al., 1993), and/or recruitment of regulatory proteins (Grant and Berger, 1999; Roth et al., 2001). The formation of open chromatin favors transcriptional activation. At the same time, the acetyl group of histones can be removed by histone deacetylase complexes (HDACs) which favors formation of closed chromatin and transcriptional repression (Yang and Seto, 2003). HATs are categorized into two groups based on their cellular localization. Type-A HATs are nuclear and acetylate histones and other chromatin-associated proteins. Type-B HATs are localized in the cytoplasm and have no direct influence on transcription. The latter are believed to function mainly to acetylate newly synthesized histones in the cytoplasm. Type-A HAT are further categorized into three groups: GNAT [GCN5 (general control of nuclear-5)-related N-acetyltransferase], p300/CBP [CREB (cAMP response element binding protein)-binding protein] and MYST [MOZ (Monocytic leukaemia zinc-finger protein), YBF2 (Yeast binding factor2)/SAS (something silencing), Tip60 (Tat interactive protein -60)] (Table 1). In addition some transcription factors and nuclear receptor coactivators have been shown to acetylate histones. For example, the nuclear receptor coactivator, Amplified in breast cancer-1 (AIB1), and transcription factor, TATA-box binding protein associated factor-250 (TAF250). Both of these proteins have been shown to acetylate histones H3 and H4.

The mechanism by which HAT complexes are recruited to the chromatin to acetylate histones is poorly understood. One possible mechanism involves the recruitment of HAT proteins as part of coactivator complexes. For example, p300/CBP HAT complexes are found to associate with polymerase II during transcription (Nakajima et al., 1997). Another plausible mechanism is through association with bromodomains containing proteins which recognize and bind to acetylated lysines (Dhalluim et al., 1999; Mujtaba et al., 2002). For example, the SWI/SNF complexes are recruited to the chromatin via their bromodomains (Hassan et al., 2002). In this case the HAT families of proteins are believed to complex with SWI/SNF complexes to acetylate histones.

The primary site for histone acetylation is the tail region which generally protrudes from the nucleosome. For example, core histones H3 and H4 can be acetylated at lysines 9, 14, 18, 23 and 5, 8, 12, 16 respectively (Roth et al., 2001) (Table 1). Histone acetylation can occur at different sites giving rise to the possibility of functional crosstalk between different acetylation marks. In fact, communication is known to occur between the same histone marks (Wang et al., 2008), between marks within the same histone tail (Duan et al., 2008), or between marks in different histone tails (Nakanishi et al., 2008). These data suggest that a single acetylation mark does not determine the state of the chromatin. Indeed, the notion of a strictly closed and open chromatin conformation has been challenged by a recent study showing that up to 51 chromatin states are possible based on the level or combination of acetylation marks (Ernst et al., 2010). For example, an active H3K4me mark and a repressive H3K27me mark have been found to co-exist in embryonic stem cells, suggesting a chromatin state that is neither open nor closed (Bernstein et al., 2006; Mikkelsen et al., 2007).

HATs	Histone Substrates
GNAT family	
• GCN5	H2B, H3-K9/14/23/27, H4-K8/16
• PCAF	H3-K14, H4-K8
P300/CBP family	
• p300	H2A-K5, H2B-K12/15/20, H3-K14/18/23, H4-K5/8/12
• CBP	H2A-K5, H2B-K12/15/20, H3-K14/18/23, H4-K5/8
MYST family	
• Tip60	H2A-K5, H3-K14, H4-K5/8/12
• MOZ	H3, H4

Table 1. HATs families and substrate specifications

As noted earlier, acetylation is a reversible process and the removal of acetyl groups is catalyzed by a class of enzymes called histone deacetylases (HDACs). Histone deacetylation is correlated with transcriptional repression. In humans, 18 isoenzymes of HDACs have been identified to date, and grouped into four classes based on their homology to yeast HDACs (Table 2). Class I (HDAC1, 2, 3 and 8) are related to yeast *RPD3* gene and are mostly located in the nuclei, except HDACs 3 and 8 which can also be cytoplasmic. Class II (HDAC 4, 5, 6, 7, 9 and 10) are related to yeast *Hda1* gene and are primarily located in the cytoplasm, but can shuttle to nucleus. Class II HDACs are further divided into two subclasses, IIa (HDAC 4, 5, 7,9) and IIb (HDAC 6, 10), based on their sequence homology and domain organization. Class III, also known as the sirtuins (SIRTIUNS (SIRT) 1-7), are related to the yeast *Sir2* gene, and are virtually unaffected by class I and II HDAC inhibitors. They are localized in the cytoplasm, mitochondria and nucleus (Table 2). Class IV (HDAC11) has a conserved domain similar to the catalytic region of Class I HDACs. Class IV is a fairly new class and needs further characterization. Classess I, II and IV share similar structural organization and a common cofactor, Zn^{2+}. Class III HDACs are structurally different from the rest and their active site is occupied by the nicotinamide adenine dinucleotide (NAD). Functionally, class II HDACs are regulated by class I HDACs and together class I and II are involved in transcriptional silencing and genomic organization during development. Class III HDACs are involved in maintenance of acetylation, as well as specific gene silencing (Denu et al., 2003).

HDAC classes		Cofactor	Localization
I			
	• HDAC 1 & 2	Zn²⁺	Nucleus
	• HDAC 3 & 8	Zn²⁺	Nucleus/cytoplasm
IIa			
	• HDAC 4, 5,7 & 9	Zn²⁺	Nucleus/cytoplasm
IIb			
	• HDAC 6 & 10	Zn²⁺	Nucleus/cytoplasm
III			
	• SIRT 1, & 2	NAD⁺	Nucleus/cytoplasm
	• SIRT 3	NAD⁺	Mitochondria/Nucleus
	• SIRT 4 & 5	NAD⁺	Mitochondria
	• SIRT 6 & 7	NAD⁺	Nucleus
IV			
	• HDAC 11	Zn²⁺	Nucleus

NAD: Nicotinamide adenine dinucleotide; SIRT: Sirtiun; Zn: Zinc

Table 2. Classes of HDACs, Cofactors and Subcellular Localization

Compared to normal cells, the interplay between acetylation and deacetylation is dysregulated in almost all cancers. HDACs have been shown to be overexpressed or mutated in many cancers (Zhu et al., 2004; Ropero et al., 2006). Under normal conditions, HDACs associate with and regulate transcription factors, tumor suupressor genes and oncogenes. HDAC1 has been shown to be in a complex with Rb and to suppress the transcriptional activation of E2F (Brehm et al., 1998). Also SIRT1 has been shown to regulate the inflammatory, stress, and survival responses of p53 (Vaziri et al., 2001). Thus, it stands to reason that loss of HDAC1 or SIRT1 could result in uncontrollable growth of cell leading to transformation. In accord with this interpretation, SIRT1 has been shown to interact with DNMT1 to affect DNA methylation patterns (Espada et al., 2007). In acute myelogenous leukemia (AML), fusion of eight-twenty-one zinc-finger nuclear protein (ETO) to AML, a transcription activator, converts the AML protein into a dominant transcriptional repressor. The AML-ETO fusion protein permanently binds to HDAC corepressor complexes and/or blocks the recruitment of coactivator complexes leading to transformation (Scandura et al., 2002). HDAC2 overexpression is a hallmark of familial-adenomatosis-polyposis-induced tumors (Zhu et al., 2004) and truncation of HDAC 2 is reported in sporadic tumors (Ropero et al., 2006). In addition, HDAC6 expression is correlated with better prognosis for breast cancer patients (Zhang et al., 2004), suggesting aberrant acetylation in breast tumors. In addition to aberrant levels of HDACs, several cancers also bear aberrant fusion proteins, mutations, or deletion of HATs and HAT releted genes (Bryan et al., 2002; Moore et al., 2004). For example, in cancer cells there is global reduction in monoacetylation at H4K16 (Fraga et al., 2005a), and HATs, such as p300 and CBP, are characterized as tumor suppressor genes since they can regulate the activity of oncoproteins, such as Jun, Fos, Myb and Rb (Yang et al., 2004). Likewise, p300 has been shown to be an interacting partner of the oncoprotein adenovirus E1A (Stein et al., 1999). CBP mutations have been shown to be involved in the initial steps of leukaemogenesis (Patrij et al., 1995). For the MYST family of HATs, mutations leading to loss of Tip60 acetyltransferase activity lead to apoptosis-resistant phenotypes and rampant cell proliferation (Ikura et al., 2000). In AML, a chimera protein is created by fusion of CPB to MOZ protein creating a protein with both p300/CBP and MYST domains (Yang et al., 2004; Borrow et al., 1996). The CBP-MOZ chimera protein exhibits gain-of-function characteristics leading to hyperacetylation and aberrant transcriptional activation. This leads to global inbalance of histone acetylation in cancer cells. Table 3 summarizes predicted impacts of acetylation and deacetylation in cancer.

Gene	Histone Mark	Genetic Defect	Tumor Type	Function	Reference
Histone acetyltransferases (HATs)					
CBP (KAT3A)	H2AK5, H2BK12, H2BK15, H3K14, H3K18, H4K5, H4K8	Deletion	ALL; lung	Loss	Shigeno et al., 2004 & Kishimoto et al., 2005
p300 (KAT3B)	H2AK5, H2BK12, H2BK15	Deletion	cervix; ALL	Loss	Ohshima et al., 2001 & Shigeno et al., 2004
p300 (KAT3B)	H2AK5, H2BK12, H2BK15	Mutation	Breast; CRC	Loss	Gayther et al. 2000
p300 (KAT3B)	H2AK5, H2BK12, H2BK15	Translocation	AML	Loss	Ida et al., 1997 & Chaffanet et al., 2000
MOZ (KAT6A)	H3K14; H4K16	Translocation	AML	Loss	Chaffanet et al., 2000 & Panagopoulos et al., 2003
Histone deacetylases (HDACs)					
HDAC2	Many acetyl residues (except H4K16)	Mutation	MSI+	Loss	Ropero et al., 2006 & Hanigan et al., 2008

ALL: Acute Lymphoblastic Leukemia; AML: Acute Myeloid Leukemia; CRC: Colorectal cancer; MSI+: Colorectal cancer with microsatellite instability.

Table 3. Aberrant Acetylation and Deacetylation Marks in Cancer

2.3.2 Histone methylations

Histone methylation occurs at either arginine or lysine residues in the tails of all histones. Two classes of enzymes catalyze the addition of methyl groups to histones: those that catalyse the addition of methyl group to arginine residues, called protein arginine methyltranferase (RHMT), and those that catalyze the addition of methyl groups to lysine residues, called histone lysine methyltransferase (HKMTs). S-adenosyl methionine (SAM) donates the methyl group in both cases of histone methylation (Pluemsampant et al., 2008). Histone methylation at arginine residues occurs at mono- or di-methylated states, while methylation at lysine residues occurs at mono-, di, and tri-methylated states. A total of 24 arginine and lysine methylation sites has been identified in all the core histones so far.

While DNA methylation generally represses transcription (except for gene body methylation), the functional impact of histone methylation is highly dependent on cellular context (Jenuwein and Allis, 2001). For example, histone methylation has been shown to cause both transcriptional activation and repression (Table 4). An emerging theme for these dual roles is explained by the fact that histone methylation creates motifs or domains that are recognized and bound by different proteins. The composition of these protein complexes determines whether the modification results in gene activation or repression. Another explanation for this phenomenon is that histone modifier genes and regulatory genes have a tissue-specific expression pattern. The composition and recruitment of tissue specific proteins determines transcriptional states. Also, there is crosstalk between histone methylation and other epigenetic modifications. For example, several histone methyltransferases have been shown to direct DNA methylation (Tachibana et al., 2008; Zhao et al., 2009) by recruiting DNMTs. DNMT3L specifically interacts with H3 tails and induces recruitment of DNMT3a, however this interaction is strongly inhibited by H3K4me (Ooi et al., 2007). Thus, the transcription state of the chromatin is also an interplay between different epigenetic modifications. In addition, the domain composition of HMTs is a determining factor of the transcriptional state. Most HMTs contain a conserved SET (SUV39 (Suppressor of variegation 3-9), Enhancer or zeste, Trithorax) domain which in combination with other domains/complexes has the ability to confer either transcriptional activation or repression. SET domain containing proteins are divided into five families: SET1, SET2, SUV39, RIZ (retinoblastoma protein interacting zinc-finger) and SMYD3 (SET and MYND-domain containing protein 3) (Table 4). The mixed lineage leukemia (MLL), SMYD3, Nuclear receptor-binding SET domain protein-1 (NSD1) and CARM1 are HMTs that activate transcription. For example, MLL-specific methylation at H3K4 is followed by recruitment of bromo domain-containing trithorax complexes which result in formation of an open chromation (Milne et al., 2002). SMYD3 in complex with RNA polymerase II and HELZ, a helicase, is recruited to the promoters of target genes where it methylates H3K4 leading to

Enzymatic Activity	Histone/Lysine	Biological Impact on Transcription
Lysine Histone Methyltransferase (KHMT)		
SET 1 family		
• SET1	H3K4	Activation
• EZH2	H3K27	Repression
• MLL 1 & 2	H3K4	Activation
SET 2 family		
• NSD1	H2K36	Activation
SUV39 family		
• SUV39H 1 &2	H3K9	Repression
	H4K20	Repression
RIZ family		
• RIZ1	H3K9	Repression
SMYD3 family		
• SMYD3	H3K4	Activation
Arginine Histone Methyltransferase (RHMT)		
• CARM1	H3R2	Repression
• PRMT 5	H3R17	Activation
	H2A/H4	Repression

Note that only a few of the HMTs are cited to illustrate their role as transcriptional activation or repression.

Table 4. Histone Methylation at Specific Lysine and Arginine Residues

transcriptional activation. NSD1 methylation at H3K36 is responsible for activation of Hox genes (Wang et al., 2007). CARM1 methylation at H3R17 has also been shown to activate transcription by complexing with hormone receptor co-activator complexes (Hong et al., 2004). On the other hand, SUV39H1, EZH2, RIZ1and PRMT5 participate in transcriptional repression. For example, EZH2 methylation at H3K27 leads to recruitment of chromo domain-containing polycomb complexes resulting in silencing of homeotic genes (Valk-Lingbeek et al., 2004). SUV39h1 trimethylation at H3K9 of the promoters of cell cycle control genes leads to recruitment of chromo domain-containing heterochromatin protein 1 (HP1) which in turn leads to transcriptional repression (Bannister et al., 2001; Lachner et al., 2001). RIZ1 methylation at H3K9 of the promoters of cell cycle control genes leads to apoptosis in breast cancer cells (He et al., 1998). Finally, methylation at H2A/H3 by PRMT negatively regulates cyclin E transcription resulting in cell cycle arrest (Fabbrizia et al., 2002). Table 4 summarizes the influence of histone methylation on transcription.

As described for histone acetylation, histone methylation is also reversible. Two classes of enzymes are responsible for removing methyl groups from histones: lysine-specific methyltransferase (KMAT) and arginine-specific methyltransferase (RMAT). KMAT includes amine oxidase domain-containing demethylases (Forneris et al., 2005) and Jumonji C (JmjC) domain containing demethylases (Tsukada et al., 2006) while RMAT includes peptidylarginine deiminase 4 (PAD4) (Cuthbert et al., 2004; Wang et al., 2004). PAD4 is the only RMAT known so far and it does not convert methylarginine to arginine, instead it converts methylarginine to citrulline. Citrullination is described as yet a unique histone modification. Several KMAT exist and the first one discovered is the lysine-specific

Gene Name	Histone Mark	Genetic Defect	Tumor Type	Function	Reference
Histone Methyltransferases (HMTs)					
DOT1L (KMT4)	H3K79	Aranslocation	AML	Loss	Okada et al., 2005
EZH2 (KMT6)	H3K27	Amplification	Prostate	Gain	Bracken et al., 2003
EZH2 (KMT6)	H3K27	Mutation	Lymphoma	Loss	Morin et al., 2010
NSD3	H3K4, H3K27	Amplification	Breast	Gain	Angrand et al., 2001
RIZ1 (KMT8)	H3K9	CpG hypermethylation	Breast, Liver	Loss	Du et al., 2001
SMYD2 (KMT3C)	H3K36	Amplification	ESCS	Gain	Komatsu et al., 2009 & Li et al., 2007
SUZ12 (HMT complex)	H3K9, H3K27	Translocation	ESS	Loss	Panagopoulos et al., 2008
Histone demethylase (HDMTs)					
LSD1	H3K4, H3K9	Amplification	Prostate, Lung, Bladder	Gain	Kahl et al., 2006 & Hayami et al., 2010
UTX	H3K4, H3K9	Mutation	Multiple cancers	Loss	Van Haaften et al., 2009
GASC	H3K9, H3K36	Amplification	Breast, Lung	Gain	Cloos et al., 2006 & Italiano et al., 2006 & Liu et al., 2009

Table 5. Aberrant histone methylation and demethylation in cancer

demethylase-1 (LSD1). LSD1 is a typical H3K4 demethylase, but can change its substrate specificity when in complex with different accessory proteins. For example, LSD1 in complex with androgen receptor is able to demethylate H3K9 (Mwtzger et al., 2005). LSD1 is also able to synergistically work with HDACs and HATs to affect transcription of target genes. For example, over expression of LSD1 in HEK293 cells leads to decreased H3K4 methylation which is in turn followed by H3 deacetylation and transcriptional repression (Lee et al., 2006). At the same time, inhibiting HDAC1 activity increases both H3 acetylation and H3K4 methylation (Lee et al., 2006).

In cancer, there is aberrant expression and composition of histone-modifier and -regulator genes. For example, silencing of the nuclear receptor SET domain protein I (NSD1) results in decreased H3K36 and H4K20 methylation, which is believed to play a role in tumors of the nervous system (Berdasco et al., 2009). CpG Island hypermethylation by the histone methyltransferase ,RIZ1, has been described in many cancers (Du et al., 2001). Suppressor of the zest 12 homolog (SUZ12) which is a component of the PCR2/EED/EZH2 complex that methylates H3K9 and H3K27 is involved in cell proliferation and survival in tumors (Li et al., 2007). In leukemias, the presence of mixed lineage leukemia (MLL) fusion oncoproteins leads to aberrant patterns of H3K79 and H3K4 methylation and altered gene expression in these tumors (Krivtsov et al., 2008; Wang et al., 2009). Some histone demethylases have also been found to be overexpressed in prostate cancer and squamous carcinomas (Shi et al., 2007). For example, LSD1 overexpression is a predictive biomarker for prostate cancer (Kahl et al., 2006)

2.3.3 Histone phosphorylation

Histone phosphorylation is described as the addition of a phosphate group (PO_3^-) to histone. So far, a small number of kinases has been shown to phosphorylate histones, and these include protein kinase B (PKB/AKT), ribosomal S6 kinase-2 (Rsk-2), mitogen- and stress-activated protein kinases 1 and 2 (Msk1/2), mixed lineage triple kinase-alpha (MLTK-α), and aurora kinases. The most interesting of the histone kinases are the aurora kinases. In normal cells, aurora kinases are involved in chromosomal segregation, condensation and orientation (Katayama et al., 2003). For example, aurora-phosphorylates both H3S10 and H3S28 during mitosis and meiosis (Andrews et al., 2003). Aurora kinases are serine/threonine kinases that include auroras A, B and C. These proteins share similar carboxyl terminal catalytic domains, but divergent amino terminals of variable length. In cancer cells, aurora kinases are frequently overexpressed and their overexpression is implicated in oncogenic transformation, as evidenced by chromosomal instability and derangement of multiple tumor suppressor and oncoprotein-regulated pathways. The mechanism through which these kinases are activated is dependent on the microenvironment of the cell. These mechanisms include, but are not limited to, activation by mitogens, cytokines, stress, signaling pathways (e.g. Ras-mitogen-activated protein kinase pathway (MAPK)) and chemical and environmental toxicants.

Functionally, histone phosphorylation alone, or when synergistically-coupled to other histone modifications (e.g. acetylation and methylation), can either facilitate or repress transcription (Cheung et al., 2000). This dichotomy is explained by the fact that histone phosphorylation can create domains that are recognized and bound by transacting factors, the composition of which determines the transcriptional state. Also histone phosphorylation can facilitate or repress further acetylation or methylation thereby regulating the transcriptional state of chromatin. For example, phosphorylation at threonine 11 has been shown to hasten removal of repressive H3K9 methylation by recruitment of the histone demethylase Jumonji C domain containing protein (JMJD2C) (Metzger et al., 2008). At this capacity, phosphorylation facilitates transcription by recruitment of histone demethylases. In addition, phosphorylation at H3 serine 10 inhibits recruitment of heterochromatin protein 1 (HP1) (Fischle et al., 2005; Hirota et al., 2005), which in turn prevents recruitment of DNMTs (DNMT1 and DNMT3a) thereby leaving chromatin in the open conformation and ready for transcription. At this level, phosphorylation prevents methylation of DNA by preventing recruitment of DNMTs. Phosphorylation can also facilitate transcription by allowing recruitment of histone acetyltransferase (HAT). For example, mutation at H3 serine 10 ablates recruitment of HATs (Chuang et al., 2000; Lo et al., 2000). Phosphorylation can also activate genes which in turn activate signaling pathways responsible for gene activation. Stimulation of inflammatory cytokine signaling activates IkB kinase α which phosphorylates histone H3 at serine 10 in the promoters of multiple nuclear factor responsive genes (Anest et al., 2003; Yamamoto et al., 2003). These phosphorylations result in expression of several inflammatory responsive genes. Lastly, it is been shown that phosphorylation of core H3 at serine 10 (cH3S10) and threonine 11 (cHT11) occur during active transcription (Chuang et al., 2000; Nowak and Cores, 2000, 2004, Metzger et al., 2008), suggesting that the negative phosphate groups added to histones might neutralize the positive charges on DNA, thus causing chromatin to unwind and allow transcription to continue. Conversely, evidence for transcriptional repression due to histone phosphorylation is mounting. For example, during mitosis, H3S10 phosphorylation is associated with condensed chromosome (Goto et al., 1999). Aurora-B kinase-mediated phosphorylation of H3S28 is also associated with condensed chromosome. Constitutive phosphorylation of H1 through the Ras-MAPK pathway leads to chromatin condensation (Chadee et al., 1995). In addition, mammalian Sterile20-like 1 (Mst1) phosphorylation of H2B-14 is associated with condensed chromatin leading to apoptosis (Cheung et al., 2003).

Gene name	Histone Mark	Genetic Defect	Tumor Type	Function	Reference
Histone phosphorylation					
Jak2	H3Y41	Point mutation	Hematogical tumors	Loss	(Dowson et al., 2009)
ATM/ATR	H2AXS139	Double stranded breaks	Melanomas	Loss	(Fernandez-Capetillo et al., 2004) and (Bassing, C.H. et al. 2003)
Aurora-kinase-B	H3S10	Chromosom al instability	Aneuploidy and Colorectal cancer	Loss	(Fischle, W. et al. 2005) and (Hirota, T. et al. 2005)
Mst1	H2BS14	Apoptosis resistance		Loss	(Hanahan and Weinberg, 2000) and (Ahn, S.H. et al. 2005)

Table 6. Aberrant Histone Phosphorylation in Cancer

Like other histone modifications, histone phosphorylation is counteracted by dephosphorylation. Phosphatases catalyze the removal of phosphate groups from histones. For example, phosphatase type 1 (PP1) interacts with aurora-B during mitosis as a feedback mechanism (Katayama et al., 2001). Also PP1 regulates Aurora-B and H3 phosphorylations during cells division (Murnion et al., 2001). In cancer cells, the balance between phosphorylation and dephosphorylation is dysregulated. For example, histone phosphorylation has been shown to play a role in cancer through modulation of the DNA repair response, chromosome instability and apoptosis. Recently JAK2, a nonreceptor tyrosine kinase, has been shown to be activated by chromosomal translocation and point mutations in hematological malignancies (Dawson et al., 2009). Also, JAK2 has been shown to phosphorylate H3Y41 which prevents the recruitment of heterochromatin protein 1α (HP1α) leading to increased expression of genes in this region. Phosphorylation at serine 139 in the highly conserved C-terminal tail (–SQEY) of H2A.X has been shown to play an important role in DNA double-strand break (DSB) repair and tumor suppression (Fernandez-Capetillo, O. et al. 2004). In addition, H3S10 and H2BS14 phosphorylations play a role in chromosomal instability and apoptosis resistance, respectively which are both hallmarks of cancer (Fischle, W. et al. 2005; Hirota, T. et al. 2005; Hanahan and Weinberg, 2000; Ahn, S.H. et., 2005).Activation of MAPK pathway by environment carcinogens leads to phosphorylation of H3 which in turn results in the induction of immediate early genes. More specifically, ultraviolet light has been shown to activate MAPK pathways resulting in phosphorylation of H3S10 by p38 kinase.

2.3.4 Histone ubiquitination and sumoylation

Ubiquitination and sumoylation involve the transfer of a polypeptide to the histone tail. The polypeptide molecules for ubiquitination and sumoylation are ubiquitin and small ubiquitin related modifier (SUMO) (Takada et al., 2007), respectively. The enzymatic cascade responsible for ubiquitination and sumoylation are similar, with three classes of enzymes involved in both instances: E1 activating enzymes, E2 conjugating enzymes and E3 ligating enzymes. In the first step of this multistep cascade, E1 adds Ubiquitin/SOMO to the target substrate in an ATP dependent manner. E2 then transfers the Ubiquitin/SOMU to E3 which associates and ligates the Ubiquitin/SOMU to histones (Nathan et al., 2003). Histone ubiquitination involves mono-ubiquitination which is different from poly-ubiquitination in that it does not result in proteosomal degradation of the target histone. Depending on the lysines that are ubiquitinated, ubiquitination can result in transcriptional activation or repression (Table 7). For example, both H2A and H2B are targets of mono-ubiquitination, and mono-ubiquitination has been shown to be a precursor to histone methylation (Gerber and Shilatified, 2003; Hampsey and Reinberg, 2003; Osley, 2004; Margueron et al., 2005). In particular, mono-ubiquitination at H2B lysine 120 (H2BK120) by E3 ligase (RNF20/RNF40) initiates methylation at H3 lysine 4 (H3K4) resulting in recruitment of homeobox genes (Zhu et al., 2005) and transcriptional activation. Conversely mono-ubiquitination at H3 lysine 119 (H3K119) by Bmi/Ring1A induces transcriptional repression (Wand et al., 2004).

It is not completely clear what role sumoylation plays on transcriptional regulation, however sumoylation has recently been shown to cause transcriptional repression (Shiio and Eisnman, 2003; Girdwood et al., 2003) (Table 1). For example, H4 sumoylation is associated with recruitment of HP1 and HDAC which is known to repress transcription. A number of oncogenes and tumor suppressor genes, including PML, Mdm2, c-Myb, c-Jun, Rb and p53, undergo SUMOylation (Muller et al., 1998; Bushmann et al., 2000; Bies et al., 2002; Schmidt et al., 2002; Huang et al., 2004; Besten et al., 2005; Ghioni et al., 2005; Ghost et al., 2005). SUMOylation of Mdm2 increases its E3 activity toward p53 tumor suppressor. SUMO negatively regulates c-Jun activity and thus restricts its oncogenic capacity. SUMOylation of

Histone Modification	Modifying Enzyme	Type of Modification	De-modifying Enzyme	Impact on transcription
Phosphorylation	Kinase e.g. JAK	Transient	Phosphatase	⬆⬇
Sumoylation	E3 Ligase	Transient	SUMO Protease e.g. SENP1	⬇
Ubiquitination	E3 Ligase	Transient	De-ubiquitinase	⬆⬇
Methylation	HMT/PRMT	Stable	PADI, JMJD	⬆⬇
Acetylation	HAT	Stable	HDAC	⬆

Red arrows indicate transcriptional activation, while black arrows indicate transcriptional repression.

Table 7. Summary, Impact of Posttranslational Modification of Histones on Transcription

c-Myb increases its stability, but negatively regulates its transactivation function of. Increasing evidence supports the notion that protein SUMOylation is important during the course of tumorigenesis and oncogenesis, and altered in human cancers, however further work is needed to determine the impact of sumoylation on cancer.

In summary, epigenetic modifications are not stand alone processes. Instead, considerable crosstalk exists among the different types of epigenetic marks. In accord with this principle, epigenetic marks by themselves, or synergistically with other epigenetic marks, function to either repress or activate transcription (Table 7). Of relevance to epigenomic regulation is that all epigenetic modifications identified to date have been shown to be reversible. Genes regulated by epigenetic modification remain intact and can therefore be returned to their original state. The reversibility of epigenetic mechanisms makes them highly susceptible to pharmacological intervention and therefore, ideal targets for cancer therapeutics.

3. Epigenetic therapies

Genetic mutations and gross structural defects permanently activate or inactivate genes; however genes modified by aberrant epigenetic modification remain structurally intact and subject to reversal of aberrant epigenetic modifications that can restore their original state. This phenomenon has made epigenetic modifications an ideal target for the treatment of many diseases, including cancer. As discussed in previous sections, cancers are plague with aberrant epigenetic modifications which have been shown to contribute to initiation and transformation. In fact, several exogenous chemicals used to treat cancers have been shown to cause unintended epigenetic modifications which in many cases have led to exacerbation of tumor progression. These factors, combined and our understanding of epigenetic modifying enzymes, pathways and accessory proteins pivotal to epigenetic modifications, have lead to the development of therapies targeting DNA methylation and DNMTs, histone modifications and histone modifying enzymes (i.e HAT, HDAC, kinases, HMT, SUMO ligase, ubiquitin ligase, etc.). Indeed, therapies targeting chromatin remodeling complexes have attracted significant interest in recent years as a means for cancer prevention, either alone or in combination with conventional cancer treatments.

3.1 DNA Methyltransferase inhibitors (DNMTis)

Inhibitors of DNA methylation (DNMTis) cause reactivation of silenced genes, inhibition of cell proliferation, apoptosis and enhancement of sensitivity to other cancer drugs. DNMTis can be grouped into nucleoside DNMTis and non-nucleoside DNMTis, based on their structure and mode of action. Nucleoside DNMTi are analogues or derivatives of the nucleoside cytidine and they include 5-azacytidine (5-Aza-CR), 5-Aza-2-deoxycytidine (5-Aza-CdR), zebularine, cytarabine and 5-Fluoro-2-deoxycytidine. The cytidine analogues (5-Aza-CR and 5-Aza-CdR) have been approved by FDA for the treatment of myeloid malignancies in the USA. The anticancer activity of these drugs is believed to be mediated by two mechanisms: (1) cytotoxicity which stems from incorporation of these drugs into DNA and/or RNA, and (2) reactivation of tumor suppressor genes by demethylation of their promoter regions (Jones and Liang, 2009). These drugs do not demethylate DNA per se, but rather with continued replication, cytidines are replaced by the cytidine analogues resulting in serial dilution of methylable cytidines. In addition, DNMTs are trapped in covalent adducts with DNA through the incorporated cytidine analogues. 5-Aza-CR and 5-Aza-CdR are taken into the cell through the concentrated nucleoside transporter 1 (hCNT1) (Rius et al., 2009). Once inside the cell, 5-Aza-CR is phosphorylated by uridine-cytidine and 5-Aza-CdR by diphosphate kinase (Stresemann et al., 2008; Issa et al., 2009) which in turn convert them into active triphosphates (i.e. 5-Aza-CTP and 5-Aza-dCTP). 5-Aza-CTP is incorporated into the DNA resulting in the formation of covalent adducts between DNMTs and DNA (Santi et al., 1984). This traps the DNMTs and prevents further methylation. In other studies, 5-Aza-dCTP was shown to be incorporated into RNA which interferes with ribosomal biogenesis and protein synthesis (Momparlar et al., 1984; Stresemann et al., 2008). In accord with these findings, Ghoshal et al. 2005 and Kuo et al. 2007 have both shown that 5-Aza-CTP and 5-Aza-dCTP hypomethylate the genome through passive dilution of cytidine and not through active demethylation. Because of the cytotoxicity and instability of 5-Aza-CR and 5-Aza-CdR, DNMTis cannot be continually given to patients. For this reason, zebularine has been developed as an alternative. Although this drug works in a manner similar to 5-Aza-CR and 5-Aza-CdR, it is more stable and less toxic than 5-Aza-CR and 5-Aza-CdR DNMTis (Zhou et al., 2002; Cheng et al., 2003). In line with these findings, zebularine has been shown to reactivate tumor suppressor genes (Flotho et al., 2009; Billam et al., 2010), enhance tumor cells' chemotherapy and radiation sensitivity (Dote et al., 2005), exert angiostatic and antimitogenic activities (Balch et al., 2005; Hellebrekers et al., 2006) and to be stable enough for oral administration (Zhou et al., 2002; Cheng et al., 2003). In addition, at low doses, zebularine can be given to patients continuously without the overt cytoxicity associated with 5-Aza-CR and 5-Aza-CdR. Another cytidine analogue, 5-fluoro-2-deoxycytidine (FdCyd) has been shown to cause demethylation in human breast and lung cancer cells (Beumer et al., 2008). In the case of FdCyd, the hydrogen atom at carbon-5 (C5) which is the methyl acceptor during the methylation reaction is replaced by a fluorine atom. When FdCyd is incorporated into DNA, the β-elimination step in which DNMT transfers the methyl group to the cytidine is inhibited. At the same time, the fluorine atom traps the DNMT to prevent elimination of the FdCyd moiety (Jones et al., 1980; Reither et al., 2003). FdCyd is currently in Phase I clinical trials for the treatment of breast and other solid tumors (Gowher et al., 2004) (Table 8). Moreover, FdCyd, in combination with other epigenetic drugs (i.e. tetrahydrouridine and dihydro-5-azacytidine (DHAC), is being evaluated in clinical studies for the treatment of malignant mesothelioma (Kratzke et al., 2008).

Although nucleoside DNMTis have proven effective for the treatment of cancers, their cytotoxicity remains a significant limitation. To address this shortcoming, non-nucleoside

DNMTis are being evaluated. Non-nucleoside DNMTis include procaine, L-trytophan derivatives, RG108, hydralazine, MG98, procainamide, and epigallocatechin-3-gallate (EGCG). Procaine is a local anesthetic drug that can also function as a DNMTi. For example, procaine has been shown to cause global demethylation and reactivation of tumor suppressor genes in human breast cancer cells (Jin et al., 2009). Unlike the nucleoside analogues, procaine competes with DNMTs for binding to CpG rich regions (Jin et al., 2001). Procainamide and hydralazine are antiarrhythmic drugs that can also function as DNMTis, and both agents have been shown to inhibit DNA methylation through interactions between the nitrogen atom of procainamide and hydralazine with the lys-162 and Arg-240 moities in the catalytic site of DNMTs (Song et al., 2009; Singh et al., 2009; Mund et al., 2006). In accord with these findings, procainamide has been shown to specifically inhibit DNMT1 (Lee et al., 2005). RG108 is a small molecule inhibitor of DNMTs that inhibits free DNMTs (Brueckner et al., 2005). This drug works by blocking the catalytic pocket of DNMTS without the formation of covalent adducts that cause cytotoxicity (Stressmann et al., 2006). Studies have also shown RG108 to cause demethylation and reactivation of tumor suppressor genes without affecting the methylation level of microsatellite regions in lung cancer cells (Suzuki et al., 2010), suggesting a specificity level in RG108 that has not been seen in other DNMTis. Table 8

DNMTi	Phase	Type of cancer	Clinical trial finding	Reference
NON-NUCLEOSIDE ANOLOGUES				
MG98	N/A	Cervical cancer	26% SD	Garzon et al., 2009
EGCG	Phase I		N/A	Brueckner et al., 2004
Procaine	Phase I	Solid Tumor	N/A	Villar-Garea et al., 2003
Procanamide	N/A	Colon cancer	N/A	Segura-Pacheco et al., 2003
Hydralazine	N/A	Cervical cancer	N/A	Song et al., 2009
RG108	N/A	Colon cancer	N/A	Suzuki et al., 2010
COMBINATION THERAPIES				
Aza-CR+Sodium Phenylbutyrate	Preclinical	Solid Tumors	50 24.2% CR; PR 11.2%	Soriano et al., 2007
Aza-CR + Valproic Acid	Phase II	MDS	62 30.7% CR; PR, 15.4%	Blum et al., 2011
Aza-CR + Lenalidomide	Phase I	MDS	44% CR, 17% HI, and 67% ORR	Jabbour et al., 2009
Aza-CR + Cytarabine	Phase I	MDS/AML	N/A	Plummer et al., 2009

DNMTi	Phase	Cancer Type	Clinical Trial Findings	Reference
NUCLEOSIDE ANOLOGUES				
5-Aza-CR	Phase II	MDS	7% CR, 16% PR, 37% HI	Yoo et al., 2008
		MDS	17% CR, 12% PR, 42% SD	Silverman et al., 2006
		MDS	10.8% CR, 9.5% PR, 20.3% HI	Santini et al., 2009
		MDS/AML	15.6% CR, 25% HI, 34.4% SD	Martin et al., 2009
5-Aza-CdR	Phase II	SM	N/A	Winquist et al., 2006
		MDS	9% CR, 13% HI, 17% ORR	Muller-Thomas et al., 2009
		MDS	34% CR	Wijermans et al., 2008
		MDS	17% CR, 18% HI, 32% ORR	Kantarjian et al., 2007
		MDS/AML	26% SD	Schrump et al., 2006
Zebularine	Phase II	MDS	13.4% CR, and 7.5% PR	Gore et al., 2006
5-FdCyd	N/A	Breast and lung	N/A	Reither et al., 2003

AML: Acute Myeloid Leukemia; CR: Complete Remission; HI: Hematologic Improvement; MDS: Myelodysplastic Syndrome; PR: Partial response; ORR: Overall Response Rate; CR: Conventional Care Regimens; N/A: Data not available; SD: Stable Disease. Note that only few DNMTis are shown here to illustrate their role in the treatment of cancers.

Table 8. DNMTis and Their Impact in Cancer

summarizes the DNMTis in clinical trial and their efficacy for cancer treatment either alone or in combination with other regimens.

3.2 Histone acetyltransferase inhibitors (HATis)

HAT inhibitors can be classified into synthetic peptide CoA base bisubstrate HATis, natural product HATis and small molecule HATis (Table 9). The synthetic bisubstrate HATis were the first to be identified based on the observation that polyamine-CoA conjugates can inhibit HAT activity in cell extracts (Cullis et al., 1982). In particular, H3-CoA-20 and Lys-CoA specifically inhibit pCAF and p300 (Lau et al., 2000) rather weakly. Introduction of a phenyl or methyl group between lysine and CoA improves the inhibition fourfold (Sagar et al., 2004). Most of the synthetic bisubstrate HATis work by mimicking the acetyl CoA-lysine intermediate complex in the HAT reactions. Crystal structure information between GCN5 and these HATis shows that GCN5 interacts with the pyrophosphate moity, the pantothanic moiety and the phosphate group of CoA. The major deficiency for this class of HATis is their impermeability to cells. Unfortunately, most of the naturally occurring HATis also suffer from a similar problem. For example, anacardic acid isolated from the shell of cashewnuts displays permeability restriction in vitro. Nevertheless, garcinol and isogarcinol were both shown to inhibit p300 and pCAF (Balasubramnyam et al., 2004; Mantelingu et al., 2007). The derivative of isogarcinol, LTK14, was shown to selectively inhibit p300, but not

HATi compound	Parental and Derivative compounds	Specificity	Reference
SYNTHETIC HATis			
	Lys-CoA: (R1 = CH₃; R2 = R3 = H)	p300	Lau et al., 2000
	H3-CoA-20: (R1 = G-G-T-S-K-R-A-T-Q-K-T-R-A-NH-COCH₃; R2 = A-P-R-K-Q-L; R3 = H)	PCAF	Lau et al., 2000
	H3-(Me)-CoA: (R1 = CH3CO-NH-A-R-T-A-R-K-S-T-G-G; R2 = A-P-R-K-Q-L; R3 = Me)	p300	Sagar et al., 2004
	Lys-Phe-Coa: (R1 = Phe, R2 = R3 = H)	p300	Sagar et al., 2004
	Lys-CoA-3'dephospho: R1 = (R1 = Phe, R2 = R3 = H)	p300	Sagar et al., 2004

NATURAL HATis	Compound	Substrate	References
	Anacardic Acid	p300, PCAF	Varier et al., 2004
	Garcinol	p300, pCAF	Balasubramanyam et al., 2004a
	Isogarcinol: (R = H)	p300 pCAF	Mantelingu et al., 2007
	LTK14: (R = CH₃)	p300	
	Curcumin	p300 CBP	Balasubramanyam et al., 2004b

SMALL MOLECULES HATis			
	γ-Butyrolactone	hGCN5	Biel et al., 2004
	Isothiazolones: (R = H, Cl; R1 = NO₂, Cl, CF₃, OCH₃, COOEt)	p300 PCAF	Mantelingu et al., 2007 & Stimson et al., 2005
	Quinolines	N/A	Mai et al., 2006

Table 9. HAT Inhibitors and Their Selectivity

pCAF (Mantelingu et al., 2007). The best characterized of the naturally occurring HATis is Curcumin, which is isolated from the *Curcuma longa* rhizome. Curcumin has shown high efficacy in the prevention and treatment of colorectal, prostate, kidney, lung, ovarian, breast, cervical and liver cancers (Balasubramnyam et al., 2004). The last group of HATis includes a number of small molecules designed to overcome the challenges in permeability of the first two groups. These include γ-butyrolactone MB-3, quinoline and isothiazolone and their derivatives. Although in their infancy, isothiazolone has been shown to inhibit the enzymatic activity of both pCAF and p300 leading to reduction in cell proliferation of human ovarian and colon cancer cell lines (Stimson et al., 2005). γ-butyrolactone MB-3 inhibits GCN5 and contains an αβ-unsaturated carbonyl group that is prone to covalently bind to the thiol group in the active site of GCN5 (Biel et al., 2004).

3.3 Histone deacetylase inhibitors (HDACis)

HDAC inhibitors (HDACis) have been classified into seven categories based on their chemical structures and mode of inhibition: short chain fatty acids, benzamides, cyclic peptides, electrophilic ketones, hydroxamine-acid-derived compounds (Espino et al., 2005; Rasheed et al., 2007), miscellaneous compounds (e.g. Depudecin and MGCD-0103) and sirtuin inhibitors (Table 10). Sirtuin or class III HDACis can be further classified structurally, but for simplicity, they are classified here into a single group. For details on class III HDACi subgroups, the reader is referred to Schemies et al., 2009. Class I, II and IV HDACis share a common metal binding domain that serves to block Zn⁺ chelation at the active site (Miller et al., 2003). Because of the presence of a different co-factor (nicotinamide (NAD)) at the active site of class III HDACs, zinc-dependent HDACis are ineffective against them. Class III

HDACi Class	Chemical Compound
Hydroxamic acid-derived compounds	TSA (trichostatin A), SAHA (suberoylanilide hydroxamic acid or Vorinostat) CBHA (*m*-carboxycinnamic acid bis-hydroxamide), ABHA (azelaic bis-hydroxamic acid), LAQ-824, LBH-589, oxamflatin, PXD-101, scriptaid, pyroxamide, SK-7041, SK-7068 and tubacin.
Cyclic peptides	Romidepsin (depsipeptide, FK-228/FR-901228), apicidin, CHAPS (cyclic hydroxamic acid-containing peptides) and trapoxin.
Short-chain fatty acids	Valproic acid, phenylbutyrate, phenylacetate and AN-9.
Benzamides	MS-275 and CI-994.
Ketones	Trifluoromethyl ketone.
Miscellaneous	Depudecin and MGCD-0103.
Sirtuin inhibitors	Nicotinamide (NAD), 2-Anilino-benzamide, Sirtinol, Dihydropyridine, Cambinol, etc.

Table 10. Histone Deacetylase Inhibitor Subgroups

HDACis are inhibited by nicotinamide, NAD$^+$ analogues, indoles, hydroxynaphthaldehyde derivatives, Splitomicins, Suramins and kinase inhibitors (Schemies et al., 2009). NAD works by specifically blocking the entry of nicotinamide adenine dinucleotide into the active site of class III HDACs. The modes of action of other satiun inhibitors are still unknown. While zinc-dependent HDACis are established anticancer drugs, and two inhibitors (Vorinostat (SAHA), Romidepsin) have been approved for cancer treatment in the United States (Johnstone et al., 2002), much less is known about the biological consequences of sirtiun inhibitors (North et al., 2004; Wesphal et al., 2007; Fatkins et al., 2008). In fact, sirtuin inhibitors shown to be effective in lower organisms, do not work on human subtypes (Biel et al., 2005; Schafer et al., 2005). In general, HDACis have shown to induce cell cycle arrest and apoptosis in G1 or G2/M. For example, in response to HDACis, p21 gene is consistently upregulated in a p53-independent manner and p21 expression is correlated with cell cycle G1 arrest (Gui et al., 2004; Vrana et al., 1999). The upregulation of p21 gene is correlated with increased acetylation of histones H3 and H4 near the p21 promoter (Hirsch et al., 2004). In addition, HDACis, such as butyrate and trichostatin A, have been shown to stabilize p21 mRNA (Hirsch et al., 2004). Moreover, HDAC inhibition represses cyclins A and D, and activates p16 and p27 to induce cell cycle arrest (Sandor et al., 2000; Wharton et al., 2000). In other studies, HDACis upregulate the expression of pro-apoptotic genes (i.e., TRAIL, DR5, Bax, Apaf-1, Bmf, Bim and TP2) and/or downregulate the expression of anti-apoptotic genes (i.e., Bcl-2, Mcl1, and XIAP) (see review by Bolden et al., 2006). The biggest advantage for many HDACis is that they can induce their effect in the nano/micromolar range, as seen for SAHA and butyric acid, respectively (Espino et al., 2005; Kelly et al., 2003). Moreover,

Class	HDACs	Relevant HDACis
I	HDACs 1 and 2	SK-7041, SK-7068, MS-275, VPA, romidepsin butyrate, trapoxin, SAHA, TSA, PXD-101, LBH-589, LAQ-824 and MGCD-0103
	HDAC 3	MS-275, VPA, butyrate, trapoxin, SAHA, TSA, PXD-101, LBH-589, LAQ-824 and MGCD-0103
	HDAC 8	VPA, butyrate, trapoxin, SAHA, TSA, PXD-101, LBH-589 and LAQ-824
IIa	HDAC 4	Romidepsin, VPA, butyrate, trapoxin, SAHA, TSA, PXD-101, LBH-589 and LAQ-824
	HDACs 5, 7 and 9	VPA, butyrate, trapoxin, SAHA, TSA, PXD-101, LBH-589 and LAQ-824
IIb	HDAC 6	Romidepsin, tubacin, SAHA, TSA, PXD-101, LBH-589 and LAQ-824
	HDCA 10	Tubacin, SAHA, TSA, PXD-101, LBH-589 and LAQ-824
III	SIRT-1, -2, -3, -4, -5, -6 and -7	Nicotinamide (NAD), 2-Anilino-benzamide, Sirtinol, Dihydropyridine, Cambinol, etc.
IV	HDAC 11	SAHA, TSA, PXD-101, LBH-589, LAQ-824 and MGCD-0103

HDAC: Histone deacetylase; SAHA: Suberoylanilide hydroxamic acid; SIRT: Sirtuin; TSA: Trichostatin A; VPA: Valproic acid.

Table 11. HDAC Classes and Relevant Inhibitors

HDACis have been shown to suppress angiogenesis and to activate and enhance the host immune system in cancer patients (Bhalla et al., 2005; Dokmanovic et al., 2005; Bolden et al., 2006).

At the clinical level, HDACis function synergistically with a host of structurally and functionally diverse cancer drugs, chemotherapeutic agents and biologically active polypeptides. In this manner, HDACis can increase the efficacy of other drugs by increasing target susceptibility. For example, in breast cancer therapy, the effectiveness of topoisomerase II inhibitors can be increased by pretreatment with SAHA (Marchion et al., 2004). In addition, HDACis have been used in combination with DNA demethylating agents in an attempt to reactivate silenced genes involved in tumor suppression. For example, three Phase I/II trials combining 5-Aza-CR or decitabine with HDAC inhibitors (phenyl butyrate or valproic acid) in patients with AML and MDS showed both tolerability and promising efficacy (Gore et al., 2006; Maslak et al., 2006; Garcia-Manero et al., 2006). Of a total of 93 patients who were treated, 14 showed complete remissions (CR), two showed partial complete remission (pCR), four showed partial response (PRs) and 6 showed hematologic improvements (HI) (Table 12). These studies combined have an overall response rate of 28%. In another phase I clinical study, the efficacy of CI-994 and various chemotherapeutic agents was examined in 104 patients. The results from these studies showed that CI-994 at doses of 4-10mg/m²/day can be safely administered to patients for 7-21 days in a 3-4 week dosing regimen (Nemunaitis et al., 2003; Undevia et al., 2004; Paur et al., 2004). In this study, two patients with esophageal and bladder cancer showed complete remission (CR) and five (three with non- small lung cancer and two with colorectal cancer) demonstrated partial remission (PR). On a related note, some leukemia and breast cancers plagued with the expression of fusion proteins (RAR–PML, RAR–PLZF or AML–ETO chimeras) that inhibit differentiation have shown improvements when HDACis in combination therapy with transretinoic acid (ATRA) is used to inhibit the function of these fusion proteins (Johnstone et al., 2003) (Table 12). Another emerging area of combination therapy is the use of HDACis with tyrosine kinase inhibitors in cancers that overexpress antiapoptic genes. For example, SAHA, LBH-589, LAQ-824 and romidepsin have demonstrated synergistic apoptotic activity in combination with imatinib and other tyrosine kinase inhibitors, such as AMN-107 in imatinib-sensitive, as well as imatinib-resistant *bcr-abl* leukemic cells (Nimmanapalli et al., 2003a, 2003b; Yu et al., 2003; Kawano et al., 2004; Fiskus et al., 2006).

HDACis	Phase	Tumor type	Patient number	Responses	Reference
Single Therapy					
Phenyl butyrate	I	Solid	75	CR(1) and SD (9)	Carducci et al., 2001; Gilbert et al., 2001; Phuphanich et al., 2005
Valporic acid	I/II	AML/MDS	18	OR(8) and PR (1)	Kuendgen et al., 2004
SAHA	I	Mesothelioma	37	PR (2)	Kelly et al., 2003
	I	Solid	13	TR (4)	Krug et al., 2006
Romsidepsin	II	CTCL	28	CR(2), PR(8), SD(16)	Whittaker et al., 2006

Combination Therapy	Phase	Tumor Type	Patient number	Response	Reference
Phenyl butyrate (+)					
5-Aza	I/II	AML/MDS	29	CR (4), PR (1), HI (6)	Gore et al., 2006
5-Aza	II	AML/MDS	10	PR (3) , SD (2)	Maslak et al., 2006
ATRA	I	APML	5	CR (1)	Zhou et al., 2002
Valproic acid (+)					
Decitabine	I/II	AML/MDS	54	CR (10) and CRp (2)	Garcia-Manero et al., 2006
ATRA	II	AML	11	CR (1) and CRi (2)	Raffoux et al., 2005
ATRA	II	AML/MDS	20	HI (6/11 evaluable)	Pilatrino et al., 2005
ATRA	II	AML	30	CR (1), CRi (1), PR (1) and SD (20)	Kuendgen et al., 2006
SAHA (+)					
Carboplatin + paclitaxel	I	Colorectal	9	PR (4) and SD (2	Ramalingam et al., 2006
CI-994 (+)					
Capecitabine	I	Solid	4	PR (1) and SD (19)	Undenvia et al., 2004
Carboplatin + paclitaxel	I	Pancreatic	30	CR (2) and PR (5)	Pauer et al., 2004

5-AZA: 5-Azacytidine; AML: Acute myeloid leukemia; APML: ATRA: All-trans-retinoic acid; CR: Complete response; CRi: Morphologic complete remission with incomplete count recovery; CRp: Complete response without complete platelet recovery; HDACi: Histone deacetylase inhibitors; MDS: Myelodysplastic syndrome; PR: Partial response; SAHA: Suberoylanilide hydroxamic acid; SD: Stable disease.

Table 12. HDACis in Clinical Trial and Combination Therapies

4. Concluding remarks

Only a handful of studies have been published examining the usefulness of drugs targeting ubiquitination, sumolyation and phosphorylation of histone as a means to combat the proliferative and differentiation deficits seen in cancer. The above discussion was not intended to provide complete coverage to a fast emerging field at rather as a means to highlight the most promising therapies investigated to date employing epigenetic-based approaches. Although these early successes establish the promise of epigenetic-based chemotherapeutic regimens in the treatment of various cancers, the degree to which gene-specific epigenetic modifications can be achieved, or the extent to which targeted therapies can be developed using epigenetic approaches remains to be fully investigated. Undeniably, the ultimate benefit to be realized from such strategies is based on the fact that the epigenetic modifications in cancer cells are reversible and subject to environmental control. Clearly, the jury is still out!

5. References

Ahn, S. H., K. A. Henderson, et al. (2005). "H2B (Ser10) phosphorylation is induced during apoptosis and meiosis in S. cerevisiae." *Cell Cycle* 4(6): 780-783.

Allfrey, V. G., R. Faulkner, et al. (1964). Acetylation and Methylation of Histones and Their Possible Role in the Regulation of *RNA Synthesis*. 51.

Andrews, P. D., E. Knatko, et al. (2003). "Mitotic mechanics: the auroras come into view." *Current Opinion in Cell Biology* 15(6): 672-683.

Anest, V., J. L. Hanson, et al. (2003). A nucleosomal function for IkappaB kinase-alpha in NF-kappaB-dependent gene expression. 423 Research Support, Non-U.S. Gov't

Angrand, P. O., F. Apiou, et al. (2001). "NSD3, a new SET domain-containing gene, maps to 8p12 and is amplified in human breast cancer cell lines." *Genomics* 74(1): 79-88.

Babushok, D. V. and H. H. Kazazian (2007) "Progress in understanding the biology of the human mutagen LINE-1." *Human Mutation* 28, 527-539.

Balasubramanyam, K., M. Altaf, et al. (2004a). Polyisoprenylated benzophenone, garcinol, a natural histone acetyltransferase inhibitor, represses chromatin transcription and alters global gene expression. *Journal Biological Chemistry* 279: 33716-33726.

Balasubramanyam, K., R. A. Varier, et al. (2004b). Curcumin, a novel p300/CREB-binding protein-specific inhibitor of acetyltransferase, represses the acetylation of histone/nonhistone proteins and histone acetyltransferase-dependent chromatin transcription. *Journal of Biological Chemistry* 279: 51163-51171.

Balch, C., P. Yan, et al. (2005). "Antimitogenic and chemosensitizing effects of the methylation inhibitor zebularine in ovarian cancer." *Molecular Cancer Therapeutics* 4(10): 1505-1514.

Bannister, A. J., E. A. Miska, et al. (2000). "Acetylation of importin-alpha nuclear import factors by CBP/p300." *Current Biology* 10(8): 467-470.

Bannister, A. J., P. Zegerman, et al. (2001). "Selective recognition of methylated lysine 9 on histone H3 by the HP1 chromo domain." *Nature* 410(6824): 120-124.

Barbacid, M. and S. Sukumar (1987). "Contribution of Ras Oncogenes to Neoplastic Development." *European Journal of Cancer & Clinical Oncology* 23(11): 1732-1732.

Bassing, C. H., H. Suh, et al. (2003). "Histone H2AX: a dosage-dependent suppressor of oncogenic translocations and tumors." *Cell* 114(3): 359-370.

Bednar, J., R. A. Horowitz, et al. (1998). Nucleosomes, linker DNA, and linker histone form a unique structural motif that directs the higher-order folding and compaction of chromatin. 95 Research Support, Non-U.S. Gov't

Berdasco, M., S. Ropero, et al. (2009). "Epigenetic inactivation of the Sotos overgrowth syndrome gene histone methyltransferase NSD1 in human neuroblastoma and glioma." *PNAS:USA* 106(51): 21830-21835.

Bernstein, B. E., T. S. Mikkelsen, et al. (2006). "A bivalent chromatin structure marks key developmental genes in embryonic stem cells." *Cell* 125(2): 315-326.

Beumer, J. H., R. A. Parise, et al. (2008). "Concentrations of the DNA methyltransferase inhibitor 5-fluoro-2'-deoxycytidine (FdCyd) and its cytotoxic metabolites in plasma of patients treated with FdCyd and tetrahydrouridine (THU)." *Cancer Chemotherapy and Pharmacology* 62(2): 363-368.

Bhalla, K. N. (2005). "Epigenetic and chromatin modifiers as targeted therapy of hematologic malignancies." *Journal of Clinical Oncology* 23(17): 3971-3993.

Biel, M., V. Wascholowski, et al. (2005). "Epigenetics--an epicenter of gene regulation: histones and histone-modifying enzymes." *Angewandte Chemie* 44(21): 3186-3216.

Bies, J., J. Markus, et al. (2002). "Covalent attachment of the SUMO-1 protein to the negative regulatory domain of the c-Myb transcription factor modifies its stability and transactivation capacity." *Journal of Biological Chemistry* 277(11): 8999-9009.

Billam, M., M. D. Sobolewski, et al. (2010). "Effects of a novel DNA methyltransferase inhibitor zebularine on human breast cancer cells." *Breast Cancer Research and Treatment* 120(3): 581-592.

Bird, A. P. (1986). "Cpg-Rich Islands and the Function of DNA Methylation." *Nature* 321(6067): 209-213.

Bird, A. P., M. H. Taggart, et al. (1987). "Nonmethylated Cpg-Rich Islands at the Human Alpha-Globin Locus - Implications for Evolution of the Alpha-Globin Pseudogene." *EMBO Journal* 6(4): 999-1004.

Blum, J. L., J. Kohles, et al. (2011). "Association of age and overall survival in capecitabine-treated patients with metastatic breast cancer in clinical trials." *Breast Cancer Research and Treatment* 125(2): 431-439.

Bolden, J. E., M. J. Peart, et al. (2006). "Anticancer activities of histone deacetylase inhibitors." *Nature Reviews* 5(9): 769-784.

Borrow, J., V. P. Stanton, Jr., et al. (1996). "The translocation t(8;16)(p11;p13) of acute myeloid leukaemia fuses a putative acetyltransferase to the CREB-binding protein." *Nature Genetics* 14(1): 33-41.

Bourc'his, D., D. Le Bourhis, et al. (2001). "Delayed and incomplete reprogramming of chromosome methylation patterns in bovine cloned embryos." *Current Biology* 11(19): 1542-1546.

Bracken, A. P., D. Pasini, et al. (2003). "EZH2 is downstream of the pRB-E2F pathway, essential for proliferation and amplified in cancer." *EMBO Journal* 22(20): 5323-5335.

Brehm, A., E. A. Miska, et al. (1998). "Retinoblastoma protein recruits histone deacetylase to repress transcription." *Nature* 391(6667): 597-601.

Brueckner, B., R. Garcia Boy, et al. (2005). "Epigenetic reactivation of tumor suppressor genes by a novel small-molecule inhibitor of human DNA methyltransferases." *Cancer Research* 65(14): 6305-6311.

Bryan, E. J., V. J. Jokubaitis, et al. (2002). "Mutation analysis of EP300 in colon, breast and ovarian carcinomas." *International Journal of Cancer* 102(2): 137-141.

Bushman, J. E., D. Palmieri, et al. (2000). "Insight into the mechanism of asparaginase-induced depletion of antithrombin III in treatment of childhood acute lymphoblastic leukemia." *Leukemia Research* 24(7): 559-565.

Cairns, B. R. (2009). "The logic of chromatin architecture and remodelling at promoters." *Nature* 461(7261): 193-198.

Carducci, M. A., J. Gilbert, et al. (2001). "A Phase I clinical and pharmacological evaluation of sodium phenylbutyrate on an 120-h infusion schedule." *Clinical Cancer Research* 7(10): 3047-3055.

Chadee, D. N., W. R. Taylor, et al. (1995). "Increased phosphorylation of histone H1 in mouse fibroblasts transformed with oncogenes or constitutively active mitogen-activated protein kinase kinase." *Journal Biological Chemistry* 270(34): 20098-20105.

Chaffanet, M., L. Gressin, et al. (2000). "MOZ is fused to p300 in an acute monocytic leukemia with t(8;22)." *Genes, Chromosomes & Cancer* 28(2): 138-144.

Chen, T. P., S. Hevi, et al. (2007). "Complete inactivation of DNMT1 leads to mitotic catastrophe in human cancer cells." *Nature Genetics* 39(3): 391-396.

Chen, Z. X., J. R. Mann, et al. (2005). "Physical and functional interactions between the human DNMT3L protein and members of the de novo methyltransferase family." *Journal Cellular Biochemistry* 95(5): 902-917.

Cheng, J. C., C. B. Matsen, et al. (2003). "Inhibition of DNA methylation and reactivation of silenced genes by zebularine." *Journal of the National Cancer Institute* 95(5): 399-409.

Cheung, P., K. G. Tanner, et al. (2000). "Synergistic coupling of histone H3 phosphorylation and acetylation in response to epidermal growth factor stimulation." *Molecular Cell* 5(6): 905-915.

Cheung, W. L., K. Ajiro, et al. (2003). "Apoptotic phosphorylation of histone H2B is mediated by mammalian sterile twenty kinase." *Cell* 113(4): 507-517.

Cho, H. S., T. Suzuki, et al. (2011). "Demethylation of RB regulator MYPT1 by histone demethylase LSD1 promotes cell cycle progression in cancer cells." *Cancer Research* 71(3): 655-660.

Chodavarapu, R. K., S. Feng, et al. (2010). "Relationship between nucleosome positioning and DNA methylation." *Nature* 466(7304): 388-392.

Chuang, L. S. H., H. I. Ian, et al. (1997). "Human DNA (cytosine-5) methyltransferase PCNA complex as a target for p21(WAF1)." *Science* 277(5334): 1996-2000.

Clapier, C. R. and B. R. Cairns (2009). "The biology of chromatin remodeling complexes." *Annual Review Biochemistry* 78: 273-304.

Cloos, P. A., J. Christensen, et al. (2006). "The putative oncogene GASC1 demethylates tri- and dimethylated lysine 9 on histone H3." *Nature* 442(7100): 307-311.

Cooper, D. N. and H. Youssoufian (1988). "The Cpg Dinucleotide and Human Genetic-Disease." *Human Genetics* 78(2): 151-155.

Cullis, P. M., R. Wolfenden, et al. (1982). "Inhibition of histone acetylation by N-[2-(S-coenzyme A)acetyl] spermidine amide, a multisubstrate analog." *Journal of Biological Chemistry* 257(20): 12165-12169.

Cuthbert, G. L., S. Daujat, et al. (2004). "Histone deimination antagonizes arginine methylation." *Cell* 118(5): 545-553.

Dawson, M. A., A. J. Bannister, et al. (2009). "JAK2 phosphorylates histone H3Y41 and excludes HP1alpha from chromatin." *Nature* 461(7265): 819-822.

de la Serna, I. L., Y. Ohkawa, et al. (2006). "Chromatin remodelling in mammalian differentiation: lessons from ATP-dependent remodellers." *Nature Reviews* 7(6): 461-473.

den Besten, W., M. L. Kuo, et al. (2005). "Myeloid leukemia-associated nucleophosmin mutants perturb p53-dependent and independent activities of the Arf tumor suppressor protein." *Cell Cycle* 4(11): 1593-1598.

Denu, J. M. (2003). "Linking chromatin function with metabolic networks: Sir2 family of NAD(+)-dependent deacetylases." *Trends in Biochemical Sciences* 28(1): 41-48.

Dhalluin, C., J. E. Carlson, et al. (1999). "Structure and ligand of a HAT bromodomain." *Nature* 399(6735): 491-496.

Doi, A., I. H. Park, et al. (2009). "Differential methylation of tissue- and cancer-specific CpG island shores distinguishes human induced pluripotent stem cells, embryonic stem cells and fibroblasts." *Nature Genetics* 41(12): 1350-U1123.

Dokmanovic, M. and P. A. Marks (2005). "Prospects: histone deacetylase inhibitors." *J. Cellular Biochemistry* 96(2): 293-304.

Dong, K. B., I. A. Maksakova, et al. (2008). "DNA methylation in ES cells requires the lysine methyltransferase G9a but not its catalytic activity." *EMBO Journal* 27(20): 2691-2701.

Dote, H., D. Cerna, et al. (2005). "Enhancement of in vitro and in vivo tumor cell radiosensitivity by the DNA methylation inhibitor zebularine." *Clinical Cancer Research* 11(12): 4571-4579.

Du, Y., T. Carling, et al. (2001). "Hypermethylation in human cancers of the RIZ1 tumor suppressor gene, a member of a histone/protein methyltransferase superfamily." *Cancer Research* 61(22): 8094-8099.

Duan, Q., H. Chen, et al. (2008). "Phosphorylation of H3S10 blocks the access of H3K9 by specific antibodies and histone methyltransferase. Implication in regulating chromatin dynamics and epigenetic inheritance during mitosis." *Journal of Biological Chemistry* 283(48): 33585-33590.

Dunn, C. A., P. Medstrand, et al. (2003). "An endogenous retroviral LTR acts as a tissue-specific promoter for the human beta 1,3-galactosyltransferase 5 gene." *American Journal of Human Genetics* 73(5): 180-180.

Ebbert, R., A. Birkmann, et al. (1999). "The product of the SNF2/SWI2 paralogue INO80 of Saccharomyces cerevisiae required for efficient expression of various yeast structural genes is part of a high-molecular-weight protein complex." *Molecular Microbiology* 32(4): 741-751.

Ernst, J. and M. Kellis (2010). "Discovery and characterization of chromatin states for systematic annotation of the human genome." *Nature Biotechnology* 28(8): 817-825.

Espada, J., E. Ballestar, et al. (2007). "Epigenetic disruption of ribosomal RNA genes and nucleolar architecture in DNA methyltransferase 1 (Dnmt1) deficient cells." *Nucleic Acids Research* 35(7): 2191-2198.

Espino, P. S., B. Drobic, et al. (2005). "Histone modifications as a platform for cancer therapy." *J. Cellular Biochemistry* 94(6): 1088-1102.

Esteller, M. (2002). "CpG island hypermethylation and tumor suppressor genes: a booming present, a brighter future." *Oncogene* 21(35): 5427-5440.

Esteller, M. (2007). "Cancer epigenomics: DNA methylomes and histone-modification maps." *Nature Reviews Genetics* 8(4): 286-298.

Esteller, M. (2008). "Molecular origins of cancer: Epigenetics in cancer." New England Journal of Medicine 358(11): 1148-1159.

Fabbrizio, E., S. El Messaoudi, et al. (2002). "Negative regulation of transcription by the type II arginine methyltransferase PRMT5." *EMBO Reports* 3(7): 641-645.

Fatkins, D. G. and W. Zheng (2008). "Substituting N(epsilon)-thioacetyl-lysine for N(epsilon)-acetyl-lysine in peptide substrates as a general approach to inhibiting human NAD(+)-dependent protein deacetylases." *International Journal of Molecular Sciences* 9(1): 1-11.

Fernandez-Capetillo, O., C. D. Allis, et al. (2004). "Phosphorylation of histone H2B at DNA double-strand breaks." *Journal of Experimental Medicine* 199(12): 1671-1677.

Fischle, W., B. S. Tseng, et al. (2005). "Regulation of HP1-chromatin binding by histone H3 methylation and phosphorylation." *Nature* 438(7071): 1116-1122.

Fiskus, W., M. Pranpat, et al. (2006). "Cotreatment with vorinostat (suberoylanilide hydroxamic acid) enhances activity of dasatinib (BMS-354825) against imatinib mesylate-sensitive or imatinib mesylate-resistant chronic myelogenous leukemia cells." *Clinical Cancer Research* 12(19): 5869-5878.

Flotho, C., R. Claus, et al. (2009). "The DNA methyltransferase inhibitors azacitidine, decitabine and zebularine exert differential effects on cancer gene expression in acute myeloid leukemia cells." *Leukemia* 23(6): 1019-1028.

Forneris, F., C. Binda, et al. (2005). "Human histone demethylase LSD1 reads the histone code." *Journal of Biological Chemistry* 280(50): 41360-41365.

Fraga, M. F., E. Ballestar, et al. (2005a). "Epigenetic differences arise during the lifetime of monozygotic twins." *PNAS:USA* 102(30): 10604-10609.

Fraga, M. F., E. Ballestar, et al. (2005b). "Loss of acetylation at Lys16 and trimethylation at Lys20 of histone H4 is a common hallmark of human cancer." *Nature Genetics* 37(4): 391-400.

Futscher, B. W., M. M. O'Meara, et al. (2004). "Aberrant methylation of the maspin promoter is an early event in human breast cancer." *Neoplasia* 6(4): 380-389.

Garcia-Manero, G., H. M. Kantarjian, et al. (2006). "Phase 1/2 study of the combination of 5-aza-2'-deoxycytidine with valproic acid in patients with leukemia." *Blood* 108(10): 3271-3279.

Gardinergarden, M. and M. Frommer (1987). "Cpg Islands in Vertebrate Genomes." *Journal Molecular Biology* 196(2): 261-282.

Garzon, R., S. Liu, et al. (2009). "MicroRNA-29b induces global DNA hypomethylation and tumor suppressor gene reexpression in AML by targeting directly DNMT3A and 3B and indirectly DNMT1." *Blood* 113(25): 6411-6418.

Gaudet, F., J. G. Hodgson, et al. (2003). "Induction of tumors in mice by genomic hypomethylation." *Science* 300(5618): 489-492.

Gayther, S. A., S. J. Batley, et al. (2000). "Mutations truncating the EP300 acetylase in human cancers." *Nature Genetics* 24(3): 300-303.

Gerber, M. and A. Shilatifard (2003). "Transcriptional elongation by RNA polymerase II and histone methylation." *Journal Biological Chemistry* 278(29): 26303-26306.

Ghioni, P., Y. D'Alessandra, et al. (2005). "The protein stability and transcriptional activity of p63alpha are regulated by SUMO-1 conjugation." *Cell Cycle* 4(1): 183-190.

Ghoshal, K., J. Datta, et al. (2005). "5-Aza-deoxycytidine induces selective degradation of DNA methyltransferase 1 by a proteasomal pathway that requires the KEN box, bromo-adjacent homology domain, and nuclear localization signal." *Molecular Cellular Biology* 25(11): 4727-4741.

Gilbert, J., S. D. Baker, et al. (2001). "A phase I dose escalation and bioavailability study of oral sodium phenylbutyrate in patients with refractory solid tumor malignancies." *Clinical Cancer Research* 7(8): 2292-2300.

Girdwood, D., D. Bumpass, et al. (2003). "P300 transcriptional repression is mediated by SUMO modification." *Molecular Cell* 11(4): 1043-1054.

Goelz, S. E., B. Vogelstein, et al. (1985). "Hypomethylation of DNA from Benign and Malignant Human-Colon Neoplasms." *Science* 228(4696): 187-190.

Goldberg, A. D., C. D. Allis, et al. (2007). "Epigenetics: a landscape takes shape." *Cell* 128(4): 635-638.

Goll, M. G., F. Kirpekar, et al. (2006). "Methylation of tRNA(AsP) by the DNA methyltransferase homolog Dnmt2." *Science* 311(5759): 395-398.

Gore, S. D., S. Baylin, et al. (2006a). "Combined DNA methyltransferase and histone deacetylase inhibition in the treatment of myeloid neoplasms." *Cancer Research* 66(12): 6361-6369.

Gore, S. D., C. Jones, et al. (2006). "Decitabine." *Nature Reviews. Drug Discovery* 5(11): 891-892.

Goto, H., Y. Tomono, et al. (1999). "Identification of a novel phosphorylation site on histone H3 coupled with mitotic chromosome condensation." *Journal of Biological Chemistry* 274(36): 25543-25549.

Gowher, H. and A. Jeltsch (2004). "Mechanism of inhibition of DNA methyltransferases by cytidine analogs in cancer therapy." *Cancer Biology & Therapy* 3(11): 1062-1068.

Grant, P. A. and S. L. Berger (1999). "Histone acetyltransferase complexes." *Sem. Cell & Developmental Biology* 10(2): 169-177.

Gui, C. Y., L. Ngo, et al. (2004). "Histone deacetylase (HDAC) inhibitor activation of p21WAF1 involves changes in promoter-associated proteins, including HDAC1." *PNAS:USA* 101(5): 1241-1246.

Hampsey, M. and D. Reinberg (2003). "Tails of intrigue: phosphorylation of RNA polymerase II mediates histone methylation." *Cell* 113(4): 429-432.

Hanahan, D. and R. A. Weinberg (2000). "The hallmarks of cancer." *Cell* 100(1): 57-70.

Hanigan, C. L., M. Van Engeland, et al. (2008). "An inactivating mutation in HDAC2 leads to dysregulation of apoptosis mediated by APAF1." *Gastroenterology* 135(5): 1654-1664 e1652.

Harikrishnan, K. N., M. Z. Chow, et al. (2005). "Brahma links the SWI/SNF chromatin-remodeling complex with MeCP2-dependent transcriptional silencing." *Nature Genetics* 37(3): 254-264.

Hassan, A. H., P. Prochasson, et al. (2002). "Function and selectivity of bromodomains in anchoring chromatin-modifying complexes to promoter nucleosomes." *Cell* 111(3): 369-379.

He, L., J. X. Yu, et al. (1998). "RIZ1, but not the alternative RIZ2 product of the same gene, is underexpressed in breast cancer, and forced RIZ1 expression causes G2-M cell cycle arrest and/or apoptosis." *Cancer Research* 58(19): 4238-4244.

Hellebrekers, D. M., K. W. Jair, et al. (2006). "Angiostatic activity of DNA methyltransferase inhibitors." *Molecular Cancer Therapeutics* 5(2): 467-475.

Hellman, A. and A. Chess (2007). "Gene body-specific methylation on active X chromosome." *Science* 315(5815): 1141-1143.

Hirota, T., J. J. Lipp, et al. (2005). "Histone H3 serine 10 phosphorylation by Aurora B causes HP1 dissociation from heterochromatin." *Nature* 438(7071): 1176-1180.

Hirsch, C. L. and K. Bonham (2004). "Histone deacetylase inhibitors regulate p21WAF1 gene expression at the post-transcriptional level in HepG2 cells." *FEBS Letters* 570(1-3): 37-40.

Ho, L. and G. R. Crabtree (2010). "Chromatin remodelling during development." *Nature* 463(7280): 474-484.

Holliday, R. and J. E. Pugh (1975). "DNA Modification Mechanisms and Gene Activity during Development." *Science* 187(4173): 226-232.

Hollstein, M., D. Sidransky, et al. (1991). "P53 Mutations in Human Cancers." *Science* 253(5015): 49-53.

Hong, L., G. P. Schroth, et al. (1993). "Studies of the DNA binding properties of histone H4 amino terminus. Thermal denaturation studies reveal that acetylation markedly reduces the binding constant of the H4 "tail" to DNA." *Journal of Biological Chemistry* 268(1): 305-314.

Huang, Y. P., G. Wu, et al. (2004). "Altered sumoylation of p63alpha contributes to the split-hand/foot malformation phenotype." *Cell Cycle* 3(12): 1587-1596.

Ida, K., I. Kitabayashi, et al. (1997). "Adenoviral E1A-associated protein p300 is involved in acute myeloid leukemia with t(11;22)(q23;q13)." *Blood* 90(12): 4699-4704.

Ikura, T., V. V. Ogryzko, et al. (2000). "Involvement of the TIP60 histone acetylase complex in DNA repair and apoptosis." *Cell* 102(4): 463-473.

Irizarry, R. A., C. Ladd-Acosta, et al. (2009). "The human colon cancer methylome shows similar hypo- and hypermethylation at conserved tissue-specific CpG island shores." *Nature Genetics* 41(2): 178-186.

Issa, J. P. and H. M. Kantarjian (2009). "Targeting DNA methylation." *Clinical Cancer Research* 15(12): 3938-3946.

Italiano, A., R. Attias, et al. (2006). "Molecular cytogenetic characterization of a metastatic lung sarcomatoid carcinoma: 9p23 neocentromere and 9p23-p24 amplification including JAK2 and JMJD2C." *Cancer Genetics & Cytogenetics* 167(2): 122-130.

Ito, T., M. Bulger, et al. (1997). "ACF, an ISWI-containing and ATP-utilizing chromatin assembly and remodeling factor." *Cell* 90(1): 145-155.

Jabbour, E., S. Giralt, et al. (2009). "Low-dose azacitidine after allogeneic stem cell transplantation for acute leukemia." *Cancer* 115(9): 1899-1905.

Jenuwein, T. and C. D. Allis (2001). "Translating the histone code." Science 293(5532): 1074-1080.

Jin, F., S. C. Dowdy, et al. (2005). "Up-regulation of DNA methyltransferase 3B expression in endometrial cancers." *Gynecologic Oncology* 96(2): 531-538.

Jin, L., E. M. Lee, et al. (2009). "Monoclonal antibody-mediated targeting of CD123, IL-3 receptor alpha chain, eliminates human acute myeloid leukemic stem cells." *Cell Stem Cell* 5(1): 31-42.

Jin, Z., G. Tamura, et al. (2001). "Adenomatous polyposis coli (APC) gene promoter hypermethylation in primary breast cancers." *British Journal of Cancer* 85(1): 69-73.

Jirtle, R. L. (1999). "Genomic imprinting and cancer." *Experimental Cell Research* 248(1): 18-24.

Jirtle, R. L. and M. K. Skinner (2007). "Environmental epigenomics and disease susceptibility." *Nature Reviews Genetics* 8(4): 253-262.

Johnstone, R. W. (2002). "Histone-deacetylase inhibitors: novel drugs for the treatment of cancer." *Nature Reviews. Drug Discovery* 1(4): 287-299.

Jones, P. A. and G. Liang (2009). "Rethinking how DNA methylation patterns are maintained." *Nature Reviews Genetics* 10(11): 805-811.

Jones, P. A. and S. M. Taylor (1980). "Cellular differentiation, cytidine analogs and DNA methylation." *Cell* 20(1): 85-93.

Kahl, P., L. Gullotti, et al. (2006). "Androgen receptor coactivators lysine-specific histone demethylase 1 and four and a half LIM domain protein 2 predict risk of prostate cancer recurrence." *Cancer Research* 66(23): 11341-11347.

Kaminsky, Z. A., T. Tang, et al. (2009). "DNA methylation profiles in monozygotic and dizygotic twins." *Nature Genetics* 41(2): 240-245.

Kantarjian, H., Y. Oki, et al. (2007). "Results of a randomized study of 3 schedules of low-dose decitabine in higher-risk myelodysplastic syndrome and chronic myelomonocytic leukemia." *Blood* 109(1): 52-57.

Katayama, H., W. R. Brinkley, et al. (2003). "The Aurora kinases: role in cell transformation and tumorigenesis." *Cancer Metastasis Reviews* 22(4): 451-464.

Katayama, H., H. Zhou, et al. (2001). "Interaction and feedback regulation between STK15/BTAK/Aurora-A kinase and protein phosphatase 1 through mitotic cell division cycle." *Journal of Biological Chemistry* 276(49): 46219-46224.

Kelly, W. K., V. M. Richon, et al. (2003). "Phase I clinical trial of histone deacetylase inhibitor: suberoylanilide hydroxamic acid administered intravenously." *Clinical Cancer Research* 9(10 Pt 1): 3578-3588.

Kim, S. C., R. Sprung, et al. (2006). "Substrate and functional diversity of lysine acetylation revealed by a proteomics survey." *Molecular Cell* 23(4): 607-618.

Kishimoto, M., T. Kohno, et al. (2005). "Mutations and deletions of the CBP gene in human lung cancer." *Clinical Cancer Research* 11(2 Pt 1): 512-519.

Komatsu, S., I. Imoto, et al. (2009). "Overexpression of SMYD2 relates to tumor cell proliferation and malignant outcome of esophageal squamous cell carcinoma." *Carcinogenesis* 30(7): 1139-1146.

Kondo, Y., L. Shen, et al. (2008). "Gene silencing in cancer by histone H3 lysine 27 trimethylation independent of promoter DNA methylation." *Nature Genetics* 40(6): 741-750.

Kornberg, R. D. (1974). "Chromatin structure: a repeating unit of histones and DNA." *Science* 184(139): 868-871.

Krivtsov, A. V., Z. Feng, et al. (2008). "H3K79 methylation profiles define murine and human MLL-AF4 leukemias." *Cancer Cell* 14(5): 355-368.

Krug, L. M., T. Curley, et al. (2006). "Potential role of histone deacetylase inhibitors in mesothelioma: clinical experience with suberoylanilide hydroxamic acid." *Clinical Lung Cancer* 7(4): 257-261.

Kuendgen, A., C. Strupp, et al. (2004). "Treatment of myelodysplastic syndromes with valproic acid alone or in combination with all-trans retinoic acid." *Blood* 104(5): 1266-1269.

Kuismanen, S. A., M. T. Holmberg, et al. (1999). "Epigenetic phenotypes distinguish microsatellite-stable and -unstable colorectal cancers." *PNAS:USA* 96(22): 12661-12666.

Kuo, H. K., J. D. Griffith, et al. (2007). "5-Azacytidine induced methyltransferase-DNA adducts block DNA replication in vivo." *Cancer Research* 67(17): 8248-8254.

Lachner, M., D. O'Carroll, et al. (2001). "Methylation of histone H3 lysine 9 creates a binding site for HP1 proteins." *Nature* 410(6824): 116-120.

Larson, R. and J. Messing (1982). "Apple-Ii Software for M13 Shotgun DNA Sequencing." *Nucleic Acids Research* 10(1): 39-49.

Lau, O. D., T. K. Kundu, et al. (2000). "HATs off: selective synthetic inhibitors of the histone acetyltransferases p300 and PCAF." *Molecular Cell* 5(3): 589-595.

Laurent, L., E. Wong, et al. (2010). "Dynamic changes in the human methylome during differentiation." *Genome Research* 20(3): 320-331.

Lee, B. H., S. Yegnasubramanian, et al. (2005). "Procainamide is a specific inhibitor of DNA methyltransferase 1." *Journal of Biological Chemistry* 280(49): 40749-40756.

Lee, D. Y., J. P. Northrop, et al. (2006). "Histone H3 lysine 9 methyltransferase G9a is a transcriptional coactivator for nuclear receptors." *Journal of Biological Chemistry* 281(13): 8476-8485.

Lee, M. G., C. Wynder, et al. (2006). "Isolation and characterization of histone H3 lysine 4 demethylase-containing complexes." *Methods* 40(4): 327-330.

Li, B., M. Carey, et al. (2007). "The role of chromatin during transcription." *Cell* 128(4): 707-719.

Li, H., X. Ma, et al. (2007). "Effects of rearrangement and allelic exclusion of JJAZ1/SUZ12 on cell proliferation and survival." *PNAS:USA* 104(50): 20001-20006.

Lin, J. C., S. Jeong, et al. (2007). "Role of nucleosomal occupancy in the epigenetic silencing of the MLH1 CpG island." *Cancer Cell* 12(5): 432-444.

Lister, R. and J. R. Ecker (2009). "Finding the fifth base: Genome-wide sequencing of cytosine methylation." *Genome Research* 19(6): 959-966.

Lo, W. S., R. C. Trievel, et al. (2000). "Phosphorylation of serine 10 in histone H3 is functionally linked in vitro and in vivo to Gcn5-mediated acetylation at lysine 14." *Molecular Cell* 5(6): 917-926.

Lopez-Serra, L. and M. Esteller (2008). "Proteins that bind methylated DNA and human cancer: reading the wrong words." *British Journal of Cancer* 98(12): 1881-1885.

Magewu, A. N. and P. A. Jones (1994). "Ubiquitous and Tenacious Methylation of the Cpg Site in Codon-248 of the P53 Gene May Explain Its Frequent Appearance as a Mutational Hot-Spot in Human Cancer." *Molecular & Cellular Biology* 14(6): 4225-4232.

Mai, A., D. Rotili, et al. (2006). "Small-molecule inhibitors of histone acetyltransferase activity: identification and biological properties." *Journal Medicinal Chemistry* 49(23): 6897-6907.

Mantelingu, K., B. A. Reddy, et al. (2007). "Specific inhibition of p300-HAT alters global gene expression and represses HIV replication." *Chemistry & Biology* 14(6): 645-657.

Marchion, D. C., E. Bicaku, et al. (2004). "Sequence-specific potentiation of topoisomerase II inhibitors by the histone deacetylase inhibitor suberoylanilide hydroxamic acid." *Journal Cellular Biochemistry* 92(2): 223-237.

Marfella, C. G. and A. N. Imbalzano (2007). "The Chd family of chromatin remodelers." *Mutation Research* 618(1-2): 30-40.

Margueron, R., P. Trojer, et al. (2005). "The key to development: interpreting the histone code?" *Current Opinion in Genetics & Development* 15(2): 163-176.

Martin, M. G., R. A. Walgren, et al. (2009). "A phase II study of 5-day intravenous azacitidine in patients with myelodysplastic syndromes." *American Journal of Hematology* 84(9): 560-564.

Maslak, P., S. Chanel, et al. (2006). "Pilot study of combination transcriptional modulation therapy with sodium phenylbutyrate and 5-azacytidine in patients with AML or myelodysplastic syndrome." *Leukemia* 20(2): 212-217.

Medina, P. P. and M. Sanchez-Cespedes (2008). "Involvement of the chromatin-remodeling factor BRG1/SMARCA4 in human cancer." *Epigenetics* 3(2): 64-68.

Melo, S. A., S. Ropero, et al. (2009). "A TARBP2 mutation in human cancer impairs microRNA processing and DICER1 function." *Nature Genetics* 41(3): 365-370.

Merlo, A., J. G. Herman, et al. (1995). "5' Cpg Island Methylation Is Associated with Transcriptional Silencing of the Tumor-Suppressor P16/Cdkn2/Mts1 in Human Cancers." *Nature Medicine* 1(7): 686-692.

Metzger, E., M. Wissmann, et al. (2005). "LSD1 demethylates repressive histone marks to promote androgen-receptor-dependent transcription." *Nature* 437(7057): 436-439.

Metzger, E., N. Yin, et al. (2008). "Phosphorylation of histone H3 at threonine 11 establishes a novel chromatin mark for transcriptional regulation." *Nature Cell Biology* 10(1): 53-60.

Mikkelsen, T. S., M. Ku, et al. (2007). "Genome-wide maps of chromatin state in pluripotent and lineage-committed cells." *Nature* 448(7153): 553-560.

Milne, J. C., P. D. Lambert, et al. (2007). "Small molecule activators of SIRT1 as therapeutics for the treatment of type 2 diabetes." *Nature* 450(7170): 712-716.

Milne, T. A., S. D. Briggs, et al. (2002). "MLL targets SET domain methyltransferase activity to Hox gene promoters." *Molecular Cell* 10(5): 1107-1117.

Miremadi, A., M. Z. Oestergaard, et al. (2007). "Cancer genetics of epigenetic genes." *Human Molecular Genetics* 16: R28-R49.

Momparler, R. L., M. Rossi, et al. (1984). "Kinetic interaction of 5-AZA-2'-deoxycytidine-5'-monophosphate and its 5'-triphosphate with deoxycytidylate deaminase." *Molecular Pharmacology* 25(3): 436-440.

Morin, R. D., N. A. Johnson, et al. (2010). "Somatic mutations altering EZH2 (Tyr641) in follicular and diffuse large B-cell lymphomas of germinal-center origin." *Nature Genetics* 42(2): 181-185.

Morrison, A. J., J. Highland, et al. (2004). "INO80 and gamma-H2AX interaction links ATP-dependent chromatin remodeling to DNA damage repair." *Cell* 119(6): 767-775.

Mujtaba, S., Y. He, et al. (2002). "Structural basis of lysine-acetylated HIV-1 Tat recognition by PCAF bromodomain." *Molecular Cell* 9(3): 575-586.

Mulero-Navarro, S. and M. Esteller (2008). "Chromatin remodeling factor CHD5 is silenced by promoter CpG island hypermethylation in human cancer." *Epigenetics* 3(4): 210-215.

Muller, S., M. J. Matunis, et al. (1998). "Conjugation with the ubiquitin-related modifier SUMO-1 regulates the partitioning of PML within the nucleus." *EMBO Journal* 17(1): 61-70.

Muller-Thomas, C., T. Schuster, et al. (2009). "A limited number of 5-azacitidine cycles can be effective treatment in MDS." *Annals of Hematology* 88(3): 213-219.

Mund, C., B. Brueckner, et al. (2006). "Reactivation of epigenetically silenced genes by DNA methyltransferase inhibitors: basic concepts and clinical applications." *Epigenetics* 1(1): 7-13.

Murnion, M. E., R. R. Adams, et al. (2001). "Chromatin-associated protein phosphatase 1 regulates aurora-B and histone H3 phosphorylation." *Journal of Biological Chemistry* 276(28): 26656-26665.

Naidu, S. R., I. M. Love, et al. (2009). "The SWI/SNF chromatin remodeling subunit BRG1 is a critical regulator of p53 necessary for proliferation of malignant cells." *Oncogene* 28(27): 2492-2501.

Nakajima, T., C. Uchida, et al. (1997). "RNA helicase A mediates association of CBP with RNA polymerase II." *Cell* 90(6): 1107-1112.

Nakanishi, S., J. S. Lee, et al. (2009). "Histone H2BK123 monoubiquitination is the critical determinant for H3K4 and H3K79 trimethylation by COMPASS and Dot1." *Journal of Cell Biology* 186(3): 371-377.

Nathan, D., D. E. Sterner, et al. (2003). "Histone modifications: Now summoning sumoylation." *PNAS* 100(23): 13118-13120.

Nemunaitis, J. J., D. Orr, et al. (2003). "Phase I study of oral CI-994 in combination with gemcitabine in treatment of patients with advanced cancer." *Cancer Journal* 9(1): 58-66.

Nimmanapalli, R., L. Fuino, et al. (2000a). "Histone deacetylase inhibitor LAQ824 both lowers expression and promotes proteasomal degradation of Bcr-Abl and induces apoptosis of imatinib mesylate-sensitive or -refractory chronic myelogenous leukemia-blast crisis cells." *Cancer Research* 63(16): 5126-5135.

Nimmanapalli, R., L. Fuino, et al. (2003b). "Cotreatment with the histone deacetylase inhibitor suberoylanilide hydroxamic acid (SAHA) enhances imatinib-induced apoptosis of Bcr-Abl-positive human acute leukemia cells." *Blood* 101(8): 3236-3239.

North, B. J. and E. Verdin (2004). "Sirtuins: Sir2-related NAD-dependent protein deacetylases." Genome Biology 5(5): 224.

Nowak, S. J. and V. G. Corces (2000). "Phosphorylation of histone H3 correlates with transcriptionally active loci." *Genes & Development* 14(23): 3003-3013.

Nowak, S. J. and V. G. Corces (2004). "Phosphorylation of histone H3: a balancing act between chromosome condensation and transcriptional activation." *Trends in Genetics* 20(4): 214-220.

Ohshima, T., T. Suganuma, et al. (2001). "A novel mutation lacking the bromodomain of the transcriptional coactivator p300 in the SiHa cervical carcinoma cell line." *Biochemical and Biophysical Research Communications* 281(2): 569-575.

Okada, Y., Q. Feng, et al. (2005). "hDOT1L links histone methylation to leukemogenesis." *Cell* 121(2): 167-178.

Okano, M., S. P. Xie, et al. (1998). "Dnmt2 is not required for de novo and maintenance methylation of viral DNA in embryonic stem cells." *Nucleic Acids Research* 26(11): 2536-2540.

Ooi, S. K., C. Qiu, et al. (2007). "DNMT3L connects unmethylated lysine 4 of histone H3 to de novo methylation of DNA." *Nature* 448(7154): 714-717.

Osley, M. A. (2004). "H2B ubiquitylation: the end is in sight." *Biochimica et Biophysica Acta* 1677(1-3): 74-78.

Panagopoulos, I., M. Isaksson, et al. (2003). "Genomic characterization of MOZ/CBP and CBP/MOZ chimeras in acute myeloid leukemia suggests the involvement of a damage-repair mechanism in the origin of the t(8;16)(p11;p13)." *Genes, Chromosomes & Cancer* 36(1): 90-98.

Panagopoulos, I., F. Mertens, et al. (2008). "An endometrial stromal sarcoma cell line with the JAZF1/PHF1 chimera." *Cancer Genetics and Cytogenetics* 185(2): 74-77.

Pauer, L. R., J. Olivares, et al. (2004). "Phase I study of oral CI-994 in combination with carboplatin and paclitaxel in the treatment of patients with advanced solid tumors." *Cancer Investigation* 22(6): 886-896.

Phuphanich, S., S. D. Baker, et al. (2005). "Oral sodium phenylbutyrate in patients with recurrent malignant gliomas: a dose escalation and pharmacologic study." *Neuro-Oncology* 7(2): 177-182.

Pilatrino, C., D. Cilloni, et al. (2005). "Increase in platelet count in older, poor-risk patients with acute myeloid leukemia or myelodysplastic syndrome treated with valproic acid and all-trans retinoic acid." *Cancer* 104(1): 101-109.

Plummer, R., L. Vidal, et al. (2009). "Phase I study of MG98, an oligonucleotide antisense inhibitor of human DNA methyltransferase 1, given as a 7-day infusion in patients with advanced solid tumors." *Clinical Cancer Research* 15(9): 3177-3183.

Raffoux, E., P. Chaibi, et al. (2005). "Valproic acid and all-trans retinoic acid for the treatment of elderly patients with acute myeloid leukemia." *Haematologica* 90(7): 986-988.

Rasheed, W. K., R. W. Johnstone, et al. (2007). "Histone deacetylase inhibitors in cancer therapy." *Expert Opinion on Investigational Drugs* 16(5): 659-678.

Reisman, D., S. Glaros, et al. (2009). "The SWI/SNF complex and cancer." *Oncogene* 28(14): 1653-1668.

Reither, S., F. Li, et al. (2003). "Catalytic mechanism of DNA-(cytosine-C5)-methyltransferases revisited: covalent intermediate formation is not essential for methyl group transfer by the murine Dnmt3a enzyme." *Journal Molecular Biology* 329(4): 675-684.

Rideout, W. M., K. Eggan, et al. (2001). "Nuclear cloning and epigenetic reprogramming of the genome." *Science* 293(5532): 1093-1098.

Riggs, A. D. (1975). "X-Inactivation, Differentiation, and DNA Methylation." *Cytogenetics and Cell Genetics* 14(1): 9-25.

Rius, M., C. Stresemann, et al. (2009). "Human concentrative nucleoside transporter 1-mediated uptake of 5-azacytidine enhances DNA demethylation." *Molecular Cancer Therapeutics* 8(1): 225-231.

Roberts, C. W. and S. H. Orkin (2004). "The SWI/SNF complex--chromatin and cancer." Nature reviews. Cancer 4(2): 133-142.

Rojas, J. R., R. C. Trievel, et al. (1999). "Structure of Tetrahymena GCN5 bound to coenzyme A and a histone H3 peptide." *Nature* 401(6748): 93-98.

Ropero, S., M. F. Fraga, et al. (2006). "A truncating mutation of HDAC2 in human cancers confers resistance to histone deacetylase inhibition." *Nature Genetics* 38(5): 566-569.

Roth, S. Y., J. M. Denu, et al. (2001). "Histone acetyltransferases." *Annual Review of Biochemistry* 70: 81-120.

Rozenblatt-Rosen, O., T. Rozovskaia, et al. (1998). "The C-terminal SET domains of ALL-1 and TRITHORAX interact with the INI1 and SNR1 proteins, components of the SWI/SNF complex." *PNAS:USA* 95(8): 4152-4157.

Ruden, D. M., L. Xiao, et al. (2005). "Hsp90 and environmental impacts on epigenetic states: a model for the trans-generational effects of diethylstibesterol on uterine development and cancer." *Human Mol. Genetics* 14 Spec No 1: R149-155.

Sagar, V., W. Zheng, et al. (2004). "Bisubstrate analogue structure-activity relationships for p300 histone acetyltransferase inhibitors." *Bioorganic & Medicinal Chemistry* 12(12): 3383-3390.

Saito, Y., G. Liang, et al. (2006). "Specific activation of microRNA-127 with downregulation of the proto-oncogene BCL6 by chromatin-modifying drugs in human cancer cells." *Cancer Cell* 9(6): 435-443.

Sandor, V., A. Senderowicz, et al. (2000). "P21-dependent g(1)arrest with downregulation of cyclin D1 and upregulation of cyclin E by the histone deacetylase inhibitor FR901228." *British Journal of Cancer* 83(6): 817-825.

Santi, D. V., A. Norment, et al. (1984). "Covalent bond formation between a DNA-cytosine methyltransferase and DNA containing 5-azacytosine." *PNAS:USA* 81(22): 6993-6997.

Santini, V. (2009). "Azacitidine in lower-risk myelodysplastic syndromes." Leukemia research 33 Suppl 2: S22-26.

Santos-Rosa, H., R. Schneider, et al. (2003). "Methylation of histone H3 K4 mediates association of the Isw1p ATPase with chromatin." *Molecular Cell* 12(5): 1325-1332.

Scandura, J. M., P. Boccuni, et al. (2002). "Transcription factor fusions in acute leukemia: variations on a theme." *Oncogene* 21(21): 3422-3444.

Schafer, S. and M. Jung (2005). "Chromatin modifications as targets for new anticancer drugs." *Archiv Pharmazie* 338(8): 347-357.

Schemies, J., W. Sippl, et al. (2009). "Histone deacetylase inhibitors that target tubulin." *Cancer Letters* 280(2): 222-232.

Schmidt, D. and S. Muller (2002). "Members of the PIAS family act as SUMO ligases for c-Jun and p53 and repress p53 activity." *PNAS:USA* 99(5): 2872-2877.

Schones, D. E., K. Cui, et al. (2008). "Dynamic regulation of nucleosome positioning in the human genome." *Cell* 132(5): 887-898.

Schrump, D. S., M. R. Fischette, et al. (2006). "Phase I study of decitabine-mediated gene expression in patients with cancers involving the lungs, esophagus, or pleura." *Clinical Cancer Research* 12(19): 5777-5785.

Seeger, R. C., G. M. Brodeur, et al. (1985). "Association of multiple copies of the N-myc oncogene with rapid progression of neuroblastomas." *New England Journal of Medicine* 313(18): 1111-1116.

Segura-Pacheco, B., C. Trejo-Becerril, et al. (2003). "Reactivation of tumor suppressor genes by the cardiovascular drugs hydralazine and procainamide and their potential use in cancer therapy." *Clinical Cancer Research* 9(5): 1596-1603.

Shen, X., G. Mizuguchi, et al. (2000). "A chromatin remodelling complex involved in transcription and DNA processing." *Nature* 406(6795): 541-544.

Shi, X. B., L. Xue, et al. (2007). "An androgen-regulated miRNA suppresses Bak1 expression and induces androgen-independent growth of prostate cancer cells." *PNAS:USA* 104(50): 19983-19988.

Shigeno, K., H. Yoshida, et al. (2004). "Disease-related potential of mutations in transcriptional cofactors CREB-binding protein and p300 in leukemias." *Cancer Letters* 213(1): 11-20.

Shiio, Y. and R. N. Eisenman (2003). "Histone sumoylation is associated with transcriptional repression." *PNAS* 100(23): 13225-13230.

Siedlecki, P. and P. Zielenkiewicz (2006). "Mammalian DNA methyltransferases." *Acta Biochimica Polonica* 53(2): 245-256.

Silverman, L. R., D. R. McKenzie, et al. (2006). "Further analysis of trials with azacitidine in patients with myelodysplastic syndrome: studies 8421, 8921, and 9221 by the Cancer and Leukemia Group B." *Journal of Clinical Oncology* 24(24): 3895-3903.

Singh, N., A. Duenas-Gonzalez, et al. (2009). "Molecular modeling and molecular dynamics studies of hydralazine with human DNA methyltransferase 1." *Chemmedchem* 4(5): 792-799.

Slamon, D. J., G. M. Clark, et al. (1987). "Human breast cancer: correlation of relapse and survival with amplification of the HER-2/neu oncogene." *Science* 235(4785): 177-182.

Song, Y. and C. Zhang (2009). "Hydralazine inhibits human cervical cancer cell growth in vitro in association with APC demethylation and re-expression." *Cancer Chemotherapy and Pharmacology* 63(4): 605-613.

Soriano, A. O., H. Yang, et al. (2007). "Safety and clinical activity of the combination of 5-azacytidine, valproic acid, and all-trans retinoic acid in acute myeloid leukemia and myelodysplastic syndrome." *Blood* 110(7): 2302-2308.

Sporn, J. C., G. Kustatscher, et al. (2009). "Histone macroH2A isoforms predict the risk of lung cancer recurrence." *Oncogene* 28(38): 3423-3428.

Stimson, L., M. G. Rowlands, et al. (2005). "Isothiazolones as inhibitors of PCAF and p300 histone acetyltransferase activity." *Molecular Cancer Therapeutics* 4(10): 1521-1532.

Stresemann, C. and F. Lyko (2008). "Modes of action of the DNA methyltransferase inhibitors azacytidine and decitabine." International journal of cancer. *Journal International du Cancer* 123(1): 8-13.

Suzuki, T., R. Tanaka, et al. (2010). "Design, synthesis, inhibitory activity, and binding mode study of novel DNA methyltransferase 1 inhibitors." *Bioorganic & Medicinal Chemistry Letters* 20(3): 1124-1127.

Szyf, M. (2007). "The dynamic epigenome and its implications in toxicology." *Toxicological Sciences* 100(1): 7-23.

Tong, J. K., C. A. Hassig, et al. (1998). "Chromatin deacetylation by an ATP-dependent nucleosome remodelling complex." *Nature* 395(6705): 917-921.

Tornaletti, S. and G. P. Pfeifer (1995). "Uv-Light as a Footprinting Agent - Modulation of Uv-Induced DNA-Damage by Transcription Factors Bound at the Promoters of 3 Human Genes." *Journal of Molecular Biology* 249(4): 714-728.

Tsukada, Y. and Y. Zhang (2006). "Purification of histone demethylases from HeLa cells." *Methods* 40(4): 318-326.

Tsukiyama, T., C. Daniel, et al. (1995). "ISWI, a member of the SWI2/SNF2 ATPase family, encodes the 140 kDa subunit of the nucleosome remodeling factor." *Cell* 83(6): 1021-1026.

Tsukiyama, T. and C. Wu (1995). "Purification and properties of an ATP-dependent nucleosome remodeling factor." *Cell* 83(6): 1011-1020.

Undevia, S. D., H. L. Kindler, et al. (2004). "A phase I study of the oral combination of CI-994, a putative histone deacetylase inhibitor, and capecitabine." *Annals of Oncology* 15(11): 1705-1711.

Valk-Lingbeek, M. E., S. W. Bruggeman, et al. (2004). "Stem cells and cancer; the polycomb connection." *Cell* 118(4): 409-418.

van Attikum, H., O. Fritsch, et al. (2004). "Recruitment of the INO80 complex by H2A phosphorylation links ATP-dependent chromatin remodeling with DNA double-strand break repair." *Cell* 119(6): 777-788.

van Haaften, G., G. L. Dalgliesh, et al. (2009). "Somatic mutations of the histone H3K27 demethylase gene UTX in human cancer." *Nature Genetics* 41(5): 521-523.

Varga-Weisz, P. D., M. Wilm, et al. (1997). "Chromatin-remodelling factor CHRAC contains the ATPases ISWI and topoisomerase II." *Nature* 388(6642): 598-602.

Varier, R. A., V. Swaminathan, et al. (2004). "Implications of small molecule activators and inhibitors of histone acetyltransferases in chromatin therapy." *Biochemical Pharmacology* 68(6): 1215-1220.

Vaziri, H., S. K. Dessain, et al. (2001). "hSIR2(SIRT1) functions as an NAD-dependent p53 deacetylase." *Cell* 107(2): 149-159.

Villar-Garea, A., M. F. Fraga, et al. (2003). "Procaine is a DNA-demethylating agent with growth-inhibitory effects in human cancer cells." *Cancer Research* 63(16): 4984-4989.

Vrana, J. A., R. H. Decker, et al. (1999). "Induction of apoptosis in U937 human leukemia cells by SAHA proceeds through pathways that are regulated by Bcl-2/Bcl-XL, c-Jun, and p21CIP1, but independent of p53." *Oncogene* 18(50): 7016-7025.

Waddington, C. H. (1939). "Preliminary Notes on the Development of the Wings in Normal and Mutant Strains of Drosophila." *PNAS:USA* 25(7): 299-307.

Waddington, C. H. (1952). "Selection of the genetic basis for an acquired character." *Nature* 169(4302): 625-626.

Wang, H., L. Wang, et al. (2004). "Role of histone H2A ubiquitination in Polycomb silencing." *Nature* 431(7010): 873-878.

Wang, H., C. Yan, et al. (2007). "Identification of an histone H3 acetylated/K4-methylated-bound intragenic enhancer regulatory for urokinase receptor expression." *Oncogene* 26(14): 2058-2070.

Wang, X. and J. J. Hayes (2008). "Acetylation mimics within individual core histone tail domains indicate distinct roles in regulating the stability of higher-order chromatin structure." *Molecular and Cellular Biology* 28(1): 227-236.

Wang, Y., J. Wysocka, et al. (2004). "Human PAD4 regulates histone arginine methylation levels via demethylimination." *Science* 306(5694): 279-283.

Wang, Z., C. Zang, et al. (2008). "Combinatorial patterns of histone acetylations and methylations in the human genome." *Nature Genetics* 40(7): 897-903.

Westphal, C. H., M. A. Dipp, et al. (2007). "A therapeutic role for sirtuins in diseases of aging?" *TIBS* 32(12): 555-560.

Wharton, W., J. Savell, et al. (2000). "Inhibition of mitogenesis in Balb/c-3T3 cells by Trichostatin A. Multiple alterations in the induction and activation of cyclin-cyclin-dependent kinase complexes." *J. Biological Chemistry* 275(43): 33981-33987.

Wijermans, P. W., M. Lubbert, et al. (2005). "An epigenetic approach to the treatment of advanced MDS; the experience with the DNA demethylating agent 5-aza-2'-deoxycytidine (decitabine) in 177 patients." *Annals of Hematology* 84 Suppl 1: 9-17.

Wilson, A. S., B. E. Power, et al. (2007). "DNA hypomethylation and human diseases." *Biochim. Biophys. Acta* 1775(1): 138-162.

Winquist, E., J. Knox, et al. (2006). "Phase II trial of DNA methyltransferase 1 inhibition with the antisense oligonucleotide MG98 in patients with metastatic renal carcinoma: a National Cancer Institute of Canada Clinical Trials Group investigational new drug study." *Investigational New Drugs* 24(2): 159-167.

Xu, F., K. Zhang, et al. (2005). "Acetylation in histone H3 globular domain regulates gene expression in yeast." *Cell* 121(3): 375-385.

Yamamoto, Y., U. N. Verma, et al. (2003). "Histone H3 phosphorylation by IKK-alpha is critical for cytokine-induced gene expression." *Nature* 423(6940): 655-659.

Yang, G., W. Khalaf, et al. (2004). "Epigenetic regulation of tumor suppressors in t(8:21)-containing AML." *Annals of Hematology* 83(6): 329-330.

Yang, X. J. and E. Seto (2003). "Collaborative spirit of histone deacetylases in regulating chromatin structure and gene expression." *Current Opinion in Genetics & Development* 13(2): 143-153.

Yin, H., X. Zhang, et al. (2009). "Epigenetic regulation, somatic homologous recombination, and abscisic acid signaling are influenced by DNA polymerase epsilon mutation in Arabidopsis." *Plant Cell* 21(2): 386-402.

Yoo, C. B., J. C. Chuang, et al. (2008). "Long-term epigenetic therapy with oral zebularine has minimal side effects and prevents intestinal tumors in mice." *Cancer Prevention Research* 1(4): 233-240.

Yoon, J. H., L. E. Smith, et al. (2001). "Methylated CpG dinucleotides are the preferential targets for G-to-T transversion mutations induced by benzo[a]pyrene diol epoxide in mammalian cells: Similarities with the p53 mutation spectrum in smoking-associated lung cancers." *Cancer Research* 61(19): 7110-7117.

Yu, C., M. Rahmani, et al. (2003). "The proteasome inhibitor bortezomib interacts synergistically with histone deacetylase inhibitors to induce apoptosis in Bcr/Abl+ cells sensitive and resistant to STI571." *Blood* 102(10): 3765-3774.

Zhang, X., W. Wharton, et al. (2004). "Activation of the growth-differentiation factor 11 gene by the histone deacetylase (HDAC) inhibitor trichostatin A and repression by HDAC3." *Molecular and Cellular Biology* 24(12): 5106-5118.

Zhao, Q., G. Rank, et al. (2009). "PRMT5-mediated methylation of histone H4R3 recruits DNMT3A, coupling histone and DNA methylation in gene silencing." *Nature Structural & Molecular Biology* 16(3): 304-311.

Zhou, L., X. Cheng, et al. (2002). "Zebularine: a novel DNA methylation inhibitor that forms a covalent complex with DNA methyltransferases." *Journal of Molecular Biology* 321(4): 591-599.

Zhu, B., Y. Zheng, et al. (2005). "Monoubiquitination of human histone H2B: the factors involved and their roles in HOX gene regulation." *Molecular Cell* 20(4): 601-611.

Zhu, P., E. Martin, et al. (2004). "Induction of HDAC2 expression upon loss of APC in colorectal tumorigenesis." *Cancer Cell* 5(5): 455-463.

Zilberman, D., D. Coleman-Derr, et al. (2008). "Histone H2A.Z and DNA methylation are mutually antagonistic chromatin marks." *Nature* 456(7218): 125-129.

Zilberman, D. and S. Henikoff (2007). "Genome-wide analysis of DNA methylation patterns." *Development* 134(22): 3959-3965.

Electrotherapy on Cancer: Experiment and Mathematical Modeling

Ana Elisa Bergues Pupo[1], Rolando Placeres Jiménez[2]
and Luis Enrique Bergues Cabrales[3]
[1]Universidad de Oriente, Facultad de Ciencias Naturales y Matemáticas, Departamento de
Física, Patricio Lumumba s/n, Santiago de Cuba
[2]Departamento de Física, Universidade Federal São Carlos, São Carlos-SP,
[3]Universidad de Oriente, Centro Nacional de Electromagnetismo Aplicado,
Departamento de Investigaciones, Ave. Las Américas s/n, Santiago de Cuba
[1,3]Cuba
[2]Brasil

1. Introduction

In this chapter are discussed the use, antitumor mechanisms and potentialities of electrotherapy of low-level direct current in cancer. We make emphasis in one of the most stimulating problems in the theme of electrotherapy-cancer as is the propose of electrode arrays that efficiently distribute the electric current density (electric field) in the tumor and its surrounding healthy tissue in order to maximize the tumor destruction with the minimum damage to the organism. A mathematical theorem is intended to obtain the analytical expressions for three-dimensional electric current density (electric field) generated by arrays of electrodes with finite length from those obtained for a point electrodes array. The importance and application of these electrode arrays in therapeutic planning are also discussed.

Electrotherapy is based on principles developed during the nineteenth and twentieth centuries following the first demonstration of "animal electricity" by Luigi Galvani in the eighteenth century. In medicine, the term electrotherapy has been applied to a range of alternative medical devices and treatments. Reputable medical and therapy Journals report that the use of electrotherapy devices has been widely researched and the advantages have been well accepted in the field of rehabilitation and in the treatment of chronic wounds, pressure ulcers, pain (improves range of joint movement) and neuromuscular dysfunction (improvement of strength, improvement of motor control, retards muscle atrophy and improves local blood flow). Also, electrotherapy has been applied in tissue repair (enhances microcirculation and protein synthesis to heal wounds and restores integrity of connective and dermal tissues), acute and chronic edema (accelerates absorption rate, affects blood vessel permeability, and increases mobility of proteins, blood cells and lymphatic flow), peripheral blood flow (induces arterial, venous and lymphatic flow), iontophoresis (delivery of pharmacological agents), urine and fecal incontinence (affects pelvic floor musculature to reduce pelvic pain and strengthen musculature and treatment may lead to complete

continence). Yet some of the treatment effectiveness mechanisms are little understood. Therefore effectiveness and best practices for their use in some instances are still anecdotal [Joa, 2010].
On the other hand, the application of electrotherapy in cancerous tissue has been found to have a beneficial effect in some cases of cancer. Many different forms of electrical current with respect to frequencies, pulse-shapes and amplitudes have been employed in biomedicine with the aim of remodeling tissues by enhancing or suppressing cell proliferation. One of the scopes is also employment of direct current as an antitumor agent [Cabrales et al., 2001; Ciria et al., 2004; Jarque et al., 2007; Ren et al., 2001; Schaefer et al., 2008; Turler, et al., 2000; Vodovnik et al., 1992; Xin et al., 2004; Yoon et al., 2007].

2. Electrotherapy on cancer

Cancer is uncontrolled cell growth and its cause is not well understood. The tumor cells are aggressive (grow and divide without respect to normal limits), invasive (invade and destroy adjacent tissues) and metastatic (spread to other locations in the body) [Cohen & Arnold, 2008]. These malignant properties of cancer differentiate of the benign tumors, which are self-limited in the growth and do not invade or metastasize.
Tumor cells have some structural and physiological characteristics that reveal their electric properties, which differ from the ones of the surrounding healthy cells. One of these properties is a smaller transmembrane potential, which happens due to the fact that sodium and water present an inward flow, while potassium, zinc, calcium and magnesium flow outwards. Another of these properties is the accumulation of an excessive amount of negative charges in the outer area, which causes the reduction of intracellular potassium and the increase of intracellular sodium that lead to a carcinogenic state in the cell. Other characteristics are the electric field decrease through the membrane, a greater electrical conductivity and permittivity, the existence of abnormal electron-transference systems, the negative bioelectrical potentials, the alteration of the normal energy production process which uses electron transport and the hydrogen ion gradient through the mitochondrial membrane, and finally, the existence of areas with a relative electron deficit [Haltiwanger, 2008; Joa, 2010].
Surgery, chemotherapy, radiation therapy, immunotherapy (vaccines, monoclonal antibody therapy, among other) are the conventional therapies for treating cancer [Haltiwanger, 2008; Vinageras et al., 2008; Xiang et al., 2008; Xin et al., 2004]. Choice of therapy depends upon tumor characteristics (location, histological variety, size and stage) and state of patient. However, these conventional therapies have major side effects, have no given a complete solution to the cancer problem, and are costly too. Hence attractive alternative, affordable, effective treatments are sought and one of the upcoming treatments is the use of electrical therapies, as electrochemotherapy [Sadadcharam et al., 2008] and electrotherapy [Cabrales et al., 2010]. The characteristics of tumor cells above mentioned may prevent the reparation and re-establishing of the normal metabolic functions of the tumor cell, but, on the other hand, they facilitate the anti-tumor action of the electrotherapy.

2.1 Preclinical and clinical studies
Electrotherapy consists in the application of a low-level direct current to the solid tumor by means of the electrodes (i.e., platinum, platinum-iridium 90/10, stainless steel). The needles are connected to an electrical device that produces a direct current, which is generated by an

applied voltage between two electrodes. The needles with a positive charge are named anodes, while the needles with a negative charge are the cathodes. Different shapes of needles are used for treatment of tumors in dependence of the size and constitution of the tumor type. Harder needles are used to treat superficial tumors (breast, skin, melanoma cancers) [Jarque et al., 2007; Xin et al., 2004] and more elastic needles are used to treat visceral tumors (lung, liver, esophageal, prostate and rectal cancers) [Chou et al., 1997; Vogl et al., 2007; Xin et al., 2004; Yoon et al., 2007]. The location of the tumor should be determined before treatment. It and the tumor size are determined by palpation with hand for the case of superficial tumors; however, in visceral tumors are determined by means of computer tomography, X ray, Imaging Nuclear Magnetic Resonance and/or ultrasound. Normally, the treatment with electrotherapy is carried out under local anesthetic and on an outpatient basis. The tumor size determines how many needle electrodes are required, which are introduced into the tumor through the skin.

Many physicians have successfully used electrotherapy, also known as electrochemical tumor therapy, Galvanotherapy and electro-cancer treatment, as a standalone treatment in thousands of cases, with some truly spectacular results. There are many potential advantages of electrotherapy over conventional treatments, such as: (1) Direct current is suitable for all types of superficial or visceral tumors, both malignant and benign. (2) This therapy is easy to perform, safe, effective, inexpensive, induces minimum damages to the organism, can be carried out on an out-patient basis and it can be applied when the conventional therapies fail or cannot be applied. (3) It may be best suitable for cancers near critical organs where surgery and/or radiation therapy have failed or could not be performed without damaging other normal parts. (4) This therapy not only reduces costs of chemotherapy, radiotherapy, hyperthermia and immunotherapy, but also improves compliance. (5) Electrotherapy may be suitable for nonresectable tumors and can save functional tissues [Jarque et al., 2007; Vogl et al., 2007; Xin et al., 2004; Yoon et al., 2007]. (6) The tumor and its surrounding healthy tissue have different electric and geometrical parameters [Aguilera et al., 2010; Cabrales et al., 2010; Foster, 2000; Foster & Schwan, 1996; Haemmerich et al., 2003; Haemmerich et al., 2009; Haltiwanger, 2008; Jiménez et al., 2011; Ng et al., 2008; Sekino et al., 2009; Seo et al., 2005; S.R. Smith et al., 1986; D.G. Smith et al., 2000], which enable electrically-mediated treatments to be more efficient for a given dose and the tumor tissue is more susceptible to damage from direct current than normal tissue, thus allowing the destruction of cancerous cells to occur when direct current is applied directly to the malignant tissue [Cabrales et al., 2001; Ciria et al., 2004; Jarque et al., 2007; Von Euler, 2003]. These are reasons for moving to direct current (electric field) method for treating cancer. Judging by the very positive therapy results, it can be assumed, that electrotherapy will become an important form of treatment for malignant diseases. In spite of these advantages, this therapy cannot be used on ascitic and hemolimphoyetic system tumors [Xin et al., 2004].

The first time that the insertion of electrodes in the base of the tumor significantly increases its destruction rate and decreases the damages to the body after the electrotherapy is published in 1997 [Chou et al., 1997]. Their report claims that this way of inserting the electrodes and alternating the sequence of cathodes and anodes induces a uniform electric field in the whole tumor, which causes a significant destruction of it. They also report that the ratio of the number of electrodes to the size of the tumor, taking into account the effective area with necrosis around the electrodes (2 cm). Since that research is conducted, most scientists have been using this type of data configuration.

Electrotherapy antitumor effectiveness can be enhanced when it is combined with intratumor injection of a chemostatic drug (i.e., bleomycin, cisplatin) [Jarque et al., 2007; Xin et al., 2004], saline solution [Jarque et al., 2007; Lin et al., 2000] and/or immunotherapy [Serša et al., 1990; Serša et al., 1992; Serša et al., 1994; Serša et al., 1996]. It has been demonstrated that intratumor bleomycin (cisplatin) treatment is more effective than intravenous treatment at the same dose and direct current potentiates the antitumor effectiveness of bleomycin several-fold [Xin et al., 2004].

In vitro and in vivo studies have demonstrated that an increase of direct current (voltage) intensity leads to an increase of electrotherapy antitumor effectiveness, as shown in Figure 1. This figure shows the Ehrlich tumor growth kinetics for the control group (CG) and different treated groups: TG1 (treated group with electrical charge of 6.7 mA for 45 min), TG2 (treated group with 11.7 mA for 45 min), and TG3 (treated group with 17 mA for 45 min). The minimum of the amount of volumetric electric charge required for the tumor destruction must be 35 coulombs/cm³; however, high antitumor effectiveness is obtained when this physical magnitude is between 80 and 100 coulombs/cm³ [Jarque et al., 2007; Ren et al., 2001; Xin et al., 2004; Yoon et al., 2007], in agreement with 92 and 80 coulombs/cm³ for which the Ehrlich (TG3 in Figure 1) and fibrosarcoma Sa-37 tumors are completely destroyed, respectively [Ciria et al., 2004].

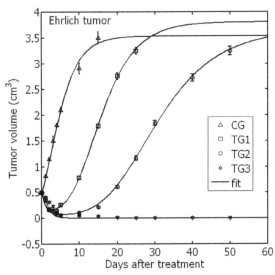

Fig. 1. Experimental data (mean ± standard deviation) and modeled growth curves of Ehrlich tumor. Each experimental group is formed by 10 mice. CG (control group), TG1 (treated group with electrical charge of 6.7 mA for 45 min), TG2 (treated group with 11.7 mA for 45 min), and TG3 (treated group with 17 mA for 45 min). When the tumors reached approximately 0.5 cm³ in BALB/c mice, a single shot electrotherapy was supplied (zero day).

In 1978 the clinical use of direct current in the treatment of malignant tumors in humans is reported for the first time when Nordenström treated patients with lung cancer and explained that the anti-tumoral effects were due to the toxic products that came from the electrochemical reactions induced on it because of the cytotoxic action of electrotherapy. Since Nordenström develops his work, the use of electrotherapy has been expanded for the treatment of patients with various histological types of cancer in other hospitals of Sweden and in different countries, as: China, Germany, Japan, Korea, Australia, Slovenia, the United States, Greece, Denmark, France, Brazil, Israel, Russia, Argentina and Cuba.

Since 1987 the electrotherapy has been used in China for the treatment of malignant and benign tumors, and so far it has been applied to over 20,000 patients. This is, therefore, the most complete clinical study to date. In the beginning, the group of researchers from China [Xin et al., 2004] changes the methodology for placing Nordenström's electrodes. Instead of placing one cathode in the tumor and one anode far from it, they insert several anodes in the center of the tumor and the same number of cathodes in the outer zone at the periphery of the tumor. Then, they modify again their electrode placing technique, and place the anodes and cathodes inside the tumor with the anodes in the center and the cathodes in the periphery. This change not only protects the normal tissue from destruction but also reinforce the effect of the therapy effect. The electrode placing technique is changed one more time by these researchers, when they place anodes and cathodes in an alternate way along the tumor volume, setting them 2 cm away from each other, just as is previously suggested by other authors [Chou et al., 1997].

In June 2005, electrotherapy is used for the first time in Cuba, under the supervision of Dr. Li Jing-Hong from the China-Japan Friendship hospital, located in China, for the treatment of patients with malignant and benign tumors [Jarque et al., 2007]. The study intends to test the electrode insertion procedures and the correct choice in electric charge amount in patients having advanced local tumors who are not recommended for conventional oncology treatment. The study also intends to evaluate the effectiveness and safety of the method. In 1997, Cabrales et al. conducted the first investigations in Cuba on the anti-tumoral effects of electrotherapy, using experimental murine tumors (Ehrlich and fibrosarcoma Sa-37 tumors) in BALB/c, NMRI and C57BL/6 mice. Studies carried out in rats are planned to evaluate the safety and the effects induced by the electrotherapy in tumors and in the body, taking into account the electric charge doses, as well as the number, polarity and orientation of the electrodes, the size and type of the murine tumor and the body characteristics [Cabrales et al., 2001; Ciria et al., 2004; Joa et al., 2010].

In clinical studies, the patient experiences a slight pressure pain or a slight tingling in the treated area during the electrotherapy application. Direct current brings about long lasting pain relief because it inhibits the activity of sensory nerve fibers. In the literature are reported different adverse events (effects), as: fever, wound infections, damages to the blood vessels when the electrodes are inserted close of these [Arsov et al., 2009; Haltiwanger, 2008; Jarque et al., 2007; Li et al., 2006; Salzberg et al., 2008; Vijh, 2006; Vogl et al., 2007; Xin et al., 2004; Yoon et al., 2007].

The underlying mechanisms more widely accepted are the toxic products from of the electrochemical reactions and change of pH. When low voltage (4 to 10 volts) and low amperage (40 to 100 mA) direct currents are administered the tumor area around the anode becomes highly acidic due to the attraction of negatively charged chloride ions and the formation of hydrochloric acid (pH < 3). The tumor areas around the cathode become highly basic (pH > 10) due to the attraction of positively charged sodium ions and the formation of sodium hydroxide. Also, chlorine gas and hydrogen gas emerge from the entry points of the anodes and cathodes, respectively. The pH change depolarizes cancer cell membranes and causes tumors to be gently destroyed [Li et al., 1997; Turjanski et al., 2009; Veiga et al., 2005;

Von Euler et al., 2003]. This suggests that the application of direct current (electric field) causes electrolysis, electrophoresis, electro-osmosis and electroporation in biological tissues, which create micro-environmental chemical changes and micro-electrical field changes [Haltiwanger, 2008; Li et al., 1997]. The chemistry of the microenvironment of healthy cells, injured cells and cancerous cells and the micro-electrical field of these cells are interrelated [Haltiwanger, 2008].

In a previous study [Li et al., 1997] is reported the existence of a group of biochemical alterations around the anode and cathode in tumors under treatment. Around the anode they find a pH of 2, acid hemoglobin, tissue hydration, hydrogen ions that are the result of water electrolysis, and oxygen and chlorine gas emissions. From these emissions they explain the formation of hydrochloric acid and the acid pH. In the cathode, meanwhile, they report a pH of 12, tissue dehydration, hydroxyl ions, which are the result of water electrolysis, and hydrogen gas emissions, from which they explain the formation of sodium hydroxide responsible for the basic pH. Halfway between the electrodes and far from them, no significant differences are observed between the pH and the water concentration in tumors treated with electrotherapy, and those in the untreated tumors. They conclude, then, that the electrochemical effects of this therapy happen around the electrodes.

Other antitumor mechanisms have been reported in the literature, such as: (1) immune system stimulation after treatment (the attraction of white blood cells to the tumor site) [Cabrales et al., 2001; Ciria et al., 2004; Jarque et al., 2007; Serša et al., 1996]; (2) lost of tissue water for electro-osmosis [Li et al., 1997; Vijh, 2004, 2006]; (3) change in the membrane potential of tumor cells, nutrient uptake by tumor cells and reduce deoxyribose nuclei acid production by tumor cells [Chou et al., 1997; Haltiwanger, 2008]; (4) both electrochemical reactions (fundamentally those in which reactive oxygen species are involved) and immune system stimulation induced by cytotoxic action of the direct current, could constitute the most important antitumor mechanisms [Cabrales et al., 2001]; (5) direct current treatment increases the expression of dihydronicotinamide adenine dinucleotide phosphate dehydrogenase (NADPH) oxidase subunits-derived reactive oxygen species which subsequently induces apoptosis of oral mucosa cancer cells [Wartenberg et al., 2008]. These authors also report that an increase of the reactive oxygen species brings about an increase of the expression of heat shock protein (Hsp 70) and Cu/Zn superoxide dismutase (anti-oxidative enzymes) and a decrease of intracellular concentration of reduced glutathione, whereas the expression of catalase remains unchanged.

Some authors evidence apoptosis as tumor dead mechanism after direct electric application [Wartenberg et al., 2008]; however, other report apoptosis and necrosis around anode and necrosis around cathode [Von Euler et al., 2003; Haltiwanger, 2008]. Our experience reveal that the morphologic pattern of necrotic cell mass is the coagulative necrosis 24 hours after direct current application [Cabrales et al., 2001; Ciria et al., 2004; Jarque et al., 2007]. Also, we observe in preclinical and clinical studies vascular congestion, peritumoral neutrophil infiltration, an acute inflammatory response, and a moderate peritumoral monocyte (and macrophages) infiltration, in agreement with other authors [Chou et al., 1997; Li et al., 1997; Serša et al., 1996; Vijh, 2004; Xin et al., 2004]. We are the opinion that apoptosis, necrosis and the electrochemical reactions into tumor (mainly around electrodes) may be explained from reactive oxygen species.

We do not reject the possibility that the electric current density induced into the tumor may affect (directly or indirectly) the cellular membrane, and intracellular and extracellular spacing that lead to irreversible damages in it. This statement may be corroborated because it has been reported that direct electric current can have significant effects on the symmetry of surface charge, resulting in a change in membrane potential. Electric fields can produce a redistribution of cell surface receptors and influence the flow of specific ions through plasma membrane ion channels [Salzberg et al., 2008; Schaefer et al., 2008]. Any change in the flow of ions through cellular ion channels can have significant effects on cellular metabolism, proliferation rate, cytoplasmic pH, mobility, cell cycle transitions, and apoptosis. Also, research shows that direct electric current application can provide electrons, helping thus to reestablish the biocurrent flows in cancer tissues that are electrically resistant, which brings about the reduction of the resistance, the reestablishing of the transmembrane potential in cancer cells, and the concentration of the sodium, potassium, chlorine and magnesium ions through cell repolarization [Haltiwanger, 2008]. On the other hand, it has been proved that some cell membrane structures can be influenced by the action of the electrical current, the electric field or the accumulated charge. These findings are also found in vitro studies [Haltiwanger, 2008; Joa, 2010; Yen et al., 1999].

Electrotherapy is not implemented in the Clinical Oncology because it is not standardized and its antitumor mechanism is poorly understood. The first reason is explained because the dosage guideline is arbitrary and dose-response relationships are not established. Also, different electrode placements are used and optimal electrode distribution has not been determined [Aguilera et al., 2010; Cabrales et al., 2010; Jiménez et al., 2011; Joa et al., 2010]. The standardization of this therapy from experimental point of view is complex, cumbersome, requires excessive handling of animals, and expensive in resources and time. That is why the mathematical modeling constitutes the core of this chapter.

2.2 Mathematical modeling on electrotherapy: electrode arrays

Computer modeling and simulation keep growing in the more important fields of mathematics and physics applied to biophysics, biology, biochemistry and bioengineering. The reasons for this growing importance are manyfold. Among them, the mathematical modeling has been shown to be a substantial tool for the investigation of complex biophysical, as the cancer. The cancer phenomenon continues to challenge oncologists. The pace of progress has often been slow, in part because of the time required to evaluate new therapies. To reduce the time to approval, new paradigms for assessing therapeutic efficacy are needed. This requires the intellectual energy of scientists working in the field of mathematics and physics, collaborating closely with biologists and clinicians. This essentially means that the heuristic experimental approach, which is the traditional investigative method in the biological sciences, should be complemented by a mathematical modeling approach [Bellomo et al., 2008; Cabrales et al., 2010].

The mathematical modeling has been little exploded in the electrotherapy-cancer topic. Some studies have been focused to propose theoretical models and computer simulations in order to describe the tumor growth kinetics [Cabrales et al., 2008; Cabrales et al., 2010; Miklavčič et al., 1995]. Predicting tumor growth is important in the planning and evaluation of screening programs, clinical trials, and epidemiological studies, as well as in the adequate selection of dose-response relationships regarding the proliferative potential of tumors. Thus, it is apparent that theoretical mathematical models are needed to study cancer [Bellomo et al., 2008; Brú et al., 2003; Jiang, 2009; Mohammadi et al., 2009; Stein et al., 2008]. A modification to the Gompertz equation, named modified Gompertz equation, is made to describe the experimental data of Ehrlich and fibrosarcoma Sa-37 tumor growth kinetics treated with different direct current intensities [Cabrales et al., 2008]. Fitting the experimental data of CG, TG1, TG2 and TG3 with this modified equation (solid line in Figure 1) suggests that it is feasible to describe the data of untreated and direct current treated tumors. This is also sustained for the small values of the sum of squares of errors (SSE), standard error of the estimate (SE), adjusted coefficient of multiple determination (r_a^2), predicted residual error sum of squares (PRESS), multiple predicted residual sum error of squares (MPRESS) and the errors of each parameter of this equation. This modified Gompertz equation establishes the analytical conditions for which are reached the four tumor responses types after treatment (progressive disease, stable disease, partial response and complete response) and it theoretically corroborates that the electrotherapy antitumor effectiveness increases with the increase of the direct current intensity, as shown in Figure 2 [Cabrales et al., 2008]. Also, this equation theoretically reveals a new antitumor response, named stationary partial response and that these different tumor responses depend on the ratio between the electric current applied to the tumor (i) and that induced in it (i_0), named i/i_0 ratio, keeping constant the other parameters of this equation, such as: the initial volume (V_0), the intrinsic growth rate of the tumor (α), the growth deceleration factor (β) related to the antiangiogenic process the growth deceleration factor related to the antiangiogenic process and the duration of the net effect induced in the solid tumor after treatment ($1/\gamma$).

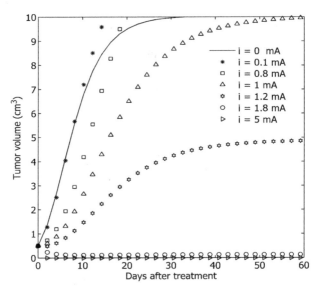

Fig. 2. Simulation of modified Gompertz equation for $\alpha = 0.6$ days^{-1}, $\beta = 0.2$ days^{-1}, $\gamma = 0.016$ days^{-1}, $i_0 = 5$ mA, $V_0 = 0.5$ cm^3 and different magnitudes of i (mA) [Cabrales et al., 2008].

From modified Gompertz equation, it is easy to verify that the complete and stationary partial responses are reached for $i/i_0 > 2$ and $i/i_0 = 2$, respectively. This suggests the existence of a threshold value of i/i_0 ratio that may be related with the tumor reversibility condition. The tumor complete remission after direct current application suggests that the tumor growth kinetic is completely reversible, as is demonstrated in a previous study. The stationary partial response is characterized first by a significant decrease of the tumor volume until a certain size, from which it remains constant in the time, fact that may be explained because the organism governs the equilibrium with this small tumor volume that survived to the direct current cytotoxic action. This tumor response type may suggest that the cancer may be a controllable chronic disease [Cabrales et al., 2010].

On the other hand, the mathematical modeling has been used to understand alterations on cellular membrane [Kotnik & Miklavčič, 2006], the role of pH in electrotherapy [Turjanski et al., 2009], the possible physicochemical reactions induced into the tumor during direct current application [Nilsson & Fontes, 2001] and the design of an one-probe two-electrode device in combination with a 3D gel model that contains the cathode and the anode very close to each other (0.1 cm) for studying pH spherical fronts and destroy a cancer cell spherical casket [Olaiz et al., 2010]. Also, the mathematical modeling constitutes a rapid way to propose an optimum electrodes array or close to it, in function of their parameters and those of tumor (localization, size, shape and consistency), using both analytical and numerical solutions. This allows the visualization of the potential, electric field intensity and electric current density distributions generated electrodes arrays in two-dimensional (2D) and three-dimensional (3D) tumors, in order to induce the highest electrotherapy effectiveness (higher tumor destruction with the minimum damage to the organism) [Aguilera et al., 2009; Aguilera et al., 2010; Čorović et al., 2007; Dev et al., 2003; Jiménez et al., 2011; Joa, 2010; Reberšek et al., 2008; Šel et al., 2003]. This later increases our understanding about the current flow inside tumor during direct current application. This is important because monitoring the current flow during aforementioned therapy is a challenging task due to the lack of available noninvasive electrical imaging techniques. We support that the direct current strength and its form of distribution, through electrodes, have potential biomedical applications and a decisive role in the electrotherapy effectiveness [Cabrales et al., 2010; Jiménez et al., 2011].

2D-electrode arrays are useful for planar tumors (basal cell carcinoma of the skin, cutaneous lymphoma, gastric cancer in its form of delinitis, and melanoma in clinical superficial extension) and the potential, electric field strength and electric current density distributions that these induce in the tumor are reported for electrodes circular array [Čorović et al., 2007; Dev et al., 2003; Šel et al., 2003] and electrodes elliptical array [Aguilera et al., 2009; Aguilera et al., 2010]. The explicit dependence of how electric current density distributions depend on the ellipse eccentricity, the ratio between the electric conductivities of the solid tumor (σ_1) and the surrounding healthy tissue (σ_2), named σ_1/σ_2 ratio, and positioning of the electrodes with respect to tumor-surrounding healthy tissue interface is shown in Figures 3 and 4 for an electrodes circular array (eccentricity = 0) and an electrodes elliptical array (eccentricity = 0.85), respectively [Aguilera et al., 2010]. In Figures 3a,d and Figures 4a,d, the electrodes are inserted in the tumor-surrounding healthy tissue interface. Electrodes inserted inside tumor are represented in Figures 3b,e and Figure 4b,e while those inserted in the surrounding healthy tissue are depicted in Figures 3c,f and Figures 4c,f. The influence of σ_1/σ_2 ratio on the electric current density distribution is evidenced for $\sigma_1/\sigma_2 = 1$ (Figures 3a-c and Figures 4a-c) and $\sigma_1/\sigma_2 = 10$ (Figures 3d-f and Figures 4d-f). The other parameters of the electrodes array are constant, such as: electrode radius (a), electrode potential (V_o), electrode polarity (red for the positive electrode, anode, and blue for the negative electrode, cathode), the angular separation between two adjacent-electrodes (θ), major radius (b_1) and minor radius (b_2) of the electrodes array, which are related by means of the eccentricity of it.

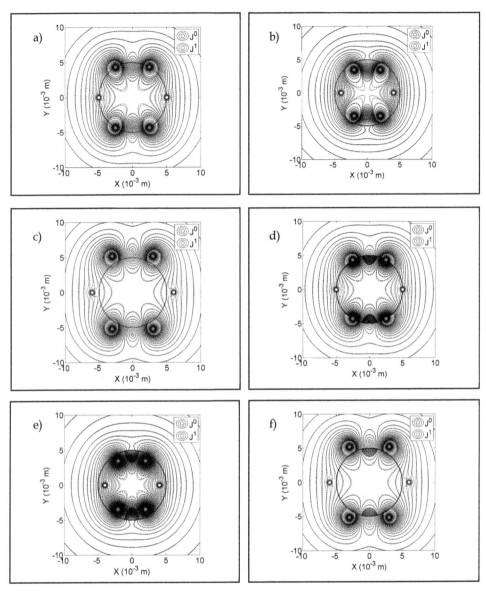

Fig. 3. Distributions of the electric current density, in leading-order, $J^0(x,y)$, and first-order term, $J^1(x,y)$, for an electrodes circular array (eccentricity = 0) for: (a) Configuration 1, $b_1 = b_2$ = 0.5 cm, and $\sigma_1/\sigma_2 = 1$; (b) Configuration 2, $b_1 = b_2$= 0.4 cm, and $\sigma_1/\sigma_2 = 1$; (c) Configuration 3, $b_1 = b_2$= 0.6 cm, and $\sigma_1/\sigma_2 = 1$; (d) Configuration 1, $b_1 = b_2$= 0.5 cm, and $\sigma_1/\sigma_2 = 10$; (e) Configuration 2, $b_1 = b_2$= 0.4 cm, and $\sigma_1/\sigma_2 = 10$; and (f) Configuration 3, $b_1 = b_2$= 0.6 cm. These simulations are made for $\theta = 60°$, $a = 0.0215$ cm, $V_o = + 0.5$ V for the electrodes 2 and 3, $V_o = - 0.5$ V for the electrodes 5 and 6, and $V_o = 0$ V for the electrodes 1 and 4. The parameters a, b_1, b_2 (in centimeter) are converted to meter.

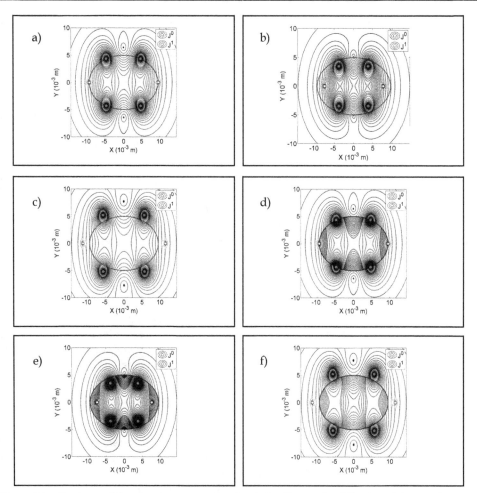

Fig. 4. Distributions of the electric current density, in leading-order, $J^0(x,y)$, and first-order term, $J^1(x,y)$, for an electrodes elliptical array with eccentricity = 0.85 for: (a) Configuration 1, b_1 = 0.9492 cm and b_2 = 0.5 cm, and σ_1/σ_2 = 1; (b) Configuration 2, b_1 = 0.7593 cm and b_2 = 0.4 cm, and σ_1/σ_2 = 1; (c) Configuration 3, b_1 = 1.1390 cm and b_2 = 0.6 cm, and σ_1/σ_2 = 1; (d) Configuration 1, b_1 = 0.9492 cm and b_2 = 0.5 cm, and σ_1/σ_2 = 10; (e) Configuration 2, b_1 = 0.7593 cm and b_2 = 0.4 cm, and σ_1/σ_2 = 10; and (f) Configuration 3, b_1 = 1.1390 cm and b_2 = 0.6 cm, and σ_1/σ_2 = 10. These simulations are made for θ = 60°, a = 0.0215 cm, V_0 = + 0,5 V for the electrodes 2 and 3, V_0 = − 0,5 V for the electrodes 5 and 6, and V_0 = 0 V for the electrodes 1 and 4. The parameters a, b_1, b_2 (in centimeter) are converted to meter.

In order to get more accurate insight of electric current density (potential and electric field intensity) distribution inside tumor with complex geometries, 3D modeling is studied because, in general, the solid tumors are volumetric. In extending both analytical solution and computational techniques for electric current density from 2D to 3D additional complexities arise, not only because of the 3D geometries but also from the physical nature of the field itself. Also, in this complexity is involved the biological characteristics of the tissues. 3D solutions are very expensive and should only be undertaken after simpler models have been explored, e.g. the 2D cross-section for the end region for a solid tumor.

There are different analytically ways to calculate the electric current density (electric field) distributions in tissues, as the method based on Green´s theorem (to obtain solutions inside defined volumes in terms of surface values of potential and the normal derivate of potential) and the Clifford analysis (it allows the matching of the electric fields across boundaries separating different conductivity regions with the help of the Clifford product) [Krüger & Menzel, 1996]. We have recently published the analytic solutions that visualize 3D stationary electric current density as a function of the electrode length, tumor size and the conductivities of the tumor (spheroid) and the surrounding healthy tissue (infinite medium) generated by a radial electrode array [Jiménez et al., 2011]. This mathematical formalism is only valid for electrodes inserted along tumor diameters. This particular electrodes configuration may be obtained from a mathematical theorem that allows the calculus of 3D electric current density generated by an array of electrodes with arbitrary shape inserted in an arbitrary region from 3D electric current density induced by a point current source. This guarantees that the electrodes may be inserted in any place of the tumor.

2.2.1 3D stationary electric current density generated by a wire from a point current source

There is a three-dimensional, conductive, heterogeneous region consisting of two linear, homogeneous, isotropic media separated by an interface Σ. Medium 1 of constant mean conductivity σ_1 (in S/m) and Medium 2 of constant mean conductivity σ_2 (in S/m) are considered as homogeneous conducting media, as shown in Figure. 5a for the point current source and in Figures. 5b,c for a wire of length L, which are inserted inside the Medium 1.

2.2.2 Point current source

We consider that current is continuous and the magnetic field associated to it may be neglected (≤ 0.02 Gauss) then the calculus of the potential φ in the point $\vec{r}$ generated by a point current source with current intensity I located inside tumor in the point $\vec{r}_0$ (Figure 5a) yield to the following boundary-value problem, named Problem 0

$$\begin{cases} \nabla^2\varphi_1 = -\dfrac{I}{\sigma_1}\delta(\vec{r}-\vec{r}_0) \\ \nabla^2\varphi_2 = 0 \end{cases} \tag{1}$$

$$\begin{cases} \varphi_1\big|_\Sigma = \varphi_2\big|_\Sigma \\ \sigma_1\dfrac{\partial\varphi_1}{\partial\hat{n}}\bigg|_\Sigma = \sigma_2\dfrac{\partial\varphi_2}{\partial\hat{n}}\bigg|_\Sigma \\ \lim_{r\to\infty}\big|\varphi_2\big| < \infty \end{cases} \tag{2}$$

where $\varphi_i\big|_\Sigma$ and $\partial\varphi_i/\partial\hat{n}\big|_\Sigma$ ($i = 1, 2$) are the potential and its normal derivative in the surface Σ that separate both mediums.

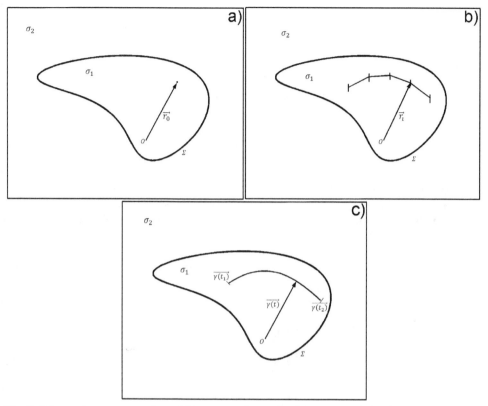

Fig. 5. Schematic representation of (a) a point electrode, (b) a wire subdivided in N small pieces of longitude δl and (c) a whole wire with ends $\vec{\gamma}(t_1)$ and $\vec{\gamma}(t_2)$ located in the Medium 1 of conductivity σ_1 surrounded of a Medium 2 of conductivity σ_2. The axis y is perpendicular to the paper (toward us out of the page).

2.2.3 Electrode in form of wire of length finite

Instead of a point current source we now assume the case of a wire of length L (Figure 5c) analytically represented for the following parametric differentiable form of the curve $\vec{\gamma}(t)$ of parameter t

$$\vec{\gamma}(t) = (x(t), y(t), z(t)), \quad t \in [t_1, t_2] \tag{3}$$

The wire is subdivided in N small pieces of longitude δl (Figure 5b), so that the first equation of the system (1) can re-write as

$$\nabla^2 \psi_1 \approx -\frac{I}{\sigma_1 L} \sum_{i=1}^{N} \delta\left(\vec{r} - \vec{\gamma}(t_i)\right) \delta l_i \tag{4}$$

with

$$L = \int_{t_1}^{t_2} \left\| \frac{d\vec{\gamma}}{dt} \right\| dt \tag{4a}$$

$$\left\| \frac{d\vec{\gamma}}{dt} \right\| = \sqrt{\left(\frac{dx}{dt}\right)^2 + \left(\frac{dy}{dt}\right)^2 + \left(\frac{dz}{dt}\right)^2} \tag{4b}$$

and

$$\delta l_i = \left\| \frac{d\vec{\gamma}}{dt} \right\|_{t=t_i} \Delta t \tag{4c}$$

where ψ_1 is the potential generated in the tumor by the wire electrode. $\|d\vec{\gamma}/dt\|$ is the modulus of the tangent to $\vec{\gamma}(t)$ in Cartesian coordinates, $\Delta t = (t_2-t_1)/N$ is the variation of t. When $\Delta t \to 0$ (in the limit N→∞) results the following boundary-value problem (named Problem 1)

$$\begin{cases} \nabla^2 \psi_1 = -\dfrac{I}{\sigma_1 L} \int_{t_1}^{t_2} \delta\left(\vec{r} - \vec{\gamma}(t_i)\right) \left\| \dfrac{d\vec{\gamma}}{dt} \right\| dt \\[2mm] \nabla^2 \psi_2 = 0 \end{cases} \tag{5}$$

$$\begin{cases} \psi_1 \big|_\Sigma = \psi_2 \big|_\Sigma \\[2mm] \sigma_1 \dfrac{\partial \psi_1}{\partial \hat{n}} \bigg|_\Sigma = \sigma_2 \dfrac{\partial \psi_2}{\partial \hat{n}} \bigg|_\Sigma \\[2mm] \lim_{r \to \infty} |\psi_2| < \infty \end{cases} \tag{6}$$

where ψ_1 and $\partial \psi_1/\partial \hat{n}$ are the potential and normal derivative of the potential in Medium 1, respectively. ψ_2 and $\partial \psi_2/\partial \hat{n}$ are these magnitudes but in Medium 2. $\hat{n}$ is the unit normal vector to the surface Σ (directed from Medium 1 to Medium 2). δ is the Dirac delta. $\vec{r}$ is the position of the spherical coordinate.

The solution of the Problem 1 may be expressed in a very simple way starting from the solution of the Problem 0 by means the following theorem

2.2.4 Theorem

Let be $\varphi_i(\vec{r}, \vec{r}_0)$, $i = 1,2$, the solution of the Problem 0. Then, the solution of the Problem 1 is

$$\psi_i(\vec{r}) = \frac{1}{L} \int_{t_1}^{t_2} \varphi_i\left(\vec{r}, \vec{\gamma}(t)\right) \left\| \frac{d\vec{\gamma}}{dt} \right\| dt \tag{7}$$

The demonstration is immediate simply if we substitute (7) in (5) and (6). Substituting (7) in (5) results

$$\nabla^2 \psi_i(\vec{r}) = \nabla^2 \frac{1}{L} \int_{t_1}^{t_2} \varphi_i\left(\vec{r}, \vec{\gamma}(t)\right) \left\| \frac{d\vec{\gamma}}{dt} \right\| dt = \frac{1}{L} \int_{t_1}^{t_2} \nabla^2 \varphi_i\left(\vec{r}, \vec{\gamma}(t)\right) \left\| \frac{d\vec{\gamma}}{dt} \right\| dt \tag{8}$$

Making $\vec{r}_0 = \vec{\gamma}(t)$ in (1) and substituting in (8) result (5). Also, it can be demonstrated that (7) satisfies the boundary conditions (6).

To illustrate the theorem above mentioned, we use the particular case of a radial electrode array proposed in a previous study [Jiménez et al., 2011]. A three-dimensional, conductive, heterogeneous region consists of two linear, homogeneous, isotropic media (tumor and the surrounding healthy tissue) separated by an interface Σ. Solid tumor (Medium 1) is considered as a homogeneous conducting sphere of radius R (in m) and constant mean conductivity σ_1 (in S/m). The surrounding healthy tissue (Medium 2) is supposed to be a homogeneous infinite medium of constant mean conductivity σ_2 (in S/m), as shown in Figure 6a.

Point electrode and wire are inserted in plane $y = 0$ m along tumor diameters and in $(r_0,0,0)$, using the system of spherical coordinates with the origin in the center of the sphere, as shown in Figures 6b (one current source) and 6c (two current sources), respectively. In the particular case that both electrode types are located in the axis z (the radial coordinate in spherical coincides with axis z of the Cartesian coordinate or $(0,0,r_0)$).

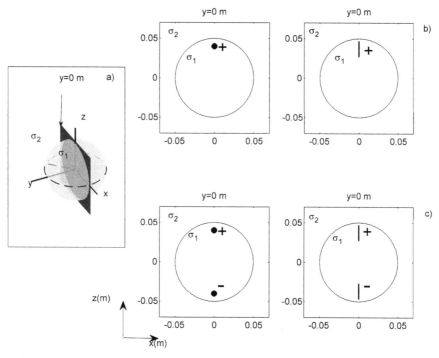

Fig. 6. (a) Spherical tumor of conductivity σ_1 (in S/m) and radius R (in m) surrounded by its healthy tissue of conductivity σ_2 (in S/m) and separated by the interface Σ. (b) A point electrode (positive) and an electrode with form of wire (positive) are inserted along tumor diameter (plane $y = 0$ cm). (c) Two point electrodes 1 (one positive and another negative) and two electrodes with form of wire (one positive and another negative) are inserted along tumor diameter (plane $y = 0$ cm).

As the point electrode is located in the tumor along the axis z (left picture in Figure 6a), the solution of the Problem 0 is given by

$$\varphi_1 = \frac{I}{4\pi\sigma_1} \frac{1}{\sqrt{r_0^2 + r^2 - 2rr_0\cos\theta}} + \sum_{n=0}^{\infty} A_n r^n P_n(\cos\theta) \tag{9}$$

$$\varphi_2 = \sum_{n=0}^{\infty} B_n r^{-(n+1)} P_n(\cos\theta) \tag{10}$$

The coefficients A_n and B_n are obtained of the boundary conditions (2), resulting

$$\varphi_1 = \frac{I}{4\pi\sigma_1} \frac{1}{\sqrt{r_0^2 + r^2 - 2rr_0\cos\theta}} + \frac{I}{4\pi}\left(\frac{\sigma_1 - \sigma_2}{\sigma_1}\right) \sum_{n=0}^{\infty} \frac{(n+1)r_0^n r^n P_n(\cos\theta)}{R^{2n+1}\left[n\sigma_1 + (n+1)\sigma_2\right]} \tag{11}$$

$$\varphi_2 = \frac{I}{4\pi} \sum_{n=0}^{\infty} \frac{(2n+1)r_0^n P_n(\cos\theta)}{r^{(n+1)}\left[n\sigma_1 + (n+1)\sigma_2\right]} \tag{12}$$

Starting from (11) and (12), corresponding to a point electrode, we can pass to the solution of the potential generated by a wire with ends in a and b inserted in the tumor along the axis z (right picture in Figure 6b). In this particular case, the parametric equations of the wire are

$$\begin{cases} x = 0 \\ y = 0 \\ z = t \end{cases} \tag{13}$$

In this case, $L = b-a$ and $\|d\vec{y}/dt\| = 1$. Substituting (13), L and $\|d\vec{y}/dt\|$ in (7), we obtain the solutions for the wire, given by

$$\psi_1 = \frac{1}{(b-a)} \int_{t_1}^{t_2} \left[\frac{I}{4\pi\sigma_1} \frac{1}{\sqrt{t^2 + r^2 - 2rt\cos\theta}} + \frac{I}{4\pi}\left(\frac{\sigma_1 - \sigma_2}{\sigma_1}\right) \sum_{n=0}^{\infty} \frac{(n+1)t^n r^n P_n(\cos\theta)}{R^{2n+1}\left[n\sigma_1 + (n+1)\sigma_2\right]} \right] dt \tag{14}$$

$$\psi_2 = \frac{1}{(b-a)} \int_{t_1}^{t_2} \frac{I}{4\pi} \sum_{n=0}^{\infty} \frac{(2n+1)t^n P_n(\cos\theta)}{r^{(n+1)}\left[n\sigma_1 + (n+1)\sigma_2\right]} dt \tag{15}$$

Integrating (14) and (15) from $t = a$ to $t = b$, we have

$$\psi_1 = \frac{I}{4\pi(b-a)} \left\{ \frac{1}{\sigma_1} \ln\left[\frac{\sqrt{b^2 + r^2 - 2br\cos\theta} + b - r\cos\theta}{\sqrt{a^2 + r^2 - 2ar\cos\theta} + a - r\cos\theta} \right] \right.$$
$$\left. + \left(\frac{\sigma_1 - \sigma_2}{\sigma_1}\right) \sum_{n=0}^{\infty} \frac{\left(b^{n+1} - a^{n+1}\right) r^n P_n(\cos\theta)}{R^{2n+1}\left[n\sigma_1 + (n+1)\sigma_2\right]} \right\} \tag{16}$$

$$\psi_2 = \frac{I}{4\pi(b-a)} \sum_{n=0}^{\infty} \frac{(2n+1)\left(b^{n+1}-a^{n+1}\right)P_n(\cos\theta)}{(n+1)r^{(n+1)}\left[n\sigma_1+(n+1)\sigma_2\right]} \tag{17}$$

The superposition principle is used when two (Figs. 6c,d) or more current sources are inserted in the tumor. From (11), (12), (16) and (17) may be determined the electric field intensity ($\vec{E}=-\nabla\varphi$) and the electric current density ($\vec{J}=-\sigma\nabla\varphi$) inside and outside the tumor for a point current source ($\left|\vec{J}_{1p}\right|$ and $\left|\vec{J}_{2p}\right|$ are the current densities inside and outside, respectively) [Jiménez et al., 2011; Joa, 2010] and a wire of length L ($\left|\vec{J}_{1w}\right|$) and ($\left|\vec{J}_{2w}\right|$ are the current densities inside and outside, respectively), which are given by

$$\left|\vec{J}_{ip}\right| = \sigma\sqrt{\left(\frac{\partial\varphi_i}{\partial r}\right)^2 + \left(\frac{\partial\varphi_i}{r\partial\theta}\right)^2} \quad (i=1,2) \tag{18}$$

with

$$\frac{\partial\varphi_1}{\partial r} = \frac{I}{4\pi}\left\{\frac{1}{\sigma_1}\frac{r-r_0\cos\theta}{\left(r_0^2+r^2-2rr_0\cos\theta\right)^{3/2}} + \left(\frac{\sigma_1-\sigma_2}{\sigma_1}\right)\sum_{n=0}^{\infty}\frac{(n+1)r_0^n r^{n-1}P_n(\cos\theta)}{R^{2n+1}\left[n\sigma_1+(n+1)\sigma_2\right]}\right\} \tag{19}$$

$$\frac{\partial\varphi_1}{r\partial\theta} = \frac{I}{4\pi}\left\{-\frac{1}{\sigma_1}\frac{r_0 sen\theta}{\left(r_0^2+r^2-2rr_0\cos\theta\right)^{3/2}} + \left(\frac{\sigma_1-\sigma_2}{\sigma_1}\right)\sum_{n=0}^{\infty}\frac{(n+1)r_0^n r^{n-1}T_n(\cos\theta)}{R^{2n+1}\left[n\sigma_1+(n+1)\sigma_2\right]}\right\} \tag{20}$$

$$\frac{\partial\varphi_2}{\partial r} = -\frac{I}{4\pi}\sum_{n=0}^{\infty}\frac{(2n+1)r_0^n P_n(\cos\theta)}{r^{(n+2)}\left[n\sigma_1+(n+1)\sigma_2\right]} \tag{21}$$

$$\frac{\partial\varphi_2}{r\partial\theta} = \frac{I}{4\pi}\sum_{n=0}^{\infty}\frac{(2n+1)r_0^n T_n(\cos\theta)}{r^{(n+2)}\left[n\sigma_1+(n+1)\sigma_2\right]} \tag{22}$$

$$T_n = -sen\theta\left[\frac{n\cos\theta\, P_n(\cos\theta)-n\, P_{n-1}(\cos\theta)}{\cos^2\theta-1}\right] \tag{23}$$

where $\partial\varphi_i/\partial r$ and $\partial\varphi_i/r\partial\theta$ are the radial and angular components of electric field vector for inside ($i=1$) and outside ($i=2$) the tumor, respectively

$$\left|\vec{J}_{iw}\right| = \sigma\sqrt{\left(\frac{\partial\psi_i}{\partial r}\right)^2 + \left(\frac{\partial\psi_i}{r\partial\theta}\right)^2} \quad (i=1,2) \tag{24}$$

with

$$\frac{\partial\psi_1}{\partial r} = \frac{I}{4\pi(b-a)}\left\{\frac{A(a,b,r,\theta)}{\sigma_1} + \left(\frac{\sigma_1-\sigma_2}{\sigma_1}\right)\sum_{n=0}^{\infty}\frac{n\left(b^{n+1}-a^{n+1}\right)r^{n-1}P_n(\cos\theta)}{R^{2n+1}\left[n\sigma_1+(n+1)\sigma_2\right]}\right\} \tag{25}$$

$$\frac{1}{r}\frac{\partial \psi_1}{\partial \theta} = \frac{I}{4\pi(b-a)}\left\{\frac{B(a,b,r,\theta)}{\sigma_1}+\left(\frac{\sigma_1-\sigma_2}{\sigma_1}\right)\sum_{n=0}^{\infty}\frac{\left(b^{n+1}-a^{n-1}\right)r^{n-1}T_n}{R^{2n+1}\left[n\sigma_1+(n+1)\sigma_2\right]}\right\} \tag{26}$$

$$\frac{\partial \psi_2}{\partial r} = -\frac{I}{4\pi(b-a)}\sum_{n=0}^{\infty}\frac{(2n+1)\left(b^{n+1}-a^{n+1}\right)P_n(\cos\theta)}{r^{(n+2)}\left[n\sigma_1+(n+1)\sigma_2\right]} \tag{27}$$

$$\frac{1}{r}\frac{\partial \psi_2}{\partial \theta} = \frac{I}{4\pi(b-a)}\sum_{n=0}^{\infty}\frac{(2n+1)\left(b^{n+1}-a^{n+1}\right)T_n}{(n+1)r^{(n+2)}\left[n\sigma_1+(n+1)\sigma_2\right]} \tag{28}$$

where

$$A(a,b,r,\theta) = \frac{\dfrac{r-b\cos\theta}{\sqrt{b^2+r^2-2br\cos\theta}}-\cos\theta}{\sqrt{b^2+r^2-2br\cos\theta}+b-r\cos\theta}-\frac{\dfrac{r-a\cos\theta}{\sqrt{a^2+r^2-2ar\cos\theta}}-\cos\theta}{\sqrt{a^2+r^2-2ar\cos\theta}+a-r\cos\theta} \tag{29}$$

$$B(a,b,r,\theta) = \frac{\dfrac{bsen\theta}{\sqrt{b^2+r^2-2br\cos\theta}}+sen\theta}{\sqrt{b^2+r^2-2br\cos\theta}+b-r\cos\theta}-\frac{\dfrac{asen\theta}{\sqrt{a^2+r^2-2ar\cos\theta}}+sen\theta}{\sqrt{a^2+r^2-2ar\cos\theta}+a-r\cos\theta} \tag{30}$$

T_n in (26) and (28) is given by (23). $\partial\psi_i/\partial r$ and $\partial\psi_i/r\partial\theta$ are the radial and angular components of electric field vector for inside (i = 1) and outside (i = 2) the tumor, respectively.

Figure 7 shows the isolines of $\left|\vec{J}_{1p}\right|$ and $\left|\vec{J}_{2p}\right|$ (Fig. 7a), and $\left|\vec{J}_{1w}\right|$ and $\left|\vec{J}_{2w}\right|$ (Figure 7b) in different planes of the sphere(y = 0.1, 2 and 4 cm) parallel to the plane that contains the electrodes (y = 0 cm) for a point current source and a wire, respectively. The point current source is located in r_0 = 4 cm (Figure 5a) whereas the wire with ends in a = 1 cm and b = 4 cm (L = 3 cm), as shown in Figure 5b. In both figures, we fix σ_1 = 0.4 S/m, σ_2 = 0.2 S/m, I = 5 mA and R = 5 cm. Figures 7a and 7b reveal that there are differences between the distributions of $\left|\vec{J}_{1p}\right|$ and $\left|\vec{J}_{1w}\right|$; however, non significant differences are observed between these distributions of $\left|\vec{J}_{1w}\right|$ and $\left|\vec{J}_{2w}\right|$ for different values of L. These differences are shown in Table 1 and are quantified by means of the maximum difference (D_{max}, in A/m²) and the Root Means Square Error (RMSE, in A/m²), given by

$$D_{max} = \max\left\|\left|\vec{J}_{wi}\right|-\left|\vec{J}_{pi}\right|\right\|, \quad (i = 1, 2) \tag{31}$$

$$RMSE = \sqrt{\sum_{i=1}^{M}\frac{\left(\left|\vec{J}_{wi}\right|-\left|\vec{J}_{pi}\right|\right)^2}{M}} \quad (i = 1, 2) \tag{32}$$

where J_{pi} are the *i-th* calculated values of $J_p(x,y)$ and J_{wi} are the *i-th* calculated values of $J_w(x,y)$ for different values of L (0.5, 1, 1.5, 2, 2.5 and 3 cm). M is the number of points where $\left|\overrightarrow{J_{1p}}\right|$ ($\left|\overrightarrow{J_{1w}}\right|$) and $\left|\overrightarrow{J_{2p}}\right|$ ($\left|\overrightarrow{J_{2w}}\right|$) are calculated.

$\Im_1$ ($\Im_1 = \sqrt{\sum_{k=1}^{m_1}\left|\overrightarrow{J_{1k}}\right|^2}$: sum of the local current density over all points in the tumor) and $\Im_2$

($\Im_2 = \sqrt{\sum_{k=1}^{m_2}\left|\overrightarrow{J_{2k}}\right|^2}$: sum of the local current density over all points in a region of the

surrounding healthy tissue) are used in the figures to compare the overall effect of changing of L on $\left|\overrightarrow{J_{1p}}\right|$ ($\left|\overrightarrow{J_{1w}}\right|$) and $\left|\overrightarrow{J_{2p}}\right|$ ($\left|\overrightarrow{J_{2w}}\right|$). $\Im_1$ and $\Im_2$ are evaluated in a set of discrete points m_1

and m_2, respectively, for both point current source and wire. $\Im_1$ is calculated in all tumor volume (m_1 = 84 050 points) except in the points where the electrodes are inserted and in their vicinities. $\Im_2$ is also calculated in the surrounding healthy tissue (m_2 = 35 301 points) comprehended in a spherical cap (between R (5 cm) and R + 2 (7 cm)). Table 2 reveals that $\Im_1$ and $\Im_2$ for the point current source are higher than those for the wire for all value of L. For the wire, it is observed that an increase of L results in a decrease of $\Im_2$ whereas inside to the tumor $\Im_1$ first decreases (up to L = 2 cm) and then increases. The behavior of $\Im_1$ with L is given in [Jiménez et al., 2011].

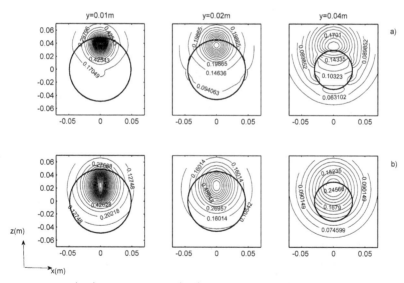

Fig. 7. Projections of $\left|\overrightarrow{J_{1p}}\right|$ (in A/m²) and $\left|\overrightarrow{J_{2p}}\right|$ (in A/m²) on planes y = 0.1, 2 and 4 cm for (a) one point electrode and (b) one electrode with form of wire ($\left|\overrightarrow{J_{1w}}\right|$, in A/m², and $\left|\overrightarrow{J_{2w}}\right|$, in A/m²). In each figure, the electrode polarity is positive (see Figure 6b).

Type of current source		Electric current density in the tumor (A/m²)		Electric current density in the surrounding healthy tissue (A/m²)	
		D_{max}	RMSE	D_{max}	RMSE
Point		0	0	0	0
Wire	L = 0.5 cm	39744.718	3.0283	0.537	0.0003
	L = 1 cm	39763.700	3.0296	0.877	0.0006
	L = 1.5 cm	39771.290	3.0302	1.103	0.0007
	L = 2 cm	39775.324	3.0305	1.262	0.0008
	L = 2.5 cm	39777.820	3.0307	1.379	0.0009
	L = 3 cm	39779.514	3.0309	1.468	0.0010

Table 1. D_{max} and RMSE of $\left|\vec{J}_{1w}\right|$ (in A/m²) and $\left|\vec{J}_{2w}\right|$ (in A/m²) for a wire of length L respect to $\left|\vec{J}_{1p}\right|$ (in A/m²) and $\left|\vec{J}_{2p}\right|$ (in A/m²) generated by a point current source. L varies from 0.5 to 3 cm.

Type of current source		$\Im_1$ (A/m²)	$\Im_2$ (A/m²)
Point		254800	63.080
Wire	L = 0.5 cm	1201.378	52.630
	L = 1 cm	1065.803	45.676
	L = 1.5 cm	1003.083	40.762
	L = 2 cm	996.252	37.128
	L = 2.5 cm	1045.207	34.344
	L = 3 cm	1182.477	32.155

Table 2. $\Im_1$ (norm of $\left|\vec{J}_{1p}\right|$ for a point electrode or $\left|\vec{J}_{1w}\right|$ for a wire) and $\Im_2$ (norm of $\left|\vec{J}_{2p}\right|$ for a point electrode or $\left|\vec{J}_{2w}\right|$ for a wire). The wire length is L (between 0.005 to 0.030 m). $\Im_1$ and $\Im_2$ are given in A/m².

The distributions of $\left|\vec{J}_{1p}\right|$, $\left|\vec{J}_{2p}\right|$, $\left|\vec{J}_{1w}\right|$ and $\left|\vec{J}_{2w}\right|$ for two point electrodes and two wires are shown in Figures 8a and 8b, respectively. The differences between these distributions are also quantified by means of D_{max} and RMSE (Table 3) and the values of $\Im_1$ and $\Im_2$ evaluated in the same discrete points m_1 and m_2 are given in Table 4. A comparison of Figures 7 and 8 reveals that an increase of the number of current sources (point or wire) results in a higher distribution of the electric current density lines in the tumor, being more evident for the electrodes in form of wire.

For the calculations of $\left|\vec{J}_{1p}\right|$, $\left|\vec{J}_{2p}\right|$, $\left|\vec{J}_{1w}\right|$, $\left|\vec{J}_{2w}\right|$, RMSE, D_{max}, $\Im_1$ and $\Im_2$, the unities of y, a, b, L and R, given in cm, are converted to meter.

The 3D-analytical expressions shown in this chapter allow the visualization of the potential, electric field strength and electric current density distributions generated for point current

Type of current source		Electric current density in the tumor (A/m²)		Electric current density in the surrounding healthy tissue (A/m²)	
		D_{max}	RMSE	D_{max}	RMSE
Point		0	0	0	0
Wire	L = 0.5 cm	39744.681	4.2824	0.564	0.0005
	L = 1 cm	39763.672	4.2845	0.918	0.0008
	L = 1.5 cm	39771.267	4.2854	1.152	0.0011
	L = 2 cm	39775.306	4.2858	1.317	0.0012
	L = 2.5 cm	39777.807	4.2861	1.440	0.0014
	L = 3 cm	39779.507	4.2863	1.537	0.0015

Table 3. D_{max} and RMSE of $\left|\vec{J}_{1w}\right|$ (in A/m²) and $\left|\vec{J}_{2w}\right|$ (in A/m²) for an array of two equal wires with different lengths L (between 0.5 to 3 cm) respect to those generated by an array of two point electrodes ($\left|\vec{J}_{1p}\right|$, in A/m², and $\left|\vec{J}_{2p}\right|$, in A/m²).

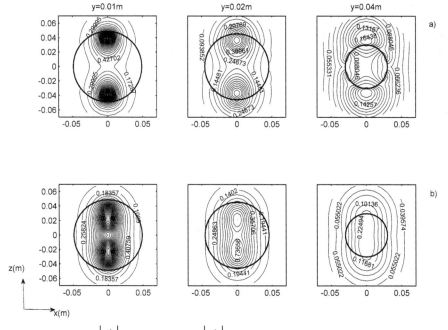

Fig. 8. Projections of $\left|\vec{J}_{1p}\right|$ (in A/m²) and $\left|\vec{J}_{2p}\right|$ (in A/m²) on planes $y = 0.1$, 2 and 4 cm for (a) two point electrodes and (b) two electrodes with forms of wire ($\left|\vec{J}_{1w}\right|$, in A/m², and $\left|\vec{J}_{2w}\right|$, in A/m²). In each figure, one electrode is positive and another is negative (Figure 6c).

Type of current source		$\Im_1\ (A/m^2)$	$\Im_2\ (A/m^2)$
Point		360340	82.912
Wire	L = 0.5 cm	1702.887	66.861
	L = 1 cm	1512.207	55.909
	L = 1.5 cm	1424.731	47.906
	L = 2 cm	1416.607	41.710
	L = 2.5 cm	1488.047	36.679
	L = 3 cm	1685.969	32.432

Table 4. $\Im_1$ (norm of $\left|\vec{J}_{1p}\right|$ for two point electrodes or $\left|\vec{J}_{1w}\right|$ for two wires) and $\Im_2$ (norm of $\left|\vec{J}_{2p}\right|$ for two point electrodes or $\left|\vec{J}_{2w}\right|$ for two wires). The wires are equals and have different lengths L (from 0.5 to 3 cm). $\Im_1$ and $\Im_2$ are given in A/m^2.

sources and radial arrays of electrodes with finite length. The results of the simulations reveal as these distributions in the tumor and its surrounding healthy tissue change in function of the tumor size, the positioning, number and polarity of the electrodes, and the difference of electrical conductivity between both tissues for, in agreement with previous theoretical studies [Aguilera et al., 2009; Aguilera et al. 2010; Čorović et al., 2007; Jiménez et al., 2011; Joa, 2010; Reberšek et al., 2008; Šel et al., 2003] and experimental reports [Chou et al., 1997; Ren et al., 2001; Serša et al., 1997; Turler et al., 2000; Xin et al., 1994; Yoon et al., 2007].

3D-analytical expressions for the potential, electric field intensity and electric current density generated by wires completely inserted in the tumor along their diameters (plane y = 0 cm) are directly obtained from the application of this mathematical theorem and the parametric form of the curve given in equation (3). This justify that equations (16) and (17) are correct from the substitution of I for $\delta I = I/(b-a)dr_0$ in equations (14) and (15) and then integrating these expressions from $r_0 = a$ to $r_0 = b$, as is suggested in a previous study [Jiménez et al., 2011].

Non-uniform current density distributions are shown in a tumor (homogeneous conductor spheroid), as shown in Figures 7 (point electrodes) and 8 (electrodes with forms of wire). Normally, needles electrodes have highly non-homogeneous fields around their tips due to the sharp geometry. There are marked differences between the electric current density (potential and electric field) patterns generated by a point electrodes array and arrays of electrodes with length L, as is expected. Electric current density near the electrodes is also imaged for both point and wire arrays. Although the electric current density is maximum near electrodes, the magnitude of it fall even more rapidly towards the tumor edges in the perpendicular direction to the plane in which are the electrodes. Tumor regions unaffected by this electric current density re-grow after treatment. The singularities observed where the electrodes contact the tumor (large electric fields at the edges) can be avoided by grading the electric field near such edges. High current densities in the vicinity of the electrodes may result in tissue damage (example, coagulative necrosis), in agreement with our observations in mice [Cabrales et al., 2001; Ciria et al., 2004] and patients [Jarque et al., 2007]. Moreover, measurement of current density distribution near the current injecting electrodes provides information on the behavior of the electrode-tissue interface. Up to now, it has not discussed as depends on the electrotherapy antitumor effectiveness in function of the homogeneity degree of the electric current density (electric field) induced in the tumor, essential aspect in the design of electrodes array and treatment planning.

The insertion of the electrodes along tumor diameters is a particular electrodes array that we have used in some patients whose tumor thickness (depth) is smaller respect to their other two dimensions (skin, breast and vulva cancers) when the conventional therapies fail or cannot be applied, as shown in Figure 9. A direct current of 10 mA for 60 min is delivered to this patient with vulva cancer through 19 electrodes inserted with alternate polarities and it is generated by ZAY-6B electric device (manufactured in Chinese). Cannulae with trocar are inserted into the tumor mass under local anesthesia and the number of these depends on the tumor size (20 cm in diameter). The cannulae are fixed with a distance (gap) between them of 1 cm and disposed along a semi-circumference because for this zone pass important blood vessels. This distance should not be further than 1.5 cm apart because the tumor killing area around the needle is about 2 cm in diameter. Then the trocar are withdrawn and electrodes are inserted into the tumor through the cannulae to ensure that the electric field will cover all the tumor mass when the direct current passes through electrodes. After insertion of the electrodes, the cannulae are withdrawn to the edge of normal tissue by palpation with hand. These cannulae in the edge are insulation tubes to protect the normal tissue from the injury due to electrolysis. This procedure guarantees that the electrodes are completely inserted into the solid tumor to maximize tumor destruction with the minimum damage in the organism. The electrodes are then connected to the cathode or anode of the ZAY-6B device to supply the direct current that pass through the solid tumor. This procedure guarantees that the electrodes are completely inserted into the tumor. We use platinum needles because these are resistant to erosion and have high electric conductivity. The diameter of the needles is 0.07 cm and length 15 cm, values that justify why we assume in this mathematical approach that the electrode cross section is neglected respect to its length [Jiménez et al., 2011]. Saline solution and bleomycin are intratumor injected before and immediately after direct current application, respectively. It is made with the aim to potentiate the electrotherapy antitumor effectiveness, fact that is theoretically verified when the tumor conductivity increases with respect to that of the surrounding healthy tissue because the electric current density lines mainly distribute inside tumor and its periphery.

We observe that as soon as direct current is connected to the electrodes, different electrochemical reactions influence the pH-value and can cause electrolysis of tumor tissue, which in turn, lead to the destruction of it. The tumor regression induced by this electrodes array is approximately 50 % one month after the application of this therapy. Minima adverse effects (events) are observed after direct current application, probably due to that the electrodes are inside tumor and this therapy is local. We are not observed immediate adverse events (first 24 hours after electrotherapy is applied); however, we have reported late adverse events (after 24 hours of applied electrotherapy), such as: necrosis on the ulcerated surface, erythema and slight edema at the area treated, inflammation because the cancerous tissue is being destroyed through this method of treatment. Immediately after treatment, we do not observe pain, fever, superinfections. The destroyed cancerous tissue is eliminated from the body and is replaced by scar tissue and then in the majority of the patients, we observe tissue granulation when the tumor is removed after this treatment [Jarque et al., 2007]. Similar results are reported in laboratory animal [Cabrales et al., 2001; Ciria et al., 2004; Haltiwanger, 2008; Mikhailovskaya et al., 2009; Sazgarnia et al., 2009; Vijh, 2006] and human [Arsov et al., 2009; Haltiwanger, 2008; Jarque et al., 2007; Li et al., 2006; Salzberg et al., 2008; Vijh, 2006; Vogl et al., 2007; Xin et al., 2004; Yoon et al., 2007].

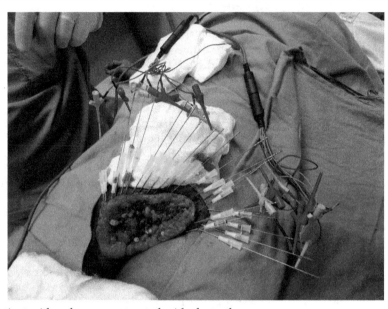

Fig. 9. Patient with vulva cancer treated with electrotherapy.

The use of this electrodes array stops the bloody flux of this patient for the vulva immediately after the electrotherapy application due to the haemostatic effect of the cathode. This fact may be explained because the cathode produces a tissue desiccation and therefore a control of the hemorrhage, in agreement with other results that demonstrate that the tumor blood flow is reduced by direct current action, fact that can be exploited to improve therapeutic outcome. It is well known that reductions in tumor blood flow can lead to an increase in hypoxia and extracellular acidification and as a result a cascade of tumor cell death will occur, due to a lack of nutrients, oxygen and an accumulation of catabolite products [Griffin et al., 1994; Haltiwanger, 2008; Xin et al., 2004]. As a result of this, this patient does not receive more blood transfusions post-treatment. This patient dies one year after the electrotherapy application due to multiple metastases in brain, lung and liver.

In electrotherapy, the electrodes are generally inserted outside of the central plane [Cabrales et al., 2001; Cabrales et al., 2010; Ciria et al., 2004; Chou et al., 1997; Jarque et al., 2007; Ren et al., 2001; Turler et al., 2000], constituting a limitation of the use of this radial electrodes array. This mathematical theorem solves the Problem 1 from the Problem 0 both harder and elastic needles. The solution of this problem becomes difficult in dependence on the complexity of this parametric form of the curve since more arduous is to solve the integral that appears in Equation (7). The simulations clearly demonstrate that analytical model is reliable and useful to search new electrode arrays that induce the highest electrotherapy effectiveness. New 3D-mathematical formalisms are obtained in dependence of the parametric curve form (Equation 3), which allow the insertion of the electrodes (hard or flexible) in any place of the tumor with arbitrary shape. This leads to solve problems more complex than that shown in a previous study [Jiménez et al., 2011] and to compare their electric current densities with those generated by other electrode arrays [Cabrales et al., 2001; Ciria et al., 2004; Chou et al., 1997; Jarque et al., 2007; Jiménez et al., 2011; Joa, 2010; Xin et al., 2004; Yoon et al., 2007].

Different authors report that there is a good correlation between the electric current density spatial distributions observed with different imaging techniques, those obtained by means of analytical and numerical solutions and experimental results [Miklavčič et al., 1998; Serša et al., 1997]. Among these techniques may be mentioned the Electric Current Density Imaging [Halter et al., 2007; Serša et al., 1997], Electrical Impedance Tomography [Saulnier et al., 2001], Magnetic Resonance Electrical Impedance Tomography [Seo et al., 2005], Magnetic Induction Tomography, Magnetoacoustic Tomography and Magnetoacoustic Tomography with Magnetic induction [Li et al., 2007]. These imaging techniques are useful to map spatial distribution of electric currents generated for any electrodes array in the tumor and its surrounding healthy tissue and to visualize the changes on electric current density patterns when the electrodes array parameters above mentioned are modified. These imaging techniques provide information on electrical conductivity inside an electrically conducting domain such as the human body and evidence that electric current density strongly depends on the placing, polarity and geometry of the electrodes, in agreement with our simulations. The quantification of the differences between the electric current densities obtained theoretically and experimentally is possible by means of an element average error (e) that can be evaluated by computing the integral over the element of the difference between the current density determined directly from the analytical expression (J_a) and the nodally averaged (interpolated) current densities over the region of support V_s (J_s), given by $e = \int_{V_S} (j_a - j_s) dV$. For this, it should be used the information provided by neighboring nodes to evaluate the magnitude of the higher order terms in the solutions that have been neglected.

These facts indicate that these imaging techniques may be used to know as change the electrical conductivity and current density distribution before, during and after electrotherapy. As a result of this fact, we have an idea of the structural, functional and pathological conditions of the tissue and therefore provide valuable diagnostic information. For this reason, we include in the electric current density the information of the electrical conductivities of the tumor and surrounding healthy tissue, whose mean values may be measured by means of such imaging techniques above mentioned [Li et al., 2007; Saulnier et al., 2001; Halter et al., 2007; Seo et al., 2005; Serša et al., 1997]. This justifies why the bulk conductivities of both tissues are assumed constant in our mathematical approach. The bulk electrical conductivity values of heterogeneous and anisotropic tissues may also be calculated, with good approximation, by means of their electric conductivity tensor mean values [Sekino et al., 2009]. We believe that the higher electric conductivity of the tumor is along of the preferential direction of growth (major diameter of tumor with ellipsoidal shape); however, an experiment should be designed to demonstrate this hypothesis. Although the majority of the solid tumors are heterogeneous, all are homogeneous for volumes ≤ 3 cm^3. Also, there are very few types of tumors (adenomas, adenocarcinomas, breast ductal carcinomas and sarcomas) with volumes > 3 cm^3 that are homogeneous, fact explained because is only observed tumor mass due to the equilibrium between the growth and the tumor cells angiogenesis. When this equilibrium is broken, the tumors make more heterogeneous due to the presence of necrosis, infiltration to tissues, among other alterations.

The fact that tumor conductivity is assumed higher than that its surrounding healthy tissue is justified because neoplasic tissues exhibit somewhat larger conductivity and permittivity values than homologous normal tissues due to that the water content is higher in the tumor

[Foster & Schwan, 1996; Haemmerich et al., 2003; Haemmerich et al., 2009; Miklavčič et al., 2006; Ng et al., 2008; S.R. Smith et al., 1986, D.G. Smith et al., 2000]. We believe that the presence of other charged particles (molecules, ions and electrons) and blood vessels (due to the angiogenic process) may also increase the tumor conductivity and therefore more current flows for the tumor, as we corroborate with the simulations shown in this chapter. These simulations have not included the effects that produce the direct current application on the tumor electric conductivity (permittivity); however, it should change during and after electrotherapy application. This may be due to that in the tumor are induced changes in the ions concentration in the intracellular and extracellular fluids [Griffin et al., 1994], structure and cellular density [Vijh, 2006; Von Euler et al., 2003], molecular composition [Von Euler et al., 2003], in the cellular membrane [Vodovnik et al., 1992; Yoon et al., 2007], among others. For instance, it has been demonstrated that the tumor conductivity changes before and after of the tumor thermal ablation [Haemmerich et al., 2009]. The changes of the electric conductivity may be one of the indicators of tissues conditions (anatomical and functional) [Seo et al., 2005]. We believe that for electric current densities (electric field intensities) below the reversible threshold value should not change significantly the tumor conductivity, not occurring thus above this threshold. This may be in correspondence with the tumor re-grow observed for $i/i_o < 2$ and the stationary partial and complete responses for $i/i_o \geq 2$, as shown in Figures 1 and 2 [Cabrales et al., 2008]. Hence, a detailed study should be carried out to know the explicit dependence between the electrical conductivity and the physiological parameters of the tumor. This may be used to establish an index for the prediction of the possible evolution of the patient during and after the direct current application (alone or combined). Also, an improved understanding of the theoretical basis of this dependence will enable structural features of the tumor tissue to be deduced from the experimental measurements.

Although it is assumed that the fields and charges are non-time varying, and the magnetic field due to the current and the reaction of this field on the current, we do not discard that magnetic field due to the direct current intensity produce bioeffects in the tumor, mainly around electrodes, in agreement with other authors [Saulnier et al., 2001; Seo et al., 2005]. It is possible that this induced magnetic field induces mechanical forces and shear stresses in the tumor that in dependence of its strength and duration may also produce a wide variety of biological effects in cells and tumor tissue, such as: electrodiffusion/osmosis (various receptors, charged membrane molecules, can be transported along the cell surface) and change in transmembrane potential (voltage-gated channels may be opened to permit the transport of ions, such as calcium, into the cell) [Hart, 2008].

It is important to point out that the images obtained with these experimental techniques are important because reveal that the spatial distribution of electric currents do not depends only on electrode array but, also on their tissue contact, which is hard to control [Foster, 1995; Serša et al., 1997]. The interaction electrode-tumor is not considered; however, it may have an important role in the skin heating. This heating is determined both by palpation with the hand and skin erythema of the patients with tumors treated with direct current [Jarque et al., 2007]. The tissue near of electrodes is heated mainly by the absorbed electrical energy, while regions further away may be heated by thermal conduction and/or some biophysic (electrochemical processes) induced into the tumor. As a consequence, the preferential heating of the tumor is governed by the electrical parameters near the electrode, whereas thermal parameters become increasingly important further away. An analysis of the energy (heat) absorbed by the tumor and its surrounding healthy tissue may be another way to select these optima parameters. The absorbed energy can be calculated by means of the expression $Q_{1,2} = \int (j_{1,2}^2 / \sigma_{1,2})dV$, where Q, j and σ are the absorbed heat quantity, electric current density and electric conductivity in the medium, respectively. The sub-indexes 1 and 2 represent to the medium 1 (tumor) and medium 2 (surrounding healthy tissue). Similar analyses of the absorbed energy quantity are carried out in radiotherapy and hyperthermia [Hall, 1988; Sadadcharam et al., 2008; Schaefer et al., 2008]. On the other hand, as the difference in electrical parameters between the tumor and its surrounding healthy tissue is substantial that might result in preferential heating of the tumor. This healing in dependence of its duration and intensity may be a result of the increase of the intratumor temperature that may provoke changes either directly or indirectly in the tissue dielectric properties and therefore irreversible damages in it [Foster, 1995]. The temperature dependence of the electrical conductivity may be related with damages in the tumor. In order to correctly mimic the absorbed energy in the tumor and its surrounding healthy tissue during electrotherapy exposure, a three dimensional model must be used.

Model tumor system as a spheroid is assumed for the following reasons: 1) the spheroid system has been applied to a number of problems in cancer and it is a model of a solid tumor in vitro and in vivo. 2) This system mimics many of these tumor characteristics and provides a rapid, useful, and economical method for screening sensitizers and chemotherapeutic agents because it is intermediate in complexity between single-cell in vitro culture and tumors in experimental animals. 3) The spheroid system is simpler, more reproducible, more economical, and easier to manipulate than animal tumors, and yet the cells can be studied in an environment that includes the complexities of cell-to-cell contact and nutritional stress from diffusion limitations that are characteristic of a growing tumor. 4) Some cells, notably several rodent tumor cell lines, such as chinese hamster V79 lung cells, mouse EMT6 mammary and R1F fibrosarcma cells, and rat 9L brain tumor cells grow as spheroids. At each successive division the daughter cells stick together, and the result is a spherical clump of cells that grows bigger and bigger with time. 5) Many types of human tumor cells can be cultured as spheroids with a wide spectrum of morphological appearance and growth rates. 6) Human tumor cell spheroids maintain many characteristics of the original tumor from the patient or of the some cells grown as xenografts. Human tumors successfully grown as spheroids include thyroid cancer, renal cancer, squamous carcinoma, colon carcinoma, neuroblastoma, human lung cancer, glioma, lymphoid tumors, melanoma, and osteosarcoma [Hall, 1988].

A feasible way to optimize 3D-electrode arrays is combining all the electrodes array parameters such that the electric current density in the tumor is the permissible maximum and that induced in the surrounding healthy tissue is smaller than 10 mA/m². For this, we suggest the following procedure: first, the parameters are automatically selected so that the electric current density in the surrounding healthy tissue is smaller than 10 mA/m². This guarantees the safety of the electrotherapy (Phase I of a Clinical Trial) and that the adverse effects in the organism are minima (Phase II of a Clinical Trial). Second, the selection of the optimum parameters depends on the electric current density (electric field strength) that induces the biggest tumor destruction (Phase III of a Clinical Trial), which may be experimentally verified by means of an experiment, in which is obtained the higher electrotherapy antitumor effectiveness, the maximum survival and life quality of the patient (laboratory animal). It evaluates the contributions of each parameter (alone or combined with other) and requires a significant consumption of calculation time for the parameters quantity involved in these equations. For the implementation of this way, we should take into account that exposure of a biological cell to electric current density (electric field) can lead to a variety of biochemical and physiological responses. For this, it is required to know what electric current density values provoke significant biological effects: below 1 mA/m² (there are not biological effects); 1-10 mA/m² (minimum biological effects, which are not significant); 10-100 mA/m² (possible biological effects without risk to the health); 100-1000 mA/m² (biological effects without possible risk to the health) and above 1000 mA/m² (biological effects with proven risks to health) [International Commission on Non-Ionizing Radiation Protection, 1998]. This is very important because the electrotherapy effectiveness is highly depend on the magnitude and spatial distribution of electric currents flowing through the tumor and its surrounding healthy tissue, in agreement with other authors [Serša et al., 1997].

The knowledge of the optimum distributions of current density vector in the tumor and its surrounding healthy tissue allows the optimum design of noninvasive electromagnetic techniques for the cancer treatment. Several authors report that the ultralow-frequency extremely weak alternating component of combined magnetic fields exhibits a marked antitumor activity [Novikov et al., 2009]. These fields will avoid the insertion of electrodes in the tumor and therefore the little trauma that this provoke in the patients treated with electrotherapy. Weak magnetic fields activate the system of antitumor immunity (i.e., production of Tumor Necrosis Factor, activation of macrophages, among other) and produce reactive oxygen species, as is also observed on electrotherapy [Cabrales et al., 2001; Serša et al., 1994; Serša et al., 1996; Watemberg et al., 2008].

Different authors have experimentally evaluated the influence of direct current intensity [Ciria et al., 2004; Cabrales et al., 2010; Chou et al., 1997, Ren et al., 2001; Xing et al., 2004] and electromagnetic field [Novikov et al., 2009] on tumor growth kinetic; however, the weight of the different parameters of an electrodes array in it has not been widely discussed. Consequently, it is possible to simultaneously know, previous treatment, the possible tumor evolution in the time and the electric current density (potential, electric field intensity) distributions in the tumor and its surrounding healthy tissue and therefore the highest electrotherapy antitumor effectiveness. This improving therapy may be obtained when the tumor reaches its complete cure (complete remission or stationary partial response) [Cabrales et al., 2008; Cabrales et al., 2010] or the higher tumor growth delay (highest survival of the patients with good life quality and/or bigger disease free interval) [Ciria et al., 2004; Chou et al., 1997; Jarque et al., 2007; Ren et al., 2001; Xin et al., 2004; Yoon et al., 2007]. The evaluation of it requires to quantify different biological parameters, such as: tumor regression percentage, mean doubling time, survival rate, antibody responses, cellular responses, apoptosis, necrosis, histological examination, immune responses, and gene expressions, among others. This will contribute to elucidate the direct current antitumor mechanism.

The tumor complete response suggests that its growth kinetic is completely reversible, as shown in Figure 10 for fibrosarcoma Sa-37 tumor [Cabrales et al., 2010]. This behaviour is obtained from the experimental data [Ciria et al., 2004] and the analysis of the first and second parts of the tumor growth kinetic by means of the use of the modified Gompertz equation [Cabrales et al., 2010]. The first part comprehends the time that elapses from the initial moment at which tumor cells are inoculated in the host (t = 0 days) up to 15 days that is the moment of direct current application, when the tumor volume reaches $V_0 = 0.5$ cm³), whereas the second part is the time that elapses from V_0 up to the end of the experiment, that is, time after direct current application. Both parts are obtained using the interpolation process and the time step is $\Delta t = 1/3$ days. The parameters i, α, β, γ and i_o are above defined and obtained from fitting the experimental data [Cabrales et al., 2008]. The analysis of these two parts reveals the existence of two tumor volumes that suggests the unavoidable tumor destruction: in the first, the tumor does not return to its state before direct current treatment, V_{id}, and therefore complete (stationary partial) response is reached. In the second, the small fraction tumor that survives to direct current action is completely destroyed by the organism, V_d, aspect that may suggest that the therapies for the cancer, including the electrotherapy, should be directed to that the tumor always reaches V_d. New investigations have been derived starting from this hypothesis.

In the case that complete remission (stationary partial response) of tumor is not reached after alone direct current stimulus, the electrotherapy should be directed to increase the survival and quality of life of patients (laboratory animals). First this, we should know the exact time in that electrotherapy may be repeated (time for which the tumor volume is between V_0 and the minimum volume observed in tumor growth, V_{min}), as shown in Figure 11 [Cabrales et al., 2010]. When the tumor volume reaches this value there is a change of both slope and sign of the first derivate of the tumor volume (corresponding to minimum value of this first derivate), aspect that may indicate a tumor response (reorganization and/or activation of the growth and protection mechanisms) to the direct current action, whose intensity is not adequate to significantly perturb to it. This fact may be explained because the biological systems, as the tumors, respond to the external perturbations in order to reach their maxima survival. As a result, the electrotherapy should be repeated or combined with other therapies when the first derivate of the tumor volume changes of slope and sign because the tumor cannot be reorganized, in agreement with the current tendency of repeating weekly (every fifteen days) this therapy of 2 to 4 times. This constitutes a novel statement because establishes that this therapy should not be applied when the tumor volume reaches V_{min}, as is implemented for the treatment of patients at present [Jarque et al., 2007; Xin et al., 2004]. It is possible a fractionated therapy may lead to the complete (stationary partial) remission.

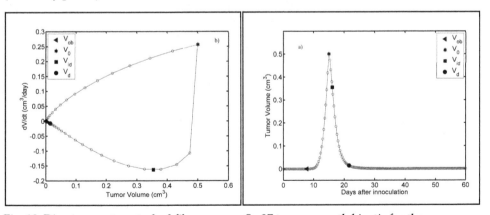

Fig. 10. Direct current-perturbed fibrosarcoma Sa-37 tumor growth kinetic for the parameters: $V_0 = 0.5$ cm^3, i = 14.8 mA, $\alpha = 0.006$ days^{-1}, $\beta = 0.207$ days^{-1}, $\gamma = 0.189$ days^{-1}, $i_o = 1.080$ mA and $\Delta t = 1/3$ days. Time dependence of tumor volume (left picture). First derivate of tumor volume versus tumor volume (right picture).

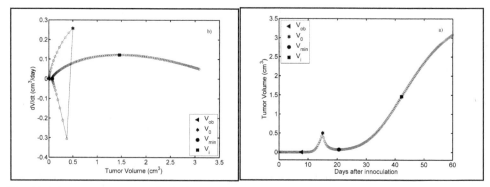

Fig. 11. Direct current-perturbed fibrosarcoma Sa-37 tumor growth kinetic for the parameters: $V_0 = 0.5$ cm³, i = 11.7 mA, $\alpha = 1.584$ days⁻¹, $\beta = 0.076$ days⁻¹, $\gamma = 0.107$ days⁻¹, $i_0 = 7.431$ mA and $\Delta t = 1/3$ days. Time dependence of tumor volume (left picture). First derivate of tumor volume versus tumor volume (right picture).

The inclusion of the other electrodes array parameters, in addition to direct current intensity, in the tumor growth kinetic may efficiently lead to complete (stationary partial) response for smaller direct current intensities.

The knowledge of these two parts of the tumor growth kinetic is important to reveal further information of it and in the therapeutic planning, as is widely discussed in a previous study. Similar results for fibrosarcoma Sa-37 tumor are also found Ehrlich tumor (results not shown) [Cabrales et al., 2010].

By optimizing the electrodes array parameters and those of the tumor growth kinetic (for instance, modified Gompertz equation), the efficiency of electrotherapy might be improved further. This procedure will have to be tested in larger animals to assess the usefulness and safety of electrotherapy in vivo for the future application to humans.

In spite of the considerable progress of electrotherapy, a number of challenges remain for the future. The future strategies include (a) increasing the volume of destroyed tissue at a single treatment session (b) the integration of electrotherapy with the other in-site tumor antitumor techniques and (c) the necessity of to incorporate realistic geometric, conductivity, and, eventually anisotropic information in order to reach the highest electrotherapy effectiveness.

3. Conclusion

In conclusion, electrotherapy of low-level direct current is promissory for cancer treatment. The electric current density (potential and electric field strength) analysis results can be used for assessing effective treatment parameters of tumor. The use of this mathematical approach and the theorem provide a rapid way to propose different optimum electrode arrays in dependence of location, depth, shape and size of the solid tumors with the purpose of obtaining the higher antitumor effectiveness and as a result to implement the electrotherapy in the Clinical Oncology.

4. Acknowledgements

This research is partially supported by the Ministry of Superior Education, Republic of Cuba. Also, the authors wish to thank to Ph.D. Carl Firley, Ph.D. Jesús Manuel Bergues Cabrales,

Ph.D. Juan José Godina Navas, MSc. Andrés Ramírez Aguilera, Bachelor Javier González Joa, Ph.D. Juan Bory Reyes, Bachelor Emilio Suárez, Ph.D. Francisco Martínez, Ph.D. Héctor Manuel Camué Ciria, MSc. Maraelys Morales González, M.D. Miguel Angel O´farril Mateus, M.D. Manuel Verdecia Jarque, M.D. Tamara Rubio González, MSc. Soraida Candida Acosta Brooks. M.D. María Cristina Céspedes Quevedo, M.D. Fabiola Suárez Palencia, M.D. Miriam Fariñas Salas, MSc. Lisset Ortíz Zamora and Ph.D. Gustavo Sierra González for their invaluable help and suggestions. Also, we thank in a special way the Editorial Board of this book, Ms Mia Devic and Ms. Masa Vidovic for the invitation to write this chapter.

5. References

Aguilera, A.R.; Cabrales, L.E.B.; Ciria, H.M.C.; Pérez, Y.S.; Oria, E.R. & Brooks, S.A. (2009). Distributions of the potential and electric field of an electrode elliptic array used in electrotherapy: Analytical and numerical solutions. *Mathematics and Computer in Simulation*, Vol.79, No.7, (March 2009), pp. 2091-2105, ISSN 0378-4754.

Aguilera, A.R.; Cabrales, L.E.B.; Ciria, H.M.C.; Pérez, Y.S.; González, F.G.; González, M.M.; Ortíz, L.Z.; Palencia, F.S.; Salas, M.F.; Bestard, N.R.; González, G.S. & Cabrales, I.B. (2010). Electric current density distribution in planar solid tumor and its surrounding healthy tissue generated by an electrode elliptic array used in electrotherapy. *Mathematics and Computer in Simulation*, Vol.80, No.9, (May 2010), pp. 1886-1902, ISSN 0378-4754.

Arsov, C.; Winter, C. & Albers, P. (2009). Value of galvanotherapy for localised prostate cancer. *Urologe*, Vol.48, No.7, (July 2009), pp. 748-754, ISSN 1433-0563.

Bellomo, N.; Li, N.K. & Maini, P.K. (2008). On the foundations of cancer modeling: selected topics, speculations, and perspectives. *Mathematical Models and Methods Applied Sciences*, Vol.18, No.4, (April 2008), pp. 593–646, ISSN 0218-2025.

Brú, A.; Albertos, S.; Subiza, J.L.; García-Asenjo, J.L. & Brú, I. (2003). The Universal Dynamics of Tumor Growth. *Biophysical Journal*, Vol.85, No.5, (November 2003), pp. 2948–2961, ISSN 0006-3495.

Cabrales, L.E.B.; Ciria, H.M.C.; Bruzón, R.N.P.; Quevedo, M.C.S.; Aldana, R.H.; González, L.M.O.; Salas, M.F. & Peña, O.G. (2001). Electrochemical treatment of mouse Ehrlich tumor with direct electric current: Possible role of reactive oxygen species and antitumoral defense mechanisms. *Bioelectromagnetics*, Vol.22, No.5, (July 2001), pp. 316-322, ISSN 0197-8462.

Cabrales, L.E.B.; Aguilera, A.R.; Jiménez, R.P.; Jarque, M.V.; Ciria, H.M.C.; Reyes, J.B.; Mateus, M.A.F.; Palencia, F.S. & Ávila, M.G. (2008). Mathematical modeling of tumor growth in mice following low-level direct electric current. *Mathematics and Computers in Simulation*, Vol.78, No.1, (June 2008), pp. 112-120, ISSN 0378-4754.

Cabrales, L.E.B.; Nava, J.J.; Aguilera, A.R.; Joa, J.A.G.; Ciria, H.M.C.; González, M.M., Salas, M.F.; Jarque, M.V.; González, T.R.; Mateus, M.A.F.; Brooks, S.C.A.; Palencia, F.S.; Zamora, L.O.; Quevedo, M.C.C.; Seringe, S.E.; Cutié, E.S.; Cabrales, I.B. & González, G.S. (2010). Modified Gompertz equation for electrotherapy murine tumor growth kinetics: predictions and new hypotheses. *BMC Cancer*, Vol.10, No.589, (October 2010), pp. 1-14, ISSN 1471-2407.

Ciria, H.M.C.; Quevedo, M.C.S.; Cabrales, L.E.B.; Bruzón, R.N.P.; Salas, M.F.; Peña, O.G.; González, T.R.; López, D.S. & Flores, J.L.M. (2004). Antitumor effectiveness of different amounts of electrical charge in Ehrlich and fibrosarcoma Sa-37 tumors. *BMC Cancer*, Vol.4, No.87, (November 2004), pp. 1-10, ISSN 1471-2407.

Chou, C.K.; McDougall, J.A.; Ahn, C. & Vora, N. (1997). Electrochemical Treatment of Mouse and Rat Fibrosarcomas with Direct Current. *Bioelectromagnetics*, Vol.18, No.1, (December 1997), pp. 14-24, ISSN 0197-8462.

Chou, C. (2007). Thirty-five years in bioelectromagnetics research. *Bioelectromagnetics*, Vol.28, No.3, (April 2007), pp. 3–15, ISSN 0197-8462.

Cohen, S.M. & Arnold, L.L. (2008). Cell Proliferation and Carcinogenesis. *Journal of Toxicology Pathology*, Vol.21, No.1, (April 2008), pp. 1-7, ISSN 0914-9198.

Čorović, S.; Pavlin, M. & Miklavčič, D. (2007). Analytical and numerical quantification and comparison of the local electric field in the tissue for different electrode configurations. *Biomedical Engineering Online*, Vol.6, No.1, (October 2007), pp. 37-50, ISSN 1475-925X.

Dev, B.S.; Dhar, D. & Krassowska, W. (2003). Electric field of a six-needle array electrode used in drug and DNA delivery in vivo: analytical versus numerical solution. *IEEE Transaction Biomedical Engineering*, Vol.50, No.11, (November 2003), pp. 1296-1300, ISSN 0018-9294.

Foster, K.R. & Schwan, H.P. (1996). Dielectric properties of tissues, In: *Handbook of Biological Effects of Electromagnetic Fields*, C. Polk & E. Postow (Ed.), 68–70 (Chapter 1), CRC Press LLC, ISBN 0-8493-06418, Boca Raton, Florida, USA.

Foster, K.R. (2000). Dielectric properties of tissues, In: *The Biomedical Engineering Handbook*, J.D. Bronzino, (Ed.), 1385-1394 (Chapter 89), CRC Press LLC, ISBN 0-8493-0461-X, Boca Raton, Florida, USA.

Griffin, D.T.; Dodd, N.F.J.; Moore, J.V.; Pullan, B.R. & Taylor, T.V. (1994). The effects of low level direct current therapy on a preclinical mammary carcinoma: tumor regression and systemic biochemical sequelae. *British Journal Cancer*, Vol.69, No.5, (May 1994), pp. 875-878, ISSN 0007-0920.

Haemmerich, D.; Staelin, S.T.; Tsai, J.Z.; Tungjitkusolmun, S.; Mahvil, D.M. & Webster, J.G. (2003). *In vivo* electrical conductivity of hepatic tumours. *Physiological Measurement*, Vol.24, No.2, (February, 2003), pp. 251-260, ISSN 0967-3334.

Haemmerich, D.; Schutt, D.J.; Wright, A.W. & Webster, J.G. (2009). Electrical conductivity measurement of excised human metastatic liver tumors before and after thermal ablation. *Physiological Measurement*, Vol.30, No.5, (May 2009), pp. 459-466, ISSN 0967-3334.

Hall, E.J. (1988). *Radiobiology for the radiologist*, In J.B. Lippincott Company/Philadelphia, ISBN 0-397-50848-4, New York, USA.

Halter, R.J.; Hartov, A.; Heaney, J.A.; Paulsen, K.D. & Schned, A.R. (2007). Electrical impedance spectroscopy of the human prostate. *IEEE Transaction Biomedical Engineering*, Vol.54, No.7, (July 2007), pp. 1321-1327, ISSN 0018-9294.

Haltiwanger, S. (April 2008). The electrical properties of cancer cells, In: *Wind Power*, 17.06.2010, Available from http://www.royalrife.com (http://www.royalrife.com/haltiwanger1.pdf).

Hart, F.X. (2008). The mechanical transduction of physiological strength electric fields. *Bioelectromagnetics*, Vol.29, No.6, (September 2008), pp. 447-455, ISSN 0197-8462.

ICNIRP. (1998). Guidelines for limiting exposure to time-varying electric, magnetic, and electromagnetic fields up to 300 GHz. International Commission on Non-Ionizing Radiation Protection). *Health Physics*, Vol.74, No.4, (April 1998), pp. 494–522, ISSN 0017-9078.

Jarque, M.V.; Mateus, M.A.O.; Jing-hong, L.; Cabrales, L.E.B.; Palencia, F.S.; Ciria, H.M.C.; Brooks, S.C.A. & Salas, M.F. (2007). Primeras experiencias clínicas en Cuba sobre el uso de la electroterapia en cuatro pacientes con tumores sólidos malignos superficiales. *Revista Electrónica MEDISAN*, Vol. 11, No.1, (January-March 2007), pp. 1-13, ISSN 1029-3019.

Jiang, Y. (2005). A Multiscale Model for Avascular Tumor Growth. *Biophysics Journal*, Vol.89, No.6, (December 2005), pp. 3884-3894, ISSN 0006-3495.

Jiménez, R.P.; Pupo, A.E.B.; Cabrales, J.M.B.; Joa, J.A.G.; Cabrales, L.E.B.; Nava, J.J.G.; Aguilera, A.R.; Mateus, M.A.O.; Jarque, M.V. & Brooks, S.C.A. (2011). 3D stationary electric current density in to spherical tumor treated with low direct current. *Bioelectromagnetics*, Vol. 32, No.2, (February 2011), pp. 120-130, ISSN 1521-186X.

Joa, J.A.G. (2010). Three-dimensional visualization of the electric current density in the tumor and its surrounding healthy tissue generated by an electrode arrays. Analytic solution. *Thesis of Bachelor in Physics*, University of Oriente, Faculty of Natural Science, Department of Physics.

Kotnik, T. & Miklavčič, D. (2006). Theoretical evaluation of voltage inducement on internal membranes of biological cells exposed to electric fields. *Biophysics Journal*, Vol.90, No.2, (January 2006), pp. 480-491, ISSN 0006-3495.

Krüger, H. & Menzel, M. (1996). Clifford analytic vector fields as models for plane electric currents, *Proceedings of the symposium on analytical and numerical methods in quaternionic and Clifford analysis*, pp. 101-111, ISBN-10: 3860120417 (ISBN-13: 978-3860120415), Seiffen, Germany, June 5-7, 1996.

Li, K.H.; Xin, Y.L.; Gu, Y.N.; Xu, B.L.; Fan, D.J. & Ni, B.F. (1997). Effects of Direct Current on Dog Liver: Possible Mechanisms for Tumor Electrochemical Treatment. *Bioelectromagnetics*, Vol.18, No.1, (December 1997), pp. 2-7, ISSN 0197-8462.

Li, J.; Xin, Y.; Zhang, W.; Liu, J. & Quan, K. (2006). Effect of electro-acupuncture in treating patients with lingual hemangioma. *Chinese Journal of Integrative Medicine*, Vol.12, No.2, (June 2006), pp. 146-149, ISSN 162-0415.

Li, X.; Xu, Y. & He, B. (2007). Imaging electrical impedance from acoustic measurements by means of magnetoacoustic tomography with magnetic induction (MAT-MI). *IEEE Transactions on Biomedical Engineering*, Vol.54, No.2, (February 2007), pp. 323-330, ISSN 0018-9294.

Lin, X.Z.; Jen, C.M.; Chou, C.K.; Chou, C.S.; Sung, M.J. & Chou, T.C. (2000). Saturated saline enhances the effect of electrochemical therapy. *Digestive Diseases and Sciences*, Vol. 45, No.3, (March 2000), pp. 509-514, ISSN 0163-2116.

Mikhailovskaya, A.A.; Kaplan, M.A.; Brodskij, R.A. & Bandurko, L.N. (2009). Evaluation of Antitumor Efficiency of Electrochemical Lysis on the Model of M-1 Sarcoma. *Bulletin of Experimental Biology and Medicine*, Vol.147, No.1, (November 2009), pp. 88-90, ISSN 0007-4888.

Miklavčič, D.; Jarm, T.; Karba, R. & Serša, G. (1995). Mathematical modelling of tumor growth in mice following electrotherapy and bleomycin treatment. *Mathematics and Computers in Simulation*, Vol.39, No.5-6, (November 1995), pp. 597-602, ISSN 0378-4754.

Miklavčič, D.; Beravs, K.; Šemrov, D.; Čemažar, M.; Demšar, F. & Serša, G. (1998). The importance of electric field distribution for effective in vivo electroporation of tissues. *Biophysical Journal*, Vol.74, No.5, (May 1998), pp. 2152-2158, ISSN 0006-3495.

Miklavčič, D.; Pavšelj, N. & Hart, F.X. (2006). Electric Properties of Tissues. In: *Wiley Encyclopedia of Biomedical Engineering* John Wiley & Sons, New York, USA.

Mohammadi, B.; Haghpanah, V. & Larijani, B. (2008). A stochastic model of tumor angiogenesis. *Computers in Biology and Medicine*, Vol.38, No.2, (October 2008), pp. 1007-1011, ISSN 0010-4825.

Ng, E.; Sree, S.; Ng, K. & Kaw, G. (2008). The Use of Tissue Electrical Characteristics for Breast Cancer Detection: A Perspective Review. *Technology in Cancer Research and Treatment*, Vol.7, No.4, (August 2008), pp. 295-308, ISSN 1533-0338.

Nilsson, E. & Fontes, E. (2001). Mathematical modelling of physicochemical reactions and transport processes occurring around a platinum cathode during the electrochemical treatment of tumors. *Bioelectrochemistry*, Vol.53, No.2, (March 2001), pp. 213-224, ISSN 1567-5394.

Novikov, V.V.; Novikov, G.V. & Fesenko, E.E. (2009). Effect of weak combined static and extremely low-frequency alternating magnetic fields on tumor growth in mice inoculated with the Ehrlich ascites carcinoma. *Bioelectromagnetics*, Vol.30, No.5, (March 2009), pp. 343-351, ISSN 0197-8462.

Olaiza, N.; Magliettia, F.; Suáreza, C.; Molinab, F.V.; Miklavčič, D.; Mir, L. & Marshall, G. (2010). Electrochemical treatment of tumors using a one-probe two-electrode device. *Electrochimica Acta*, Vol.55, No.20, (August 2010), pp. 6010-6014, ISSN 0013-4686.

Reberšek, M.; Čorović, S.; Serša, G. & Miklavčič, D. (2008). Electrode commutation sequence for honeycomb arrangement of electrodes in electrochemotherapy and corresponding electric field distribution. *Bioelectrochemestry*, Vol.74, No.1, (November 2008), pp. 26-31, ISSN 1567-5394.

Ren, R.L.; Vora, N.; Yang, F.; Longmate, J.; Wang, W.; Sun, H.; Li, J.R.; Weiss, L.; Staud, C.; McDougall, J.A. & Chou, C.K. (2001). Variations of dose and electrode spacing for rat breast cancer electrochemical treatment. *Bioelectromagnetics*, Vol.22, No.3, (April 2001), pp. 205-211, ISSN 0197-8462.

Sadadcharam, M.; Soden, D.M. & O'sullivan, G.C. (2008). Electrochemotherapy: An emerging cancer treatment. *International Journal of Hyperthermia*, Vol.24, No.3, (January 2008), pp. 263-273, ISSN 0265-6736.

Salzberg, M.; Kirson, E.; Palti, Y. & Rochlitza, C. (2008). A Pilot Study with Very Low-Intensity, Intermediate-Frequency Electric Fields in Patients with Locally Advanced and/or Metastatic Solid Tumors. *Onkologie*, Vol.31, No.7, (July 2008), pp. 362-365, ISSN 0378-584X.

Saulnier, G.J.; Blue, R.S.; Newell, J.C.; Isaacson, D. & Edic, P.M. (2001). Electrical impedance tomography. *IEEE Signal Processing Magazine*, Vol.18, No.6, (November 2001), pp. 31-43, ISSN 1053-5888.

Sazgarnia, A.; Bahreyni, T.S.; Shirin, S.M.; Bayani, R.S.; Khouei, A.L.; Esmaeili, H.E. & Homaei, F. (2009). Treatment of colon carcinoma tumors by electrolysis: effect of electrical dose and polarity. *Iranian Journal of Medical Physics*, Vol.5, No.2(20-21), (Winter 2009), pp. 39-51, ISSN 1735-160X.

Schaefer, N.; Schafer, H.; Maintz, D.; Wagner, M.; Overhaus, M.; Hoelscher, A.H. & Türler A. (2008). Efficacy of Direct Electrical Current Therapy and Laser-Induced Interstitial Thermotherapy in Local Treatment of Hepatic Colorectal Metastases: An Experimental Model in the Rat. *Journal of Surgical Research*, Vol.146, No.2, (May 2008), pp. 230-240, ISSN 0022-4804.

Sekino, M.; Ohsaki, H.; Yamaguchi-Sekino, S.; Iriguchi, N. & Ueno, S. (2009). Low-frequency conductivity tensor of rat brain tissues inferred from diffusion MRI. *Bioelectromagnetics*, Vol.30, No.6, (September 2009), pp. 489-499, ISSN 0197-8462.

Šel, D.; Mazeres, S.; Teissié, J. & Miklavčič, D. (2003). Finite-element modeling of needle electrodes in tissue from the perspective of frequent model computation. *IEEE Transaction Biomedical Engineering*, Vol.50, No.11, (November 2003), pp. 1221-1232, ISSN 0018-9294.

Seo, J.K.; Kwon, O. & Woo, E.J. (2005). Magnetic resonance electrical impedance tomography (MREIT): conductivity and current density imaging. *Journal of Physics: Conference Series*, Vol.12, No.1, (June 2004), pp. 140-155, ISSN 1742-6588.

Serša, G. & Miklavčič, D. (1990). Inhibition of Sa-1 tumor growth in mice by human leucocyte interferon alpha combined with low-level direct current. *Molecular Biotherapy*, Vol.2, No.3, (September 1990), pp. 165-168, ISSN 0952-8172.

Serša, G.; Miklavčič, D.; Batista, U.; Novakovič, S.; Bobanovič, F. & Vodovnik, L. (1992). Antitumor effect of electrotherapy alone or in combination with interleukin-2 in mice with sarcoma and melanoma tumors. *Anti-Cancer Drugs*, Vol.3, No.3, (June 1992), pp. 253-260, ISSN 0959-4973.

Serša, G.; Golouh, R. & Miklavčič, D. (1994). Antitumor effect of tumor necrosis factor combined with electrotherapy on mouse sarcoma. *Anti-Cancer Drugs*, Vol.5, No.1, (February 1994), pp. 69-74, ISSN 0959-4973.

Serša, G.; Kotnik, V.; Cemazar, M.; Miklavčič, D. & Kotnik, A. (1996). Electrochemotherapy with bleomycin in SA-1 tumor bearing mice-natural resistance and immune responsiveness. *Anti-Cancer Drugs*, Vol.7, No.7, (September 1996), pp. 785-791, ISSN 0959-4973.

Serša, I.; Beravs, K.; Dodd, N.J.F.; Zhao, S.; Miklavčič, D. & Demsar, F. (1997). Electric current density imaging of mice tumors. *Magnetic Resonance in Medicine*, Vol.37, No.3, (March 1997), pp. 404-409, ISSN 1522-2594.

Smith, S.R.; Foster, K.R. & Wolf, G.L. (1986). Dielectric properties of VX-2 carcinoma versus normal liver tissue. *IEEE Transaction Biomedical Engineering*, Vol.33, No.5, (May 1986), pp. 522-254, ISSN 0018-9294.

Smith, D.G.; Potter, S.R.; Lee, B.R.; Ko, W.W.; Drummond, W.R.; Telford, J.K. & Partin, A.W. (2000). In vivo measurement of tumor conductiveness with the magnetic bioimpedance method. *IEEE Transaction Biomedical Engineering*, Vol.47, No.10, (October 2000), pp. 1403-1405, ISSN 0018-9294.

Stein, W.D.; Figg, W.D.; Dahut, W.; Stein, A.D.; Hoshen, M.B.; Price, D.; Bates, S.E. & Fojo, T. (2008). Tumor Growth Rates Derived from Data for Patients in a Clinical Trial Correlate Strongly with Patient Survival: A Novel Strategy for Evaluation of Clinical Trial Data. *The Oncologist*, Vol.13, No.10, (October 2008), pp. 1046-1054, ISSN 1083-7159.

Turjanski, P.; Olaiz, N.; Abou-Adal, P.; Suarez, C.; Risk, M. & Marshall, G. (2009). pH front tracking in the electrochemical treatment (EChT) of tumors: Experiments and simulations. *Electrochimica Acta*, Vol.54, No.26, (November 2009), pp. 6199-6206, ISSN 0013-4686.

Turler, A.; Schaefer, H.; Schaefer, N.; Wagner, M.; Maintz, D.; Qiao, J.C. & Hoelscher, A.H. (2000). Experimental low-level direct current therapy in liver metastases: influence of polarity and current dose. *Bioelectromagnetics*, Vol.21, No.5, (July 2000), pp. 395-401, ISSN 0197-8462.

Veiga, V.F.; Nimrichter, L.; Teixeira, C.A.; Morales, M.M.; Alviano, C.S.; Rodrigues, M.L. & Holandino, C. (2005). Exposure of Human Leukemic Cells to Direct Electric

Current: Generation of Toxic Compounds Inducing Cell Death by Different Mechanisms. *Cell Biochemical Biophysics*, Vol.42, No.1, (February 2005), pp. 61-74, ISSN 1085-9195.

Vijh, A. (2004). Electrochemical treatment (ECT) of cancerous tumours: necrosis involving hydrogencavitation, chlorine bleaching, pH changes, electroosmosis. *International Journal of Hydrogen Energy*, Vol.29, No.6, (May 2004), pp. 663-665, ISSN 0360-3199.

Vijh, A.K. (2006). Phenomenology and Mechanisms of Electrochemical Treatment (ECT) of Tumors. In. *Modern Aspects of Electrochemistry*, C.G. Vayenas, R.E. White, M.E. Gamboa-Adelco (Ed.), 231-274 (Vol. 39), Springer, ISBN-10: 0-387-23371-7 (ISBN-13: 978-0387-23371-0, ISBN: 0-387-31701-5), New York, USA.

Vinageras, E.N.; de la Torre, A.; Rodríguez, M.O.; Ferrer, M.C.; Bravo, I.; del Pino, M.M.; Abreu, D.A.; Brooks, S.C.A.; Rives, R.; Carrillo, C.C.; Dueñas, M.G.; Viada, C.; Verdecia, B.G.; Ramos, T.C.; Marinello, G.G. & Dávila, A.L. (2008). Phase II Randomized Controlled Trial of an Epidermal Growth Factor Vaccine in Advanced Non–Small-Cell Lung Cancer. *Journal of Clinical Oncology*, Vol.26, No.9, (March 2008), pp. 1452-1458, ISSN 0732-183X.

Vodovnik, L.; Miklavčič, D. & Serša, G. (1992). Modified cell proliferation due to electrical currents. *Medical & Biological Engineering & Computing*, Vol.30, No.4, (July 1992), pp. CE21-CE28, ISSN 0140-0118.

Vogl, T.J.; Mayer, H.P.; Zangos, S.; Bayne, J.; Ackermann, H. & Mayer, F.B. (2007). Prostate Cancer: MR Imaging–guided Galvanotherapy-Technical Development and First Clinical Results. *Radiology*, Vol.245, No.3, (December 2007), pp. 895-902, ISSN 0033-8419.

Von Euler, H.; Olsson, J.M.; Hultenby, K.; Thorne, A. & Lagerstedt, A.S. (2003). Animal models for treatment of unresectable liver tumours: a histopathologic and ultra-structural study of cellular toxic changes after electrochemical treatment in rat and dog liver. *Bioelectrochemistry*, Vol.59, No.1-2, (April 2003), pp. 89-98, ISSN 1567-5394.

Wartenberg, M.; Wirtz, N.; Grob, A.; Niedermeier, W.; Hescheler, J.; Peters, S.C. & Sauer, H. (2008). Direct current electrical fields induce apoptosis in oral mucosa cancer cells by NADPH oxidase-derived reactive oxygen species. *Bioelectromagnetics*, Vol.29, No.1, (January 2008), pp. 47-54, ISSN 0197-8462.

Xiang, S.D.; Scalzo-Inguanti, K.; Minigo, G.; Park, A.; Hardy, C.L. & Plebanski, M. (2008). Promising particle-based vaccines in cancer therapy. *Expert Reviews of Vaccines*, Vol.7, No.7, (September 2008), pp. 1103-1119, ISSN 1476-0584.

Xin, Y.; Zhao, H.; Zhang,W.; Liang, C.; Wang, Z. & Liu, G. (2004). *Electrochemical Therapy of Tumors*, Bioelectromagnetic Medicine, Marcel Dekker Inc., ISBN 709-726, New York, USA.

Yen, Y.; Li, J.R.; Zhou, B.S.; Rojas, F.; Yu, J.; Chou, C.K. (1999). Electrochemical treatment of human KB cells in vitro. *Bioelectromagnetics*, Vol.20, No. 1, (January 1999), pp. 34-41, ISSN 0197-8462.

Yoon, D.S.; Ra, Y.M.; Ko, D.G.; Kim, Y.M.; Kim, K.W.; Lee, H.Y.; Xin, Y.L.; Zhang, W.; Li, Z.H. & Kwon, H.U. (2007). Introduction of Electrochemical Therapy (EChT) and Application of EChT to the breast Tumor. *Journal of Breast Cancer*, Vol.10, No.2, (June 2007), pp. 162-168, ISSN 1738-6756.

Permissions

The contributors of this book come from diverse backgrounds, making this book a truly international effort. This book will bring forth new frontiers with its revolutionizing research information and detailed analysis of the nascent developments around the world.

We would like to thank Assoc. Prof. Dr. Öner Özdemir, for lending his expertise to make the book truly unique. He has played a crucial role in the development of this book. Without his invaluable contribution this book wouldn't have been possible. He has made vital efforts to compile up to date information on the varied aspects of this subject to make this book a valuable addition to the collection of many professionals and students.

This book was conceptualized with the vision of imparting up-to-date information and advanced data in this field. To ensure the same, a matchless editorial board was set up. Every individual on the board went through rigorous rounds of assessment to prove their worth. After which they invested a large part of their time researching and compiling the most relevant data for our readers. Conferences and sessions were held from time to time between the editorial board and the contributing authors to present the data in the most comprehensible form. The editorial team has worked tirelessly to provide valuable and valid information to help people across the globe.

Every chapter published in this book has been scrutinized by our experts. Their significance has been extensively debated. The topics covered herein carry significant findings which will fuel the growth of the discipline. They may even be implemented as practical applications or may be referred to as a beginning point for another development. Chapters in this book were first published by InTech; hereby published with permission under the Creative Commons Attribution License or equivalent.

The editorial board has been involved in producing this book since its inception. They have spent rigorous hours researching and exploring the diverse topics which have resulted in the successful publishing of this book. They have passed on their knowledge of decades through this book. To expedite this challenging task, the publisher supported the team at every step. A small team of assistant editors was also appointed to further simplify the editing procedure and attain best results for the readers.

Our editorial team has been hand-picked from every corner of the world. Their multi-ethnicity adds dynamic inputs to the discussions which result in innovative outcomes. These outcomes are then further discussed with the researchers and contributors who give their valuable feedback and opinion regarding the same. The feedback is then collaborated with the researches and they are edited in a comprehensive manner to aid the understanding of the subject.

Apart from the editorial board, the designing team has also invested a significant amount of their time in understanding the subject and creating the most relevant covers. They scrutinized every image to scout for the most suitable representation of the subject and create an appropriate cover for the book.

The publishing team has been involved in this book since its early stages. They were actively engaged in every process, be it collecting the data, connecting with the contributors or procuring relevant information. The team has been an ardent support to the editorial, designing and production team. Their endless efforts to recruit the best for this project, has resulted in the accomplishment of this book. They are a veteran in the field of academics and their pool of knowledge is as vast as their experience in printing. Their expertise and guidance has proved useful at every step. Their uncompromising quality standards have made this book an exceptional effort. Their encouragement from time to time has been an inspiration for everyone.

The publisher and the editorial board hope that this book will prove to be a valuable piece of knowledge for researchers, students, practitioners and scholars across the globe.

List of Contributors

Luigi Aurisicchio and Gennaro Ciliberto
Takis, via di Castel Romano, 100, 00128 Rome, Italy

Luigi Aurisicchio
Biogem scarl, via Camporeale, 83131 Ariano Irpino (AV), Italy

Gennaro Ciliberto
Dipartimento di Medicina Sperimentale e Clinica, Università degli studi di Catanzaro "Magna Graecia" Campus Germaneto, 88100 Catanzaro, Italy

V.I. Seledtsov
Immanuel Kant Baltic Federal University, Kaliningrad, Russia

A.A. Shishkov and G.V. Seledtsova
Institute of Clinical Immunology SB RAMS, Novosibirsk, Russia

Jennifer Wu
University of Washington, USA

Xuanjun Wang
Yunnan Agriculture University, China

Shinichiro Akiyama and Hiroyuki Abe
Kudan Clinic Immune Cell Therapy Center, Japan

M. Eichbaum, C. Mayer, E. Bischofs, J. Reinhardt, J. Thum and C. Sohn
Departments of Obstetrics and Gynecology, University of Heidelberg, Heidelberg, Germany

Seshadri Sriprasad
Consultant Urological Surgeon - Darent Valley Hospital, Dartford, Kent, UK

Howard Marsh
Consultant Urological Surgeon- Medway Maritime Hospital, Gillingham, Kent, UK

Dariush Sardari
College of Engineering, Islamic Azad University Science and Research Branch, Tehran, Iran

Nicolae Verga
Carol Davila University of Medicine and Pharmacy, Bucharest, Romania

Walid Touati, Philippe Beaune and Isabelle de Waziers
UMR-S 775 Université Paris Descartes INSERM, France

Ramaswamy Bhuvaneswari, Malini Olivo and Soo Khee Chee
National Cancer Centre Singapore, 11 Hospital Drive, Singapore

Malini Olivo
School of Physics, National University of Ireland Galway, University Road, Galway, Ireland
Department of Pharmacy, National University of Singapore, Singapore
Singapore Bioimaging Consortium, Biomedical Sciences Institutes, Singapore

Gan Yik Yuen
Natural Sciences and Science Education, National Institute of Education, Nanyang Technological University, Singapore

Pasano Bojang, Jr. and Kenneth S. Ramos
Department of Biochemistry and Molecular Biology, University of Louisville, Louisville, KY, USA

Ana Elisa Bergues Pupo
Universidad de Oriente, Facultad de Ciencias Naturales y Matemáticas, Departamento de Física, Patricio Lumumba s/n, Santiago de Cuba, Cuba

Rolando Placeres Jiménez
Departamento de Física, Universidade Federal São Carlos, São Carlos-SP, Brasil

Luis Enrique Bergues Cabrales
Universidad de Oriente, Centro Nacional de Electromagnetismo Aplicado, Departamento de Investigaciones, Ave. Las Américas s/n, Santiago de Cuba, Cuba

Printed in the USA
CPSIA information can be obtained
at www.ICGtesting.com
JSHW011450221024
72173JS00004B/1017

9 781632 410733